124.00

D1558409

ROYAL VICTORIA HOSPITAL
MEDICAL LIBRARY

Inherited Disorders and the Eye

BIBLIOTHEQUE MEDICALE

DEC 12 2006

HOPITAL ROYAL VICTORIA

OPHTHALMOLOGY MONOGRAPHS

A series published by Oxford University Press in cooperation
with the American Academy of Ophthalmology

Series Editor: Richard K. Parrish II, Bascom Palmer Eye Institute

American Academy of Ophthalmology Advisory Board:
Thomas J. Liesegang, Mayo Clinic
Gregory L. Skuta, Dean A. McGee Eye Institute

A COMPENDIUM OF
Inherited Disorders and the Eye

by Elias I. Traboulsi

Published by Oxford University Press
IN COOPERATION WITH
The American Academy of Ophthalmology

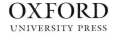
UNIVERSITY PRESS

2006

OXFORD
UNIVERSITY PRESS

Oxford University Press, Inc., publishes works that further
Oxford University's objective of excellence
in research, scholarship, and education.

Oxford   New York
Auckland   Cape Town   Dar es Salaam   Hong Kong   Karachi
Kuala Lumpur   Madrid   Melbourne   Mexico City   Nairobi
New Delhi   Shanghai   Taipei   Toronto

With offices in
Argentina   Austria   Brazil   Chile   Czech Republic   France   Greece
Guatemala   Hungary   Italy   Japan   Poland   Portugal   Singapore
South Korea   Switzerland   Thailand   Turkey   Ukraine   Vietnam

Copyright © 2006 by Oxford University Press, Inc.

Published by Oxford University Press, Inc.
198 Madison Avenue, New York, New York 10016

www.oup.com

Oxford is a registered trademark of Oxford University Press

All rights reserved. No part of this publication may be reproduced,
stored in a retrieval system, or transmitted, in any form or by any means,
electronic, mechanical, photocopying, recording, or otherwise,
without the prior permission of Oxford University Press.

Library of Congress Cataloging-in-Publication Data
Traboulsi, Elias I.
   A compendium of inherited disorders and the eye / by Elias
   Traboulsi, with contributions by Lourdes Garcia . . . [et al.].
      p. ; cm. — (Ophthalmology monographs ; 18)
   Includes bibliographical references.
   ISBN-13 978-0-19-517096-2
   ISBN 0-19-517096-2
   1. Eye—Diseases—Genetic aspects.   2. Genetic disorders—Complications.
   3. Ocular manifestations of general diseases.
   [DNLM: 1. Eye Diseases, Hereditary—genetics.   WW 140 T758c   2005]
   I. Title   II. Series.
   RE48.T697   2005
   617.7'042—dc22   2004012390

9 8 7 6 5 4 3 2 1

Printed in China
on acid-free paper

The American Academy of Ophthalmology provides the opportunity for material to be presented for educational purposes only. The material represents the approach, ideas, statement, or opinion of the author, not necessarily the only or best method or procedure in every case, nor the position of the Academy. Unless specifically stated otherwise, the opinions expressed and statements made by various authors in this monograph reflect the author's observations and do not imply endorsement by the Academy. The material is not intended to replace a physician's own judgment or give specific advice for case management. The Academy does not endorse any of the products or companies, if any, mentioned in this monograph.

Some material on recent developments may include information on drug or device applications that are not considered community standard, that reflect indications not included in approved FDA labeling, or that are approved for use only in restricted research settings. This information is provided as education only so physicians may be aware of alternative methods of the practice of medicine, and should not be considered endorsement, promotion, or in any way encouragement to use such applications. The FDA has stated that it is the responsibility of the physician to determine the FDA status of each drug or device he or she wishes to use in clinical practice, and to use these products with appropriate patient consent and in compliance with applicable law.

The Academy and Oxford University Press (OUP) do not make any warranties as to the accuracy, adequacy, or completeness of any material presented here, which is provided on an "as is" basis. The Academy and OUP are not liable to anyone for any errors, inaccuracies, or omissions obtained here. The Academy specifically disclaims any and all liability for injury or other damages of any kind for any and all claims that may arise out of the use of any practice, technique, or drug described in any material by any author, whether such claims are asserted by a physician or any other person.

Each author states that he or she has no significant financial interest or other relationship with the manufacturer of any commercial product discussed in the chapters that he or she contributed to this publication or with the manufacturer of any competing commercial product.

PREFACE

The idea for this monograph was conceived more than 20 years ago by Irene Maumenee of Johns Hopkins Hospital. Drs. Linn Murphree, Maumenee, and I worked on an atlas that contained structured entries on many of the disorders included in this book, but the project became dormant for many years. Over the last two decades, our understanding of the molecular genetics of inherited eye diseases and their classification and management has witnessed a huge expansion; the field of human genetics has benefited from technological advances and from increased interest by physicians and scientists in all fields of medicine. The amount of clinical and basic scientific information on inherited systemic and eye diseases has become so large that general ophthalmologists, ophthalmic subspecialists, and physicians in other fields of medicine have found it hard to keep up with.

This monograph is intended to be a practical and reasonably comprehensive catalog of genetic diseases that involve the eye. After an introduction that reviews basic clinical and molecular genetic principles, individual diseases or groups of diseases are listed alphabetically, with the aim of making searching for an entry as simple as possible. The structured presentation of the information in each entry is also intended to make the book a quick shelf reference for health care professionals who need access to its information. Although the material in each entry is a synthesis of numerous articles and reviews on the subject, only key references are listed. These represent the original description of the disease or a review of the subject, or they contain excellent illustrative photographs. Many entries contain at least one high-quality illustration of the disorder under discussion. Tables are used judiciously, primarily for groups or categories of diseases that would have otherwise required a very large amount of text for adequate coverage, an endeavor beyond the scope of this monograph. I have also tried to list at least one Web site of a patient support group or other organization related to the disease under discussion in each entry; the World Wide Web, especially sites devoted to the discussion of the clinical and molecular genetics of human diseases, has become an invaluable tool in our daily practice of medicine and was one of my sources of information as I prepared this monograph. Finally, the hard copy of the book is accompanied by a Web site (www.oup.com/us/aao/traboulsi/genetic) that contains electronic copies of all the illustrations, allowing academicians to use them in the preparation of lectures on the subject.

I would like to thank all the individuals who have helped in the preparation and production of this book, especially Pearl Vapnek, formerly on staff at the American Academy of Ophthalmology, Dr. Lourdes Garcia and Sue Crowe at the Cole Eye Institute, and the superb editorial and production staff at Oxford University Press. I finally would like to acknowledge the encouragement and support of Dr. Sprague Eustis and of my wife Mayya in carrying out this most instructive project.

CONTENTS

Please see the companion Web site at
www.oup.com/us/aao/traboulsi/genetic

M. Lourdes Garcia, M.D., Ph.D.
Research Fellow
The Cole Eye Institute
The Cleveland Clinic Foundation

Irene H. Maumenee, M.D.
Professor of Ophthalmology and Professor of Medicine and Pediatrics
Wilmer Eye Institute
The Johns Hopkins Hospital

A. Linn Murphree, M.D.
Professor of Ophthalmology and Professor of Pediatrics
Childrens Hospital of Los Angeles
Doheny Eye Institute
University of Southern California, Keck School of Medicine

Kang Zhang, M.D., Ph.D.
Assistant Professor of Ophthalmology
Investigator Program in Human Molecular Biology and Genetics
Program in Human Genetics
Department of Ophthalmology and Visual Science
The University of Utah, School of Medicine

Fundamentals of Genetics

Evidence that many common and rare diseases are genetically determined has emerged over the past two centuries through the clinical description of families, the mapping of genes to specific chromosomal loci, and the identification of the genes' structure and function. The elucidation of biochemical and molecular pathways of embryologic development and cellular functions has paralleled these discoveries.

Two major groups of genetic eye diseases can be identified. In the first or monogenic group, a specific gene defect leads to the interruption of a biochemical or developmental pathway and to the dysfunction of a group of cells that affect a predominant function. A number of retinal dystrophies, such as retinitis pigmentosa, Stargardt disease, and Leber congenital amaurosis, fall into this category. The genes that are involved in the retinal dystrophies are predominantly or uniquely expressed in the retina, and their mutations cause photoreceptor dysfunction and death. Furthermore, adjacent tissues, such as other types of retinal neurons, the retinal pigment epithelium, and the choroid, become secondarily affected, and changes in these layers cause the characteristic ophthalmoscopic signs of the individual disorder. Ocular malformations, such as aniridia and anterior segment dysgenesis, can also be classified in this group of monogenic disorders. They result from mutations in transcription factors that determine the fate of embryonal cells and the orderly differentiation of fetal structures. Other monogenic ocular diseases include all the corneal dystrophies, the inherited types of infantile cataracts, and many syndromic conditions such as the neuronal ceroid lipofuscinoses and the Usher syndromes.

In the second group of genetic eye disorders, multiple genes or a combination of genes and environmental factors cause the disease phenotype. Aside from the digenic form of retinitis pigmentosa and the multigenic forms of Bardet-Biedl syndrome are some of the more common conditions encountered in the clinical practice of ophthalmology, such as age-related macular degeneration and adult-onset open-angle glaucoma. A single gene may cause a significant predisposition to the disease, while other genes or environmental factors may lead to the development of disease manifestations. For example, mutations in the gene for myocilin, a cause of juvenile glaucoma, are more common in patients with adult-onset open-angle glaucoma, and mutations in the *ABCA4* gene, a cause of Stargardt disease, have been implicated in some cases of age-related macular degeneration. Some mutation-carrying family members of patients with these diseases do not develop the disease, lending support to the presence of modifier genes or epigenetic factors in these individuals. The presymptomatic detection of mutation carriers in such diseases will allow the institution of rigid screening protocols and early therapy, preventing severe complications and vision loss.

Technological Advances

The use of automated high-throughput DNA sequencers, powerful laboratory molecular biologic tools, and supercomputers has allowed scientists to completely decipher the entire human genome sequence with its approximately 40,000 genes through a massive effort sponsored by the National Institutes of Health, the U.S. Department of Energy, and private industry. The generated data have allowed scientists to move at a much faster pace in matching diseases and genes, and to direct future efforts to the identification of cellular and systemic effects of gene mutations and the means of early detection and modification of such effects.

Assays of micromolecular biologic reactions for the detection of mutations or gene products will allow quick screening of patients for abnormalities in panels of genes that have been linked to the genesis of their disease. So-called microarray DNA chip technology is already in wide use in the experimental setting and will be in use in diagnostic laboratories. Physicians will be able to order diagnostic DNA tests on patients with, among other diseases, cataracts, glaucoma, macular degeneration, and retinal dystrophies. They will also be able to choose modalities of therapy based on this information. Such therapy could include medications that are more effective in certain molecular genetic disease subtypes, micronutrient supplements that are effective in some diseases, or direct replacement of the gene product with local or systemic administration. A theoretic possibility is early surgical intervention in patients with types of glaucoma that are known to be resistant to medical therapy. These modalities of treatment are expected to become available in this century. Another application for rapid sequencing technology will be the detection of mutations in large genes, such as the retinoblastoma gene, allowing precise prognostication of the risk of developing additional retinal and systemic tumors; and of mutations in the fibrillin and collagen genes, allowing precise diagnosis of Marfan syndrome, other connective tissue diseases, and the vitreoretinopathies.

The biotechnology industry has played, and will continue to play, a major role in the development of effective and well-tolerated medications that will target specific biochemical and genetic pathways. Some of these medications will selectively and specifically treat disease subtypes. This selectivity may alleviate some of the uncertainties in therapeutic responses that physicians and patients experience today, with diseases still being lumped into large groups with common clinical findings but different pathophysiologic and genetic mechanisms. The great cost of developing such therapies will hopefully be justified in the long run by the availability of safe, effective, and cost-effective medications that will reduce the burden of blindness on society and enhance work productivity.

It will be possible in the not too distant future for a patient newly diagnosed with a common disease, such as glaucoma or macular degeneration, to have a blood sample drawn in the ophthalmologist's office, DNA extracted, serum proteins isolated, and a battery of tests performed to examine for abnormalities in DNA or protein markers responsible for the various types of individual diseases. The results of the tests would then be made available to the physician, who would prescribe the most appropriate therapy.

Gene Identification and Mapping

McKusick's first printed edition of *Mendelian Disorders in Man* listed 1468 inherited diseases. The number of entries in the online version of the book, *Online Mendelian Inheritance in Man* (www.ncbi.nlm.nih.gov/omim), as of April 2005 was 15,991, of which 13,705 had an established gene locus and 2286 had only a phenotype description (www.ncbi.nlm.nih.gov/omim/stats.mimstats.html). Table 1, based on data from January 2004, gives a breakdown of the entries by inheritance pattern. A large number of autosomal dominant, autosomal recessive, X-linked, and mitochondrial ocular diseases have been mapped and their individual genes cloned. Screening some of these genes for

TABLE 1. Number of Entries in *Mendelian Inheritance in Man* as of January 2004

	Mode of Inheritance			
	Autosomal	**X-Linked**	**Y-Linked**	**Mitochondrial**
Established locus	10,547	572	46	37
Phenotype description	1326	110	0	23
Other entries	2233	156	2	0
Total	14,107	838	48	60

mutations has allowed definitive diagnosis in many patients and has provided the opportunity to correlate disease manifestations with individual mutations and gain insight into the function of the gene and its molecular biophysiology.

Single-gene ocular disorders are responsible for up to 50% of blindness in children in the developed world and for a large proportion of significant visual impairment in developing countries. Many common ophthalmologic disorders, such as refractive errors, strabismus, age-related macular degeneration, and glaucoma, are clearly familial in a large proportion of cases, and several genetic loci have been established for some of these diseases.

The next sections review the structure of chromosomes and DNA and recapitulate the basic principles of inheritance.

Chromosomes

Normal human somatic cell nuclei contain 22 pairs of autosomes and one pair of sex chromosomes. The nucleus also contains the enzymes and products needed for gene duplication, chromosome formation, mitosis, meiosis, gene regulation, transcription, imprinting, X-chromosomal inactivation, and intron removal from messenger ribonucleic acid (mRNA). The 22 pairs of autosomes are *homologs*; that is, they contain an identical number and sequence of genes. Each parent contributes one of the chromosomes in a homologous pair. Genes on

the same chromosome are *syntenic*, that is, located together. The exchange of genetic material between sister chromatids in meiosis, called *crossing over*, explains how syntenic genetic material may be rearranged in the offspring. The closer together two genes are on the same chromosome, the less likely it is that crossing over will separate them. Syntenic genes are *linked* if their loci are so close together that there is a significantly less than 50% chance of independent assortment of the two genes. *Linkage analysis* is the study of the proximity of syntenic genes based on whether or not they assort independently.

DNA, RNA, and Genes

Deoxyribonucleic acid (DNA) is a double-helical structure composed of nucleotides, each of which contains a deoxyribose sugar linked by phosphate to a nitrogenous base. There are four bases: adenine (A) and guanine (G) are purines; thymine (T) and cytosine (C) are pyrimidines. Nucleotides polymerize into chains through the formation of covalent phosphodiester bonds between the 5′ carbon of one deoxyribose and the 3′ carbon of the next sugar in the sequence; these chains form each of the two strands of the DNA double helix. The two polynucleotide chains are held together by hydrogen bonds between A in one chain and T in the other or between G and C. Because of this obligatory pairing, the strands are complementary. *Histones* are basic proteins that bind with DNA to form the stable structure of chromosomes. Their structure is highly conserved among distant species. There is an equal weight amount of histones and of DNA in chromosomes. Some histones may be involved in gene regulation. Chromosomes also contain nonhistone proteins involved in organizing long regions or domains of DNA.

The gene is the basic unit of heredity and is composed of a stretch of DNA within a chromosome. The number of gene loci in humans is estimated to be about 30,000–40,000 pairs, and the human genome contains approximately 3.2 billion base pairs (bp). The position of a specific gene on a chromosome is referred to as its *locus*. Alternative genes found at the same locus and coding for the same type of polypeptide are known as *allelic genes*. The human *gene map* depicts the positions of the genes whose loci are known.

The components of a gene are arranged linearly on chromosomes (Fig. 1). They consist of a 5′ untranslated region that contains the promoter and other regulatory elements, such as the enhancer, inducer, and inhibitor. These elements serve as targets for transcription factors that activate genes and regulate their transcription. The promoter turns the gene on, depending on developmental and tissue-specific needs. The first codon of the coding region of the gene is called the *initiation codon* and is followed by the *open reading frame*, which is composed of exons encoding a protein. *Exons* are contained in the mature, processed mRNAs, and *introns* are composed of sequences that are spliced out during the processing of the transcribed mRNA. The last component of the gene in the last exon is called the *3′ untranslated region*. It serves, at least in part, a regulatory function and can be the site of mutations that inactivate the gene. Introns may have evolved in higher organisms to confer evolutionary benefits. Some introns contain small nucleolar RNAs, which play a role in ribosome assembly; others contain completely separate genes, which may be mutated in certain diseases or may influence the expression of other genes. The expansion of unstable repeats within introns can cause abnormal splicing and result in genetic disease. Mutations in introns close to intron and exon junctions may also cause abnormal splicing of mRNA and hence induce disease.

Approximately 97% of base sequences in human DNA do not encode proteins or RNAs that have well-defined functions. Some of these sequences may code for regulatory signals or may participate in normal genome repair. Some are repetitive and form telomeric DNA, which is essential to the maintenance of chromosomes. Loss of telomeric DNA correlates with cellular aging and with carcinogenesis. Other repetitive sequences include satellites, minisatellites, microsatellites, short interspersed elements (SINEs), and long interspersed elements (LINEs). The most common of these repetitive sequences is the 300 bp *Alu* sequence, a SINE that occurs about 500,000 times in the human genome. *Alu* sequences can cause disease if they insert within and disrupt a gene, as is the case in some patients with neurofibromatosis type 1.

From DNA to Protein and DNA Replication

In the cell nucleus, and in order to produce an identical copy of a DNA sequence, the DNA double helix separates into two strands, each of which serves as a template for a complementary strand. The enzyme DNA polymerase then catalyzes a reaction through which bases are linked together and form the complementary strand of DNA. The strand of DNA called the *sense strand* is not transcribed into RNA by RNA polymerase. It contains the correct sequence of information. A template of mRNA forms along the *antisense strand*, which is complementary to the sense strand. Hence, the mRNA contains the same 5′ to 3′ sequence as the sense DNA strand. The primary structure of RNA is similar to that of DNA, except that it is single-stranded, the sugar ribose replaces deoxyribose, and uracil (U) replaces thymine (T). After splic-

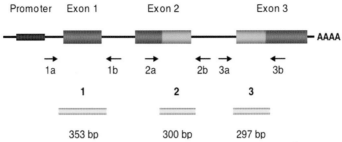

Figure 1. Norrie disease gene structure shows promoter, exons, introns, and poly-A tail. 1a, 1b, 2a, 2b, 3a, and 3b show sites of attachment of PCR primers that will amplify fragments 1 (353 bp), 2 (300 bp), and 3 (297 bp) of DNA from the three exons.

ing out of unnecessary sequences, the transcribed RNA template takes the genetic blueprint from the nucleus to the ribosomal complex in the cell cytoplasm for production of the designated polypeptide.

A code composed of 64 trinucleotides, 61 of which specify 1 of 20 amino acids, determines the unique amino acid sequence and thus the protein product. One codon, ATG, which codes for methionine, initiates translation, and three codons—UGA, UAA, and UAG1/M—stop translation. The genetic code is universal; that is, the same amino acids are specified by the same codons (three bases) in all species and genera (Table 2). The polypeptide that is generated at the ribosomal complex may be the final gene product or may be processed further, depending on the nature of the necessary end-product molecule and its function.

Mutations

A *mutation* is a permanent change in the genetic material (see Table 3 for types of mutations). Mutations in *germ cells* (spermatozoa and ova) affect all cells and tissues of the fetus and can be passed to successive generations. Mutations in other cells are called *somatic mutations*; they occur at any time after the first postzygotic mitosis. The individual will thus have two genotypically different cell popula-

tions, a condition called *mosaicism*. When a postzygotic mutation occurs in a germ cell, the individual has a condition called *germ-line mosaicism* and is at risk for passing on the mutation to his or her children.

The spontaneous mutation rate averages 10^{-6} to 10^{-5} per locus per gamete. Of all persons born, 3% to 5% have some tangible genetic defect and all persons are heterozygous for at least three to five lethal recessive genes. Another important factor in mutagenesis is advanced paternal age because of the increased risk of new dominant mutations in aging sperm cells. Some dominant diseases, such as achondroplasia, are more common in children of older fathers. Advanced maternal age leads to chromosomal nondisjunction in aged ova and to conditions such as trisomy 21 (Fig. 2), 13, and 18.

The finding of a nucleotide sequence change in a candidate gene in an individual with a genetic disease does not necessarily indicate that the sequence change is responsible for the disease. The sequence change is likely to be the disease-causing mutation if three conditions prevail: (*1*) if it does not occur in the normal population; (*2*) if it alters protein function or expression; and (*3*) if it segregates with the disease in a given family and is absent in nonaffected family members. Additional evidence of pathogenicity includes alteration of gene sequences that are conserved among different species throughout evolution, increased preva-

TABLE 2. Genetic Code

Amino Acid	Three-Letter Symbol	One-Letter Symbol	Trinucleotide Code
Alanine	Ala	A	GTC, GCC, GCA, GCG
Arginine	Arg	R	AGA, AGG, CGT, CGC, CGA, CGG
Asparagine	Asn	N	AAT, AAC
Aspartic acid	Asp	D	GAT, GAC
Asn and/or Asp	Asx	B	—
Cysteine	Cys	C	TGT, TGC
Glutamine	Gln	Q	CAA, CAG
Glutamic acid	Glu	E	GAA, GAG
Gln and/or Glu	Glx	Z	—
Glycine	Gly	G	GGT, GGC, GGA, GGG
Histidine	His	H	CAT, CAC
Isoleucine	Ile	I	ATT, ATC, ATA
Leucine	Leu	L	TTA, TTG, CTT, CTC, CTA, CTG
Lysine	Lys	K	AAA, AAG
Methionine	Met	M	ATG
Phenylalanine	Phe	F	TTT, TTC
Proline	Pro	P	CCT, CCC, CCA, CCG
Serine	Ser	S	TCT, TCC, TCA, TCG
Threonine	Thr	T	ACT, ACC, ACA, ACG
Tryptophan	Trp	W	TGG
Tyrosine	Tyr	Y	TAT, TAC
Valine	Val	V	GTT, GTC, GTA, GTG

lence of the mutation among patients compared to the normal population, and production of a stop codon or absence of the protein product.

Mendelian Inheritance

The principles of hereditary transmission of physical characteristics were formulated in 1865 by Gregor Johann Mendel. The Czech monk bred hybrid garden peas that resembled one parent rather than being a blend of both parents. He theorized that "hereditary units," now called *genes*, expressed dominant or recessive characteristics. Mendel's laws are summarized in Table 4. Diseases or physical characteristics that are produced by the effects of one or both genes in a single gene pair are referred to as *monogenic* or *Mendelian* (Table 5).

AUTOSOMAL DOMINANT INHERITANCE

Dominant traits and diseases result from the effects of mutations in one of a pair of allelic genes of a *somatic chromosome* (autosome) as opposed to a *sex chromosome* (X or Y). Mutations in both alleles of an autosomal dominant gene pair (*homozygosity*) have severe consequences and may be incompatible with life. If two forms of a dominant disease gene occur in an individual and if the presence of both mutations is compatible with life, both are expressed (*codominance*). In autosomal dominant disorders, both sexes are equally affected be-

TABLE 3. Types of Mutations

Type of Mutation	Change
Polymorphism	Any variation in DNA sequence that occurs at a rate of 1% or more in the normal population
Missense or nonsense	Single base change that produces either a stop codon directly or a frameshift with creation of a stop codon downstream; mutations may also cause loss or gain of a donor or acceptance of a splice junction site, resulting in loss of exons or inappropriate incorporation of introns into spliced mRNA
Conserved	Single base mutation that codes for the same amino acid or a tolerable change in amino acid sequence
Null	Results in no active gene product; includes missense and nonsense mutations
Gain of function	Results in a new function of a protein product, which may be beneficial (such as antibiotic resistance in bacteria) or detrimental (such as ligand mutations that produce tight binding to target receptor proteins)
Transition	Replacement of a purine by another purine
Transversion	Replacement of a pyrimidine by a purine or vice versa
Insertion	Insertion of any number of bases, with an effect on translation of a sequence
Deletion	Deletion of any number of bases, with an effect on translation of a sequence
Complex rearrangements of chromosomal material	Inversion, duplication, or translocation of segments of DNA

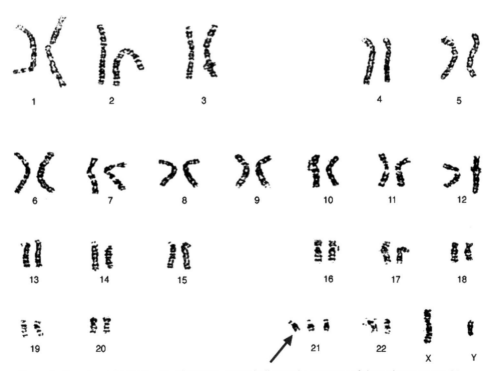

Figure 2. Karyotype of patient with trisomy 21. Arrow indicates the presence of three chromosomes 21.

TABLE 4. Mendel's Laws

Mendelian Principle	Explanation
Law of uniformity	The hereditary unit remains unaltered in passage from generation to generation
Law of segregation	All genes are paired (except for those on sex chromosomes); two members of a single gene pair always separate during gametogenesis and thus are normally never found together in mature ova or sperm or, consequently, in the offspring
Law of independent assortment	The determination of each gene pair's segregation (the daughter cell to which each gene will go) is made independently

cause the abnormal gene is on an autosome. Approximately 50% of the offspring of an affected individual will have the disease because one of the gene pair is abnormal. If the child is unaffected, the disease cannot be transmitted to his or her offspring unless there is *nonpenetrance*, that is, nonexpression of the abnormal gene in an individual carrying the mutation. Systemic dominant disorders usually affect more than one organ or tissue (*pleiotropy*), because very few tissues in the body contain unique structural material. Autosomal dominant disorders exhibit vertical transmission within pedigrees (Fig. 3); that is, affected individuals will appear in each generation. Male-to-male transmission of a disease in a pedigree that contains male and female affected individuals in multiple generations is strong evidence for autosomal dominant inheritance. *Pseudodominant* inheritance refers to the instance in which a recessive disorder appears to be transmitted as a dominant one because of the union of affected individuals with unaffected carriers of mutations in one allele and the birth of affected children to such couples.

The characteristics of autosomal dominant inheritance with complete penetrance are as follows:

TABLE 5. Some Terms Used in Mendelian Genetics

Term	Explanation
Genotype	The actual type or variant of a gene in a subject; usually refers to a single gene but may refer to the whole organism
Phenotype	The visible effects of one gene or a given set of genes
Phenocopy	An environmentally induced mimic of a genetic disease
Penetrance	The power of a gene and its ability to express itself in the phenotype; penetrance is expressed as the ratio of individuals who carry the mutated gene and express its effects over the total number of gene carriers in a population
Expressivity	The variation in the severity or degree to which the trait or disease is expressed; variable expressivity is characteristic of autosomal dominant traits and is unusual in recessive diseases
Pleiotropy	The production of multiple effects by a mutant gene
Genetic heterogeneity	The production of identical or very similar phenotypes by mutations of allelic or nonallelic genes; the classic example is retinitis pigmentosa, which may result from mutations in genes such as rhodopsin, peripherin/retinal degeneration slow, and others

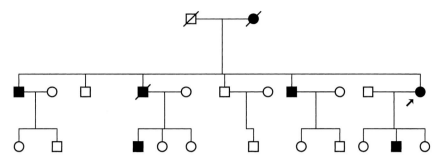

Figure 3. Pedigree with autosomal dominant transmission. Note vertical transmission of the disease trait (filled symbols). There is male-to-male transmission, and males as well as females are affected.

- The trait appears in multiple generations (*vertical transmission*).
- Affected males and females are equally likely to transmit the trait to male and female offspring. Thus, male-to-male transmission occurs.
- Each affected individual has an affected parent unless the condition arose by a new mutation in the given individual.
- Males and females are affected in equal proportions.
- Unaffected persons do not transmit the trait to their children; the trait is expressed in the heterozygote but is more severely affected in the homozygote.

- On average, the age of fathers of *isolated cases* (new mutations) is advanced compared to that of other fathers having children in the same year.
- The more severely the trait interferes with survival and reproduction, the greater the proportion of isolated cases, that is, new mutations.
- Variability in expression of the trait from generation to generation and between individuals in the same generation is expected.
- On average, affected persons transmit the trait to 50% of their offspring.
- Sex limitation can occur, for example, breast cancer and Stein-Leventhal syndrome.

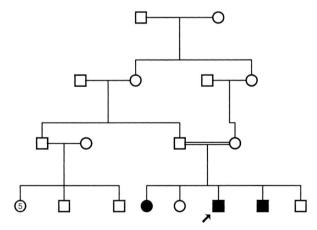

Figure 4. Autosomal recessive pedigree. Note consanguineous (double lines) marriage of unaffected parents and multiple affected male and female children. Arrow indicates proband (i.e., individual who brought the family to medical attention).

AUTOSOMAL RECESSIVE INHERITANCE

In general, one normal copy of a recessive gene produces sufficient substrate to permit the normal expected function. A mutation in one of a pair of recessive allelic genes (*heterozygosity*) does not usually cause clinical disease. Mutations of both alleles (*compound heterozygosity* if the mutations are different or *homozygosity* if the mutations are identical) result in the expression of the disease. Autosomal recessive disorders affect the sexes equally. Both parents are carriers of the mutant gene either somatically or germinally. There is a 25% chance of homozygosity or compound heterozygosity in the fetus in each subsequent pregnancy. Hence, the recurrence risk in siblings of an individual with an autosomal recessive disease is one in four. The other possibilities for each fetus are a 50% chance of carrying one abnormal gene and one normal allele and a 25% chance that both alleles are normal. Consanguineous marriages are more likely to result in autosomal recessive disorders in the offspring because of the higher likelihood that each parent shares some mutant recessive genes from a common ancestor. Autosomal recessive diseases usually appear in only one generation, as opposed to successive generation in autosomal dominant disorders (Fig. 4).

The characteristics of autosomal recessive inheritance are as follows:

- The mutant gene usually does not cause clinical disease in heterozygotes.
- Individuals (homozygotes) inheriting both genes of the altered type express the disorder.
- Typically, the trait appears only in siblings, not in their parents, offspring, or other relatives.
- The ratio of normal to affected in a sibship is 3:1. The larger the sibship, the more likely more than one child will be affected.
- The sexes are affected in equal proportions.
- Parents of the affected person may be genetically related (*consanguinity*); this is increasingly likely the more rare the trait.

- Approximately 50% of the children of carrier parents are carriers, and 25% are normal without risk of transmitting the disease.
- Affected individuals have children who, although phenotypically normal, are carriers (heterozygotes) of the mutant gene.

X-LINKED RECESSIVE AND DOMINANT INHERITANCE

X-linked disorders result from mutant genes on the X chromosome. X-linked recessive diseases and traits are more likely to affect males because males have only one X chromosome. Thus, a mutant recessive gene will have an immediate effect because of the absence of a normal polypeptide-enzyme product from another X chromosome. X-linked dominant mutations cause disease in women and are generally lethal in men. Some examples of interest to the ophthalmologist include incontinentia pigmenti, Goltz syndrome, and Aicardi syndrome. Because the only way a father can produce a son is by contributing his Y chromosome, there is no male-to-male transmission of X-linked diseases (Fig. 5). None of the sons of a male with an X-linked disease can inherit the gene for the condition, but all of the daughters will be carriers. Similarly, half of the sons of a female carrier will be affected, and half of the daughters will be carriers.

According to the Lyon principle, early in the development of female fetuses, one of the X chromosomes of each somatic cell is randomly inactivated and moved to the edge of the nucleus, where it remains inert for the remainder of the cell's life, detected as the Barr body. Successive generations of cells have the same inactive X chromosome. This process accounts for the clinical mosaicism seen in certain tissues of female carriers of X-linked diseases. For example, the ocular fundus of female carriers of X-linked ocular albinism has blotches and streaks of depigmented retinal pigment epithelium and choroid alternating with streaks of normal pigmentation (see entry on albinism). Similarly, the corneal epithelium of carriers of Fabry disease

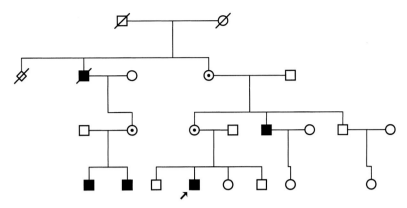

Figure 5. X-linked inheritance with affected males (filled square symbols) born to carrier females (circles with central dot). Arrow indicates proband.

has streaks and whorls of opacities, causing cornea verticillata (see entry on Fabry disease).

The characteristics of X-linked inheritance are as follows:

- Males are affected, and carrier females rarely manifest signs and symptoms of the disease if Lyonization results in more of the normal gene being inactivated and more of the abnormal gene being expressed.
- An affected male transmits the gene to all of his daughters but none of his sons.
- A heterozygous female transmits the gene to half of her daughters and half of her sons with equal frequency.

In X-linked dominant inheritance, females will express the disease. Males are usually severely affected, and in some diseases male fetuses are aborted or die at or shortly after birth. Examples of X-linked dominant diseases include incontinentia pigmenti and Aicardi syndrome.

MITOCHONDRIAL INHERITANCE
Mitochondrial DNA (mtDNA) is inherited exclusively with the mother's ovum, which contains about 100,000 copies of circular mtDNA. Mitochondria in sperm do not fuse with the pronucleus. Somatic cells contain 1000 to 10,000 of these circular strands of mtDNA, which constitute 0.3% of cellular DNA. Each

circular DNA strand is 16,569 bases in length. It contains 37 genes for respiratory chain polypeptides, as well as those for 22 mitochondrial transfer RNAs and 2 mitochondrial ribosomal RNAs. There are no introns in the coding region of the mtDNA, which determines the production of 13 of the more than 69 peptides of the mitochondrial respiratory chain, such as 3 of the subunits of cytochrome oxidase, 2 of adenosine triphosphate (ATP) synthase, 7 of reduced nicotinamide adenine dinucleotide–coenzyme (NADH-CoQ) reductase, and 1 of CoQ-cytochrome-*c* reductase. The genetic code for mtDNA is slightly different from that of nuclear DNA. The mutation rate for mtDNA is 10 to 20 times higher than that of nuclear DNA because of the absence of repair enzymes and the high oxygen concentration in mitochondria. Mitochondria use DNA polymerase γ for DNA synthesis, as opposed to polymerases α, β, δ, and ε, which are used by nuclear DNA. *Heteroplasmy* is the term signifying that only some of the mtDNA rings carry a gene mutation, while others are normal.

Because diseases caused by abnormalities of mtDNA can be passed on only by carrier females in their eggs and not by affected males, they do not follow Mendelian laws of inheritance. Pedigrees of mitochondrial diseases cannot have transmission of the disease through male lines. A carrier female will give the mutated mtDNA to all her offspring. The pheno-type and severity of mitochondrial disease de-pend on the nature of the mutation, the pres-ence and degree of heteroplasmy, and the oxidative needs of the tissues involved. Alter-ations of mtDNA accumulate with age. There is a preferential replication of smaller mtDNA, and deletions favor the predominance of cells that are homoplasmic for the abnormal mtDNA. Disease appears when energy produc-tion by the abnormal electron transport system becomes insufficient to maintain the function of cells or tissues.

Leber hereditary optic neuropathy (LHON) is caused by point mutations in mtDNA and is expressed preferentially in males, while carrier females manifest the disease only if they have enough copies of abnormal mtDNA in their tis-sues. About 60% of carrier males and less than 20% of carrier females will manifest the disease. Other diseases, such as chronic external oph-thalmoplegia (CPEO) that includes the so-called Kearns syndrome, are caused by deletions of mtDNA and can affect males and females equally (see Table 6).

MULTIFACTORIAL INHERITANCE

Multifactorial traits are thought to result from the interaction of multiple genes or their prod-ucts. Environmental factors play additional roles in modifying these traits. Multifactorial inheritance accounts for much of the normal variation in physical characteristics and con-tributes to a large number of common diseases, such as diabetes mellitus, cardiovascular dis-ease, psychiatric disorders, and some congeni-tal malformations.

Although the words *multifactorial* and *poly-genic* are commonly used interchangeably, *poly-genic* denotes conditions resulting only from genetic factors, while *multifactorial* indicates en-vironmental as well as genetic influences.

Some examples of common multifactorial traits are as follows:

- Anencephaly/spina bifida
- Cleft lip/palate
- Clubfoot (pes equinovarus)
- Common psychoses (schizophrenia, affec-tive disorder)
- Congenital heart disease (some forms)
- Congenital scoliosis
- Coronary heart disease (some forms)
- Diabetes mellitus (some forms)
- Hirschsprung disease
- Hydrocephalus, nonspecific neural-tube defects
- Hypertension
- Mental retardation
- Open-angle glaucoma (some forms)

TABLE 6. Categories of Diseases Resulting from Alterations in Mitochondria DNA (mtDNA)

Category	Diseases
Large rearrangements of mtDNA	Chronic progressive external ophthalmoplegia (CPEO) Kearns syndrome Pearson marrow and pancreas syndrome
Mutations in mitochondrial ribosomal ribonucleic acid (mtrRNA)	Sensorineural deafness Aminoglycoside-induced deafness
Mutations in mitochondrial transfer ribonucleic acid (mttRNA)	Mitochondrial encephalopathy, lactic acid, and stroke-like episodes (MELAS) Myoclonus with epilepsy and ragged red fibers (MERRF) Adult-onset diabetes and deafness 30% of cases of CPEO
Missense or nonsense mutations	Leber hereditary optic neuropathy (LHON) Neuropathy, ataxia, and retinitis pigmentosa (NARP)

- Pyloric stenosis
- Refractive errors
- Strabismus (some forms)
- Urinary tract malformations

The empiric recurrence risks for polygenic disorders are as follows:

- Increased risk compared to the general population among first- and second-degree relatives of the affected person.
- Baseline 3% to 5% risk for first-degree relatives of the affected person (*proband*), and about half of that risk for second-degree relatives.
- Increased risk with increasing numbers of affected genetic relatives, especially first- and second-degree relatives.
- Increased risk if the affected person is of the less commonly affected sex.
- Increased risk with increased severity of the trait.

Cancer Genetics

Several genetic mechanisms have been implicated in cancer biogenesis, the most common being the activation of oncogenes or the loss of tumor-suppressor gene activity. *Oncogenes* or *proto-oncogenes* code for intracellular signals that are able to activate cellular growth or differentiation in response to external signals (*signal transduction factors*). A proto-oncogene can be activated to oncogene by losing its mechanisms of regulation. Oncogene expression becomes constitutive and results in unrestrained cell growth and tumor development. Usually, a single mutated allele of the oncogene gene is enough to result in cancer.

Tumor-suppressor genes, or *antioncogenes*, control cell proliferation. They may have different functions in the cell. Based on a statistical model, Knudson hypothesized that two mutations are needed for retinoblastoma to develop from a normal cell. This is now known as *Knud-*

son's two-hit hypothesis. The molecular explanation is as follows: When one allele is mutated, the wild-type allele of the tumor-suppressor gene is still able to prevent tumor development in most cases. If a mutation takes place in the second allele (loss of heterozygosity, or LOH), tumors will develop. Retinoblastoma results from loss of activity of the two copies of the Rb tumor-suppressor gene on 13q14.

Identification of Disease Genes

The ultimate understanding of the pathophysiology of any genetic disease depends on the identification of the responsible gene, its physical structure, the function of its product, and the alteration of this product and its effect on the individual's tissues. In one approach to the identification of disease genes, the gene's chromosomal locus is determined first, followed by its cloning and a search for mutations in patients with the disease in question (Fig. 6). A gene's locus can be inferred from the consistent occurrence of a disease in patients with identical or overlapping chromosomal rearrangements. This may occur within a family or in unrelated individuals. Such deletions or chromosomal rearrangements involving a number of genes located next to each other on a chromosome segment result in *contiguous gene syndromes.* For example, the gene for retinoblastoma was localized to chromosome 13q14 after numerous reports of retinoblastoma in unrelated patients with deletions involving this region. Other examples include the WAGR (Wilms' tumor, aniridia, genitourinary defects, and retardation) syndrome as a consequence of deletions of 11p13 and choroideremia with deafness.

The genetic localization of animal diseases, especially in the mouse, has also helped in the assignment of human disease genes. There is homology, or correspondence, between chromosomal regions, presumably carrying genes of identical nature between animals of different

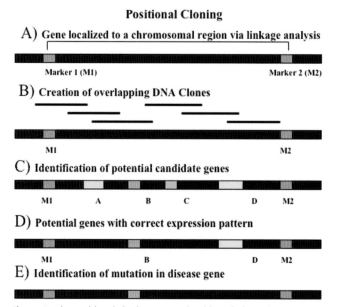

Figure 6. The positional cloning approach. This technique does not rely on the knowledge of a particular gene, but rather involves the process of narrowing down the disease-causing gene by continuously analyzing and eliminating DNA fragments surrounding the disease locus on a chromosome. The specific steps in this approach are as follows. (A) Genetic linkage analysis which localizes the disease gene to a specific chromosomal region. (B) Creation of overlapping DNA clones covering entire region containing the disease gene. (C) Identification of several potential genes that may be the disease gene. (D) Limitation of potential genes to only those with an expression pattern consistent with the disease. (E) Identification of the disease gene with a mutation found only in patients with the disease phenotype and not in normal controls. (Reprinted from Zhang K, et al: Genetic and molecular studies of macular dystrophies: recent developments. Survey of Ophthalmology 1995;40:51–61, with permission.)

genera and species. For example, the mouse gene for rhodopsin is localized to the distal half of mouse chromosome 1, which is syntenic (carries a similar sequence of genes, hence "equivalent to" or syntenic) to human chromosome 3q, where the human rhodopsin gene is located. Homologous human and murine genes, however, may have different tissue-specific expression, and mutations in one may not have the same or all of the effects in the two organisms. For example, mutations in murine *Myosin 7a*, located on mouse chromosome 7, cause deafness and vestibular dysfunction in the *shaker1* mouse. Mutations in the homologous human

MYO7A, which localizes to the homologous chromosome 11q13 region, cause type IB Usher syndrome, which includes not only deafness and vestibular dysfunction, but also retinitis pigmentosa. *MYO7A* became a candidate gene for Usher syndrome type IB (USHIB) after the disease was found to map to 11q13 and was known to share clinical features with *shaker1*.

Mutant genes can be assigned to specific chromosomes or segments thereof if their function is determined to be reduced or absent in artificially created somatic cell lines that lack these chromosomal regions.

It is important to differentiate the association

of two clinical traits in the same patient because of a predisposing or protective role of one over the other from clinical traits that result from the effects of syntenic genes (genes located on the same chromosome). For example, individuals with the type O blood group are more predisposed to peptic ulcer disease, although the *ABO* gene and a gene for peptic ulcer disease are neither identical nor located on the same chromosome.

GENE DOSAGE AND HAPLOINSUFFICIENCY

Some diseases are produced by the complete absence of one copy of the gene and hence the absence of half the amount of the message. This is called *haploinsufficiency*. Most dominantly inherited ocular malformations result from haploinsufficiency. Because one-half of the quantity of the transcription factor that determines normal ocular development is not sufficient to determine normal differentiation, the development of ocular structure malformations, such as aniridia or anterior segment dysgenesis, occurs.

GENE MAPPING AND LINKAGE ANALYSIS

The Human Genome Project has provided the base sequence of all DNA sequences in the human genome. These discoveries were made possible by dividing the chromosomes into smaller fragments, which were characterized and ordered (*mapped*) to correspond to their respective locations on the chromosomes. After mapping was completed, the base sequence of each of the ordered DNA fragments was determined. Another goal of the Human Genome Project is to develop tools for using this information in the study of human biology and medicine.

Many genes responsible for genetic eye diseases have been mapped to specific chromosomal locations since Bell and Haldane assigned congenital color deficiency to the X chromosome when they recognized the association of color blindness with hemophilia and the preferential occurrence of both in males. A *genome map* describes the order of genes or other DNA markers and the spacing between them on each chromosome. *Genetic linkage maps* depict the relative chromosomal locations of DNA markers (genes and other identifiable DNA sequences) by their patterns of inheritance. *Physical maps* describe the chemical characteristics of the DNA molecule itself.

Genetic markers can be expressed DNA regions (genes) or DNA segments that have no known coding function but whose inheritance pattern can be followed with laboratory assays. DNA sequence *variants*, or *polymorphisms*, are especially useful markers because of their large numbers and known locations in the genome. To be useful in gene mapping, markers have to be polymorphic; that is, alternative forms must exist among individuals so that they are detectable among different members in family studies (Fig. 7). Polymorphisms are variations in DNA sequence that occur on average once in every 300 to 500 bp. Most variations occur within introns or outside a gene and have little or no effect on an organism's appearance or function, yet they are detectable at the DNA level and can be used as markers (Table 7).

The basic principle of mapping an inherited trait rests on the frequency of its inheritance with one marker or a set of markers of known chromosomal location. Two markers located near each other on the same chromosome will tend to be passed together from parent to child. During gametogenesis, DNA strands occasionally break and rejoin in different places on the same chromosome or on the other copy of the same chromosome. This process, called *meiotic recombination* (or *crossing over*), results in the separation of two markers originally on the same chromosome. The closer together physically the marker and the disease trait are to each other, the less likely a recombinational event will separate them. Recombination frequency is used as an estimate of the distance between two markers. This distance is measured in centimorgans (cM). Two markers are 1 cM apart if they are separated by recombination 1% of the time (one cM is roughly equal to 1 million base

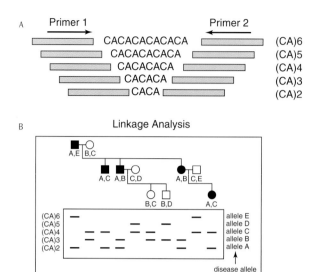

Figure 7. The polymerase chain reaction (PCR). PCR allows for the quick and efficient analysis of specific regions of DNA (genetic markers). In this example the PCR technique is used to demonstrate the presence of a genetic marker segregating with a disease phenotype. (A) DNA from a patient's blood is collected and amplified using PCR and two oligonucleotide primers (#1, #2). The primers flank the genetic markers designated (CA)2, (CA)3, (CA)4, (CA)5, and (CA)6. The genetic markers are called short tandem repeats (STRs) because they occur in pairs and in repeat, that is, from two to six times. These differences in size can be revealed by polyacrylamide gel electrophoresis (bottom of figure), where the smallest STR (CA)2 travels to the bottom of the gel and the largest STR (CA)6 remains near the top of the gel. (B) The allele A is associated with the disease phenotype and is defined by the STR designated (CA)2. In this family, each allele is designated A, B, C, D, or E and corresponds to the STR genetic markers (CA)2, (CA)3, (CA)4, (CA)5, and (CA)6, respectively. Family members affected with the disease are designated by a filled box (male) or filled circle (female). Note that allele A is associated with each family member who is affected with the disease, indicating that the genetic marker (CA)2 is linked to the disease, information that is useful in determining family members potentially susceptible to the development of the disease phenotype. (Reprinted from Zhang K, et al: Genetic and molecular studies of macular dystrophies: recent developments. Survey of Ophthalmology 1995;40:51–61, with permission.)

pairs of DNA). Hence, an inherited disease can be located on the map by following the inheritance of a DNA marker present in affected individuals (but absent in unaffected individuals), even though the molecular basis of the disease may not yet be understood or the responsible gene identified. Statistical analysis is then applied to the data obtained and a *logarithm of the* *likelihood ratio* (LOD) score is calculated. A LOD score higher than 3 is considered indicative of linkage and means that the probability of these two markers being linked is 1000 times higher than the probability that they are not, for a *P* value of .05. A LOD score of 2 or 3 is suggestive of linkage. A LOD score of less than –2 excludes linkage between the disease-trait lo-

TABLE 7. Types of Markers

Type of Marker	Explanation
Restriction fragment length polymorphisms (RFLPs)	Sequence variations in DNA sites that can be cleaved by specific DNA restriction enzymes
Single nucleotide polymorphisms (SNPs)	Polymorphic variations at single nucleotide locations
Variable number of tandem repeat sequences (VNTRs)	Short repeated sequences that vary in the number of repeated units and therefore in length, making them easy to measure

cus and the marker for which the calculation is done.

PHYSICAL MAPPING

Physical maps of the human genome vary in their degree of resolution. The lowest-resolution map is the *cytogenetic* (or *chromosomal*) *map*, which is based on the distinctive banding patterns observed by light microscopy of stained chromosomes. A complementary DNA (cDNA) map shows the location of expressed DNA regions (exons) on the chromosomal map. The more detailed *cosmid contig map* depicts the order of overlapping DNA fragments spanning the genome. A *macrorestriction map* describes the order of and distance between enzyme cutting (*cleavage*) sites. The highest-resolution physical map is the complete DNA base-pair sequence of each chromosome in the human genome. (Chromosomal maps are covered in more detail below.)

In a chromosomal map, genes or other identifiable DNA fragments are assigned to their respective chromosomes, with distances measured in base pairs. Markers can be physically associated with particular bands (identified by cytogenetic staining) primarily by in situ hybridization, a technique that involves tagging the DNA marker with a fluorescent or radioactive label. The location of the labeled probe can be detected after it binds to its complementary DNA strand in an intact chromosome.

The technique of *fluorescent in situ hybridization* (FISH) has allowed the detection of variations (for example, submicroscopic deletions) in DNA sequences as small as 100,000 bp,

but typically in the range of 2 to 5 Mbp (million base pairs). Classic karyotyping techniques with chromosomal banding only resolve down to 10 Mbp deletions.

A cDNA map shows the position of expressed DNA regions (exons) relative to particular chromosomal regions or bands. (Expressed DNA regions are those transcribed into mRNA.) Complementary DNA is synthesized in the laboratory using the mRNA molecule as a template. The cDNA is then mapped to genomic regions. A cDNA map can provide the chromosomal location for genes whose functions are currently unknown. For disease-gene hunters, the map can also suggest a set of candidate genes to test when the approximate location of a disease gene has been mapped by genetic linkage techniques.

At present, there are two approaches to high-resolution physical mapping: top-down (producing a macrorestriction map) and bottom-up (resulting in a contig map). With either strategy, the maps represent ordered sets of DNA fragments that are generated by cutting genomic DNA with restriction enzymes. The fragments are then amplified by cloning or by polymerase chain reaction methods. Electrophoretic techniques are used to separate the fragments according to size. The use of purified chromosomes separated either by flow sorting from human cell lines or by hybrid cell lines allows a single chromosome to be mapped. The original order of the DNA fragments is then reconstructed with techniques based on the ability of single strands of DNA and/or RNA to hybridize and form double-stranded segments by hydrogen bonding between complementary bases. The extent of sequence homology between the two strands can be inferred from the length of the double-stranded segment. Fingerprinting uses restriction-map data to determine which fragments have a specific sequence (*fingerprint*) in common and therefore overlap. Another approach uses linking clones as probes for hybridization to chromosomal DNA cut with the same restriction enzyme.

Tools of Molecular Genetics

1. *Restriction enzymes.* Restriction enzymes are isolated from bacteria and cut DNA molecules at specific sites, where they recognize short sequences of DNA. In nature, these enzymes protect bacteria by attacking viral and other foreign DNA. On average, restriction enzymes with 4-base recognition sites yield DNA pieces 256 bases long, those with 6-base recognition sites yield pieces 4000 bases long, and those with 8-base recognition sites yield pieces 64,000 bases long. Because hundreds of different restriction enzymes have been characterized, DNA can be cut into many different small fragments. If a mutation has altered the binding site of a restriction enzyme, the enzyme will not be able to cut the DNA and hence the mutation can be detected.

2. *Southern, Northern, and Western blotting.* After enzyme digestion, different DNA fragments can be separated by electrophoresis on a gel (*Southern blotting*). If gel electrophoresis is used to separate fragments of mRNA, the process is called *Northern blotting.* The analog for proteins is called *Western blotting.*

3. *Pulsed-field gel electrophoresis.* While conventional gel electrophoretic methods separate DNA pieces less than 40 kbp (1000 base pairs) in size, pulsed-field gel electrophoresis separates molecules of up to 10 Mbp, allowing the application of both conventional and new mapping methods to larger genomic regions.

4. *Flow sorting.* Flow sorting technique uses flow cytometry to separate, according to size, chromosomes isolated from cells during cell division, when they are condensed and stable. Chromosomes are differentiated by size with a laser beam, which analyzes the amount of DNA present. Individual chromosomes are then directed to specific collection tubes.

5. *Somatic cell hybrid.* In somatic cell hybridization, human and rodent tumor cells are fused. With cell division and over time, human chromosomes are lost preferentially from a hybrid cell until only one or a few remain. This technique has generated a number of hybrid cell lines, each with a specific single human chromosome.

6. *Cloning or in vivo DNA amplification.* Cloning uses recombinant DNA technology to propagate DNA fragments within a foreign host. The fragments are isolated from chromosomes with restriction enzymes and are ligated to a carrier vector. The DNA fragments are then introduced into suitable host cells, in which they reproduce along with the host cell DNA. *Vectors* are DNA molecules derived from viruses, bacteria, and yeast cells. They accommodate foreign DNA fragments of various sizes, ranging from 12,000 bp for bacterial vectors (*plasmids* and *cosmids*) to 1 Mbp for yeast vectors (*yeast artificial chromosomes,* or YACs). Bacteria are most often the hosts for these inserts, but yeast and mammalian cells are also used. Cloning provides unlimited material for experimental studies. A random or unordered set of cloned DNA fragments is called a *library.* Sets of overlapping fragments encompassing an entire genome are called *genomic libraries.* Also available are *chromosome-specific libraries,* which consist of fragments derived from source DNA enriched for a particular chromosome,

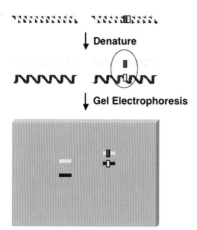

Figure 8. Single-strand conformation polymorphism technique allows separation of DNA strands differing by single base pairs (top panel) through their modified pattern of migration on a gel (bottom panel)

and *whole organ* (or *tissue-specific*) *libraries*, such as retina or brain libraries.

7. *Polymerase chain reaction (PCR).* The technique of PCR can amplify a desired DNA sequence of any origin hundreds of millions of times in hours. Polymerase chain reaction is especially valuable because it is highly specific, easily automated, and capable of amplifying a minute amount of a sample. The technique is based on a polymerase enzyme that can synthesize a complementary strand to a given DNA strand in a mixture containing the 4 DNA bases and 2 DNA primers, each about 20 bases long, that flank the target sequence. The mixture is heated to separate the strands of double-stranded DNA containing the target sequence and then cooled to allow the primers to find and bind to their complementary sequences on the separated strands, and the polymerase to extend the primers into new complementary strands. Repeated heating and cooling cycles multiply the target DNA exponentially as each new double strand separates to become two templates for further synthesis. In about 1 hour, 20 PCR cycles can amplify the target sequence a million-fold.

8. *Single-stranded conformational polymorphism (SSCP).* The SSCP technique consists of the electrophoresis of single-strand DNA fragments in a nondenaturing gel. As the DNA migrates, it folds according to its sequence. DNA fragments of the same size migrate differently if their sequence is not the same (Fig. 8). Sometimes, differences in as little as 1 bp can result in different folding and different migration in the gel, thus allowing the identification of a mutated fragment. DNA fragments of less than 300 bp are preferred for this technique.

9. *Denaturing gradient gel electrophoresis (DGGE).* In the DGGE technique, electrophoresis of double-stranded DNA on a gel with a gradient of a denaturing agent, like urea, can also be used to detect mutations. The migration of the DNA is altered if there is a mutation in the sequence. A GC base–rich nucleotide sequence (GC clamp) is frequently added to primers for PCR to improve the sensitivity of the technique.

10. *Sequencing.* There are two basic sequencing approaches: the Maxam-Gilbert (or chemical-degradation) method and the Sanger (or chain-termination or dideoxy) method. The two methods differ primarily in the way the nested DNA fragments are produced. Both are based on the fact that gel electrophoresis produces high-resolution separation of DNA molecules that differ by as little as a single nucleotide. All steps in these sequencing methods are now automated. The latest-generation capillary-based sequencing technologies have been used to sequence the entire human genome.

11. *Allele-specific oligonucleotides.* Allele-specific oligonucleotides are designed to recognize by hybridization a specific DNA sequence. They can be synthesized to recognize the normal allele or a known point mutation.

Putting It All Together

Correlating sequence information with genetic-linkage data and disease-gene research will reveal the molecular basis for human variation. Altered protein gene products are compared with normal proteins to identify the cause of the disease under study. Efforts can then be directed to the correction of the defective process.

MAPPING DATABASES

The Genome Database (GDB, initially established at Johns Hopkins University in Baltimore, Maryland, and currently hosted by the Bioinformatics Supercomputing Center of the Hospital for Sick Children in Toronto, Canada; http://gdbwww.gdb.org) provides location, ordering, and distance information for human genetic markers, probes, and contigs linked to known human genetic disease. The GDB is presently working on incorporating physical mapping data. The *Online Mendelian Inheritance in Man* database (http://www.ncbi.nlm.nih.gov/omim, also started at Johns Hopkins and now based at the National Institutes of Health) is a catalog of inherited human traits and diseases and gives clinical details, responsible gene mutations, and extensive references.

The Human and Mouse Probes and Libraries Database (located at the American Type Culture Collection in Rockville, Maryland; http://www.atcc.org) and the GBASE mouse database (located at Jackson Laboratory, Bar Harbor, Maine; http://www.informatics.jax.org) include data on restriction fragment length polymorphisms (RFLPs), chromosomal assignments, and probes from the laboratory mouse.

SEQUENCE DATABASES

Public databases containing the complete nucleotide sequence of the human genome and sequences of selected model organisms are one of the most useful products of the Human Genome Project. Five major public databases now store nucleotide sequences: GenBank (http://www.ncbi.nlm.nih.gov/Genbank) and the Genome Sequence DataBase (GSDB; http://wehih.wehi.edu.au/gsdb/gsdb.html) in the United States; the European Molecular Biology Laboratory (EMBL; http://www.embl-heidelberg.de/); the Nucleotide Sequence Database in the United Kingdom (http://www.ebi.ac.uk/embl/); and the DNA Data Bank in Japan (DDBJ; http://www.cib.nig.ac.jp/). The databases collaborate to share sequences, which are compiled from direct submissions from the Human Genome Project Consortium and journal scans. Although human sequences predominate, more than 8000 species are represented.

The major protein sequence databases have recently joined forces and can be accessed through a centralized Internet portal called United Protein Databases (http://pir.georgetown.edu/uniprot/).

A COMPENDIUM OF

Inherited Disorders and the Eye

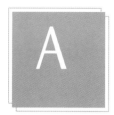

Abetalipoproteinemia

Also called Bassen-Kornzweig syndrome

OMIM NUMBER
200100

INHERITANCE
Autosomal recessive

GENE/GENE MAP
Microsomal triglyceride transfer protein deficiency

4q22–q24

Normotriglyceridemic abetalipoproteinemia is due to mutations in the apolipoprotein B gene

EPIDEMIOLOGY
Most cases with this extremely rare disease have been in Eastern European (Ashkenazi) Jews, but it has been reported in other populations.

CLINICAL FINDINGS
Lipid malabsorption in infancy results in a deficiency of the fat-soluble vitamins A, E, and, less commonly, K. Although lipid is able to enter the intestinal mucosal epithelium, its exit is blocked. Fat-soluble vitamins cannot be normally incorporated into chylomicrons for transportation to the liver from the intestine.

Steatorrhea with abdominal distension, failure to thrive, malnutrition, and spinal curvature beginning in the first few months of life are all present.

Patients develop spinocerebellar ataxia, areflexia, and weakness accompanying a diffuse neuromuscular disease that resembles Friedreich ataxia.

There are crenated or "thorny" red cells on blood smear (acanthocytosis). Plasma cholesterol level is less than 100 mg/dL. There is complete absence of apolipoprotein (apo) B and lipoproteins from plasma, and absence of apo-LDL (low-density lipoprotein) from plasma confirms the diagnosis.

OCULAR FINDINGS
Night blindness develops, with retinal degeneration and later onset of pigmentary changes secondary to vitamin A deficiency. White dots are present throughout the fundus and are most numerous in the periphery. A retinitis pigmentosa–like picture eventually ensues.

Angioid streaks have been reported in a few cases and can be complicated by subretinal neovascularization.

Reduced electroretinographic responses are present early in the course of the disease.

Ptosis, ophthalmoplegia, strabismus, and nystagmus are less common findings.

THERAPEUTIC ASPECTS
Serum vitamin A levels should be determined. One oral dose of 200,000 IU of vitamin A palmitate maintains serum levels in the normal range for several months. Additional doses are given, depending on serum levels of vitamin A.

Vitamin K supplementation may be necessary to prevent bleeding.

Vitamin E supplementation has been shown to arrest neuropathy and myopathy.

Life expectancy is reduced, and death often occurs from cardiac arrhythmias.

REFERENCES

Cogan DG, Rodrigues M, Chu FC, et al: Ocular abnormalities in abetalipoproteinemia: a clinicopathologic correlation. *Ophthalmology* 1984;91: 991–998.

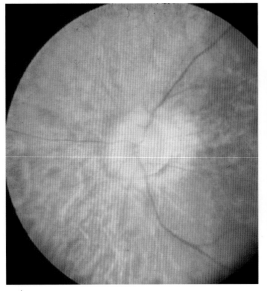 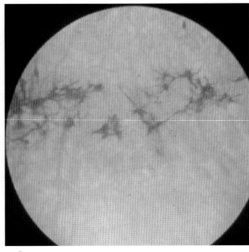

A   B

Abetalipoproteinemia (A) Posterior pole of a patient with abetalipoproteinemia showing a pale optic nerve head, attenuated blood vessels, and atrophic retina. (B) Midperipheral bony spicule pigmentary changes in same patient as in (A). (Courtesy of W.R. Green, M.D.)

Duker JS, Belmon J, Bosley TM: Angioid streaks associated with abetalipoproteinemia. *Arch Ophthalmol* 1987;105:1173–1174.

Luckenbach MW, Green WR, Miller NR, et al: Ocular clinicopathologic correlation of Hallervoden-Spatz syndrome with acanthocytosis and pigmentary retinopathy. *Am J Ophthalmol* 1983;95:369–382.

Runge P, Muller PR, McAlliter J, et al: Oral vitamin E supplements can prevent the retinopathy of abetalipoproteinemia. *Br J Ophthalmol* 1986;70:166–173.

Sperling MA, Hiles DA, Kennerdell JS: Electroretinographic responses following vitamin A therapy in A-beta-lipoproteinemia. *Am J Ophthalmol* 1972;72:342–351.

Wetterau JR, Aggerbeck LP, Bouma ME, et al: Absence of microsomal triglyceride transfer protein in individuals with abetalipoproteinemia. *Science* 1992;258:999–1001.

RESOURCES

National Tay-Sachs and Allied Diseases Association
www.ntsad.org
Yahoo! Abetalipoproteinemia Group
groups.yahoo.com/group/abetalipoproteinemia

Ablepharon-Macrostomia Syndrome

OMIM NUMBER
200110

INHERITANCE
Autosomal recessive

GENE/GENE MAP
Unknown

EPIDEMIOLOGY
Very few patients have been reported.

CLINICAL FINDINGS
Macrostomia (large mouth), abnormal nose and auricles
Forehead hypertrichosis
Skin alterations, persistent lanugo hair, and other abnormalities, such as absent nipples and ambiguous genitalia
Psychomotor retardation

OCULAR FINDINGS

Severe malformation of lids, with vertical shortening due to absence of lid

THERAPEUTIC ASPECTS

Continuous ocular surface lubrication should be instituted from birth to prevent damage from corneal exposure.

Surgical intervention to correct vertical lid shortening and accompanying entropion or ectropion should be performed as soon as feasible after birth.

REFERENCE

Hornblass A, Reifler DM: Ablepharon macrostomia syndrome. *Am J Ophthalmol* 1985;99:552–556.

RESOURCE

FACES: The National Craniofacial Association www.faces-cranio.org

Achromatopsia

See Retinal Dystrophies and Degenerations

Adenomatous Polyposis of Colon

Also called familial adenomatous polyposis *or* Gardner syndrome*; includes* Turcot syndrome

OMIM NUMBERS

175100
276300

INHERITANCE

Autosomal dominant

GENE/GENE MAP

APC (adenomatous polyposis coli), a tumor-suppressor gene
5q11–q22

EPIDEMIOLOGY

1 in 13,500 in Denmark
1 in 50,000 in Northern England

CLINICAL FINDINGS

Hundreds of adenomatous colonic polyps, with inevitable progression to colon cancer if colectomy is not performed.

Called *Gardner syndrome* when extracolonic manifestations are present. These include benign soft-tissue and bony tumors, jaw lesions, desmoid tumors (10%), and pigmented ocular fundus lesions (POFLs).

Higher risk of developing extracolonic cancers of the thyroid, adrenal glands, and liver.

Turcot syndrome is a variant of familial adenomatous polyposis (FAP) with brain tumors such as glioblastoma multiforme and astrocytoma. Turcot syndrome can also result from mutations in the mismatch repair genes *MLH1* or *PMS2*.

OCULAR FINDINGS

Multiple and bilateral asymptomatic patches of congenital hypertrophy (with or without hyperplasia) of the retinal pigment epithelium (CHRPE). The presence of four or more POFLs is a reliable presymptomatic, highly specific (>90%), and relatively sensitive (70% to 80%) clinical marker for FAP. This biologic marker is especially helpful in families where multiple affected individuals have numerous POFLs because of the intrafamilial consistency of expression of the ocular trait. The absence of the ocular trait, however, does not rule out the disease in any family. The number of POFLs appears to be consistent among members of individual families. Pigmented ocular fundus lesions are absent in some families with FAP. They do not interfere with vision. Some patients with Turcot syndrome have multiple POFLs.

Mutations in exons 1 to 8 of the *APC* gene are associated with a POFL-negative phenotype, while those in exons 10 to 15 are generally associated with a POFL-positive phenotype. Mutations in exons 4, 5, 9, and distal 15 are associated with an attenuated phenotype, while those between codons 1250 and 1464 lead to a more severe phenotype. Mutations lead to a truncated protein product and loss of protein function.

Orbital osteomas have been reported in a few patients with Gardner syndrome.

Epidermal cysts of the lid skin may occur in some patients.

THERAPEUTIC ASPECTS

Determination of disease status in children is done by ocular examination, panoramic X-rays of the mandible to detect opaque jaw lesions, testing of the *APC* gene for mutations or its protein product for truncation, or a combination of these.

Examination of the colon for polyps should be performed annually, commencing at 10 years of age, in patients at risk for the disease.

Colectomy before the development of colon cancer remains the mainstay of treatment.

Six months of twice-daily treatment with 400 mg celecoxib, a cyclooxygenase-2 inhibitor, leads to a reduction in the number of colorectal polyps.

REFERENCES

Blair NP, Trempe CL: Hypertrophy of the retinal pigment epithelium associated with Gardner's syndrome. *Am J Ophthalmol* 1980;90:661–667.

Olschwang S, Tiret A, Laurent-Puig P, et al: Restriction of ocular fundus lesions to a specific subgroup of *APC* mutations in adenomatous polyposis coli patients. *Cell* 1993;75:959–968.

Steibach G, Lynch P, Phillips RK, et al: The effect of celecoxib, a cyclooxygenase-2 inhibitor, in familial adenomatous polyposis. *N Engl J Med* 2000;342:1946–1952.

Traboulsi EI, Krush AJ, Gardner EJ, et al: Prevalence and importance of ocular fundus lesions in Gardner's syndrome. *N Engl J Med* 1987;316:661–667.

Traboulsi EI, Murphy SF, Maumenee IH, et al: A clinico-pathologic study of the eyes in familial adenomatous polyposis with extracolonic manifestations (Gardner's syndrome). *Am J Ophthalmol* 1990;110:550–561.

Wallis YL, Macdonald F, Hulten M, et al: Genotype–phenotype correlation between position of constitutional *APC* gene mutation and CHRPE expression in familial adenomatous polyposis. *Hum Genet* 1994; 94:543–548.

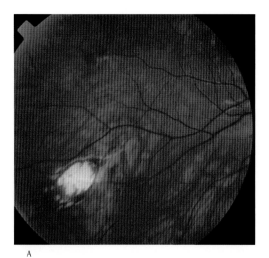

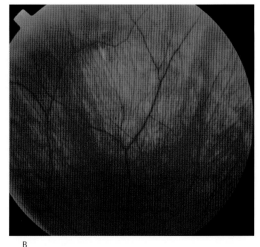

A   B

Adenomatous polyposis of colon (A) Fundus photograph of multiple pigmented ocular fundus lesions in a patient with familial adenomatous polyposis. One of the lesions is round with two smaller satellite lesions. The larger lesion is mostly depigmented but has the characteristic droplet shape. A very small lesion is seen at the superior edge of the photo. (B) Fundus photograph of a typical peripheral elongated lesion with a trail of depigmentation.

RESOURCES

Familial Polyposis Registry
  Department of Colorectal Surgery
  Cleveland Clinic Foundation
  9500 Euclid Ave.
  Cleveland, OH 44195-5001
  216-444-6470
Hereditary Colon Cancer Association
  3601 N. 4th Ave., Suite 201
  Sioux Falls, SD 57104
  605-373-2067
  800-264-6783
  hcc@dtgnet.com

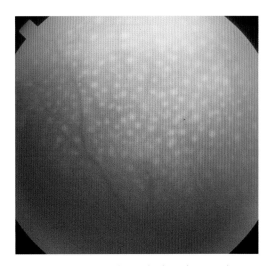

Neonatal adrenoleukodystrophy (NALD) Leopard-spot retinopathy in an infant with NALD. (Courtesy of Sprague Eustis, M.D.)

Adrenoleukodystrophy, Neonatal (NALD)

OMIM NUMBER
202370

INHERITANCE
Autosomal recessive

GENE/GENE MAP
Caused by mutations in *PTS1* receptor gene (*PXR1*, OMIM 600414), peroxin-1 gene (*PEX1*, OMIM 602136), peroxin-10 gene (*PEX10*, OMIM 602859), and peroxin-13 gene (*PEX13*, OMIM 601789)

EPIDEMIOLOGY
Very rare

CLINICAL FINDINGS
Onset is in the first few days of life, with severe psychomotor retardation, opisthotonus, and seizures.

There is extensive demyelination of the brain.

Patients have adrenal insufficiency and later become deaf and blind.

Death occurs between the ages of 1 and 9 years.

There are increased serum levels of very long chain fatty acids (VLCFAs) and decreased plasmalogen levels.

OCULAR FINDINGS
Abnormal retinal pigmentation, with "leopard spots" and optic atrophy.

The electroretinogram is nonrecordable.

Other ocular findings include neonatal polar cataracts and strabismus.

THERAPEUTIC ASPECTS
No specific treatment

REFERENCES

Al-Hazzaa SA, Ozand PT: Peroxisomal bifunctional enzyme deficiency with associated retinal findings. *Ophthalmic Genet* 1997;18:93–99.

Cohen SM, Green WR, de la Cruz ZC, et al: Ocular histopathologic studies of neonatal and childhood adrenoleukodystrophy. *Am J Ophthalmol* 1983;95:82–96.

Folz SJ, Trobe JD: The peroxisome and the eye. *Surv Ophthalmol* 1991;35:353–368.

RESOURCE

United Leukodystrophy Foundation
  www.ulf.org

Adrenoleukodystrophy, X-Linked

OMIM NUMBER
300100

INHERITANCE
X-linked

GENE/GENE MAP
ALDP (adrenoleukodystrophy protein) involved in peroxisome biogenesis: very long chain fatty acid coenzyme A (VLCFA CoA) synthetase

Belongs to ATP-binding superfamily of transporters

Xq28

EPIDEMIOLOGY
1 in 15,000 to 1 in 20,000

CLINICAL FINDINGS
A defect in peroxisomal VLCFA metabolism leads to increased concentrations of hexacosanoate (C26:0) and other VLCFAs in plasma and their accumulation in brain white matter and adrenal cortex.

The phenotype is extremely variable. There are six types of presentation. The most common is (1) the childhood cerebral form, which occurs in 50% of patients. Onset is between 4 and 8 years of age. The first symptoms are behavioral disturbances and scholastic failure or increased skin pigmentation, often precipitated by a viral illness. The disease course worsens over several years and is characterized by dementia, visual loss, hearing loss, and motor disturbances, including spastic paraplegia, ataxia, sphincter disturbances, impotence, and peripheral neuropathy. Primary adrenal insufficiency leads to skin hyperpigmentation and symptoms of hypoadrenalism. The main pathologic finding is a severe, progressive demyelination in the occipital and posterior parietal areas, with caudorostral spread of the lesions.

Other forms of the disease include (2) adolescent cerebral (5%), (3) adult cerebral (3%), and (4) adrenomyeloneuropathy (AMN) (25%), in which patients present in the third decade of life with progressive spastic paraparesis, peripheral neuropathy, and bowel and bladder disturbances. The adrenal insufficiency is severe, and gonadal function may be impaired. Adrenomyeloneuropathy shows the same ultrastructural and biochemical abnormalities as childhood ALD, and the two disorders have occurred in the same kindred and even in siblings. Visual abnormalities have not been reported in AMN.

The last two types are (5) isolated adrenal insufficiency (Addison disease) and (6) an asymptomatic form (10%). Some of these types convert to other phenotypes with time.

OCULAR FINDINGS
Visual disturbances are extremely common and include loss of visual acuity, homonymous hemianopia, and visual agnosia. They rarely precede other neurologic deficits.

Optic atrophy eventually occurs in all patients with the childhood cerebral form. Optic nerve hypoplasia has been reported in one patient.

Horizontal gaze abnormalities simulating congenital motor apraxia may occur. Exotropia is frequent.

Loss of corneal sensation can result from peripheral neuropathy.

THERAPEUTIC ASPECTS
Unsuccessful therapeutic approaches include dietary restriction of VLCFAs, administration of carnitine and clofibrate, immunosuppression, plasma exchange, and systemic corticosteroids.

REFERENCES
Cohen SM, Green WR, de la Cruz ZC, et al: Ocular histopathologic studies of neonatal and childhood adrenoleukodystrophy. *Am J Ophthalmol* 1983;95: 82–96.

Moser HW, Smith KD, Moser AB: X-linked adrenoleukodystrophy. In: Scriver CR, Beaudet AL, Sly WS, et al, eds: *The Metabolic and Molecular Bases of Inherited Disease.* New York: McGraw-Hill; 1995:2325–2349.

Traboulsi EI, Maumenee IH: Ophthalmologic manifestations of X-linked childhood adrenoleukodystrophy. *Ophthalmology* 1987;94:47–52.

RESOURCE

United Leukodystrophy Foundation
www.ulf.org

Aicardi Syndrome

OMIM NUMBER
304050

INHERITANCE
X-linked with lethality in hemizygous males
All cases are the result of new mutations

GENE/GENE MAP
Xp22

EPIDEMIOLOGY
200 cases in world literature

CLINICAL FINDINGS
A definite diagnosis requires the presence of all three major features:
1. Infantile flexion spasms
2. Structural brain abnormalities, the most consistent of which is partial or complete absence of the corpus callosum
3. Typical lacuna-shaped chorioretinal lesions

A number of other congenital malformations may also be present, including costovertebral defects in the form of hemivertebrae or butterfly vertebrae, absent or abnormal ribs, cleft lip and/or palate, hiatal hernia, hip dysplasia, postaxial polydactyly (personal observation), and precocious puberty.

A few patients have developed tumors: choroid plexus papillomas in five, teratoma of the soft palate in one, and embryonal carcinoma of the cheek in one.

OCULAR FINDINGS
The chorioretinal lesions of Aicardi syndrome are characteristic, and their presence often leads to the correct diagnosis. The lesions are round, well-defined, and excavated (lacunar), have minimal pigmentation along their edges, and are most frequently found around the optic nerve head and at the posterior pole. The lesions decrease in size and number toward the peripheral fundus. Some patients may have only a few small lesions.

Ocular histopathologic studies have shown abnormalities of retinal architecture, with anterior displacement of retinal insertion, areas of atrophy of the retinal pigment epithelium, and hyperplasia and migration of the retinal pigment epithelium. There are areas of retinal dysplasia with photoreceptor rosette formation. The sensory retina may be completely absent in the "lacunae."

Electroretinographic studies are normal or minimally abnormal.

Other associated ocular malformations include microphthalmos with or without cyst, typical chorioretinal colobomas at the disc or elsewhere in the inferior fundus, gliosis at the nerve head, persistence of the hyaloid system of blood vessels, persistence of the pupillary membrane, posterior synechiae, and retinal detachment.

Nystagmus and sixth cranial nerve palsy have also been reported.

THERAPEUTIC ASPECTS
Treatment consists of antiepileptic medications and general supportive measures.

Most patients die in the first decade of life, usually from recurrent pneumonia and debilitation.

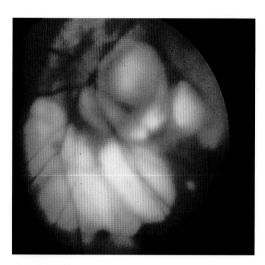

Aicardi syndrome Typical retinal "lacunar" lesions in the inferior part of the posterior fundus surrounding an optic nerve with colobomatous defects.

REFERENCES

Aicardi J, Lefebvre J, Lerique-Koechlin A: A new syndrome: spasms in flexion, callosal agenesis, ocular abnormalities. *Electroencephalogr Clin Neurophysiol* 1965;19:609–610.

Del Pero RA, Mets MB, Tripathi RC, et al: Anomalies of retinal architecture in Aicardi syndrome. *Arch Ophthalmol* 1986;104:1659–1664.

Donnenfeld AE, Packer RJ, Zackai EH, et al: Clinical, cytogenetic, and pedigree findings in 18 cases of Aicardi syndrome. *Am J Med Genet* 1989;32:461–467.

Lorenz B, Hasenfratz G, Laub MC, et al: Retrobulbar cysts in Aicardi's syndrome. *Ophthalmic Genet* 1991;12:105–110.

Menezes AV, Enzenauer RW, Buncic JR: Aicardi syndrome: the elusive mild case. *Br J Ophthalmol* 1994;78:494–496.

RESOURCE

Aicardi Syndrome Foundation
www.aicardisyndrome.org

Alagille Syndrome

Also called arteriohepatic dysplasia

OMIM NUMBER
118450

INHERITANCE
Autosomal dominant

GENE/GENE MAP
Jagged 1 encodes ligand of transmembrane notch receptor
20p12

EPIDEMIOLOGY
1 in 70,000 to 1 in 100,000 live births

CLINICAL FINDINGS
Three of the five main clinical criteria are needed for diagnosis:

1. Neonatal jaundice: cholestasis is nonprogressive and usually improves with age
2. Pulmonic valvular and peripheral arterial stenosis
3. Posterior embryotoxon
4. Distinctive facies with broad forehead, prominent mandible, and bulbous tip of nose
5. Skeletal abnormalities of spine (butterfly vertebrae), ribs, and limbs

The diagnosis should be suspected in a child with neonatal jaundice and posterior embryotoxon.

There is hypoplasia of the interlobular bile ducts in the liver. The extrahepatic biliary duct

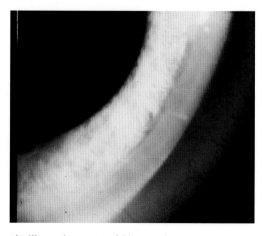

Alagille syndrome Axenfeld anomaly.

may also be involved. This results in hypercholesterolemia and hypertriglyceridemia. Serum liver enzyme levels may be chronically elevated.

Other clinical findings include renal dysplasia, endocrine abnormalities, growth retardation, absent deep tendon reflexes, learning disability, and (rarely) tumors such as hepatocarcinoma and papillary thyroid carcinoma.

OCULAR FINDINGS

Mild anterior segment dysgenesis, with prominence and anterior displacement of Schwalbe's line (posterior embryotoxon), is common. This is present in 50% to 75% of patients. Circulus juvenilus can result from the hypercholesterolemia.

Pigmentary changes and chorioretinal atrophy occur in 57% to 69% of cases. Electroretinogram and electrooculogram abnormalities are nonspecific.

Anomalous optic discs are found in 75% of cases, with optic nerve drusen (50% bilateral, 90% unilateral).

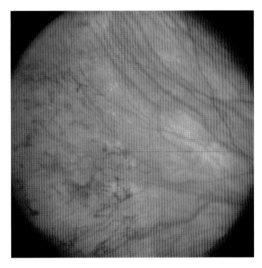

Alagille syndrome Pigmentary retinopathy.

Less common are vascular tortuosity, choroidal folds, infantile myopia, band keratopathy, keratoconus, and posterior subcapsular cataracts.

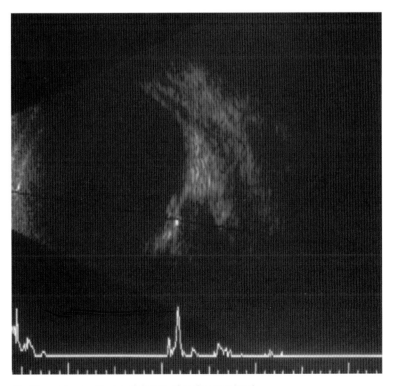

Alagille syndrome B-scan of drusen of optic nerve head.

THERAPEUTIC ASPECTS

Early supplementation with fat-soluble vitamins is recommended to prevent pigmentary retinopathy.

Symptomatic treatment for pruritus is helpful.

Liver transplantation in selected patients is advisable.

Twenty-five percent of patients die before age 5 years from cardiovascular or hepatic complications.

REFERENCES

Alagille D, Odievre M, Gautier M, et al: Hepatic ductular hypoplasia associated with characteristic facies, vertebral malformations, retarded physical, mental and sexual development, and cardiac murmur. *J Paediatr* 1975;86:631.

Brodsky MC, Cunniff C: Ocular anomalies in the Alagille syndrome (arteriohepatic dysplasia). *Ophthalmology* 1993;100:1767–1774.

Hingorani M, Nischal KK, et al: Ocular abnormalities in Alagille syndrome. *Ophthalmology* 1999; 106:330–337.

Oda T, Elkahloun AG, Pike BL, et al: Mutations in the human *Jagged I* gene are responsible for Alagille syndrome. *Nat Genet* 1997;16:235–242.

Puklin JE, Riely CA, Simon RM, et al: Anterior segment and retinal pigmentary abnormalities in arteriohepatic dysplasia. *Ophthalmology* 1981;88: 337.

RESOURCE

The Alagille Syndrome Alliance
www.alagille.org

Albinism

OMIM NUMBERS

OCA1: 203100
OCA2: 203200
OCA3: 203290
OCA4: 606574
Albinism, ocular (OA1): 300500
Hermansky-Pudlak syndrome (HPS): 203300
Chediak-Higashi syndrome (CHS1): 214500

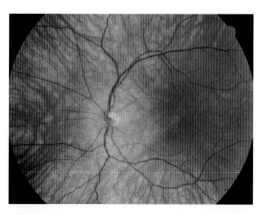

Albinism Ocular fundus hypopigmentation and foveal hypoplasia in tyrosinase-positive oculocutaneous albinism.

INHERITANCE

All autosomal recessive, except Nettleship-Falls ocular albinism, which is X-linked recessive

GENE/GENE MAP

See Table 8.

EPIDEMIOLOGY

Prevalence varies with the racial makeup in any particular geographic area. Frequency is 1 in 18,000 among U.S. whites, 1 in 10,000 among U.S. blacks, and 1 in 20,000 in the United States overall.

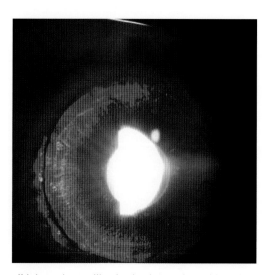

Albinism Iris transillumination in a patient with oculocutaneous albinism.

TABLE 8. Types of Albinism and Genetic Defects

Clinical Type of Albinism	Abbreviation	OMIM No.	Defective Gene	Gene Map
Tyrosinase-negative oculocutaneous albinism	OCA1a	203100	Tyrosinase	11q14–q21
Yellow-type oculocutaneous albinism	OCA1b	606952	Tyrosinase	11q14–q21
Tyrosinase-positive oculocutaneous albinism	OCA2	203200	*P* gene or tyrosinase	15q11.2–q12 11q14–q21
Rufous albinism (xanthism)	ROCA	278400	*TYRP1* Tyrosinase-related protein	9p23
Brown albinism	BOCA or OCA3	203290	*P* gene	15q11.2–q12
Oculocutaneous albinism type IV	OCA4	606574	*MATP*	5p
Nettleship-Falls ocular albinism, X-linked ocular albinism	OA1	300500	Melanosomal G protein-coupled receptor	Xp22.3
Hermansky-Pudlak syndrome	HPS1 HPS2	203300 603401	Transmembrane component of cytoplasmic organelles	10q23.1–q23.3
Chediak-Higashi syndrome	CHS	214500	*CHS/LYST* Important in lysosomal and granular cell compartmentalization	1q43

CLINICAL FINDINGS

Albinism comprises a heterogeneous group of inherited disorders characterized by the reduction or total absence of pigment in the eyes, hair, and skin.

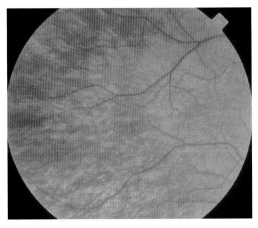

Albinism Posterior pole in female carrier of X-linked ocular albinism with pigment mottling

Albinism has been classified as total or partial by the degree and distribution of hypopigmentation and as ocular versus oculocutaneous.

With the identification of the underlying molecular mechanisms, albinism can now be more accurately classified according to the specific genetic defect in each clinical subtype (Table 9).

OCULAR FINDINGS

Ocular abnormalities are present in all forms of albinism. Signs and symptoms vary in severity.

Signs include nystagmus, hypopigmentation of the uveal tract and retinal pigment epithelium, iris transillumination, foveal hypoplasia, and abnormal decussation of optic nerve fibers at the chiasm.

Strabismus and high refractive errors are common.

Symptoms include decreased visual acuity, reduced or absent stereoacuity, and photophobia.

TABLE 9. Melanogenesis Disorders

Feature	1A	1B	2	4	XLOA	Hermansky-Pudlak	Chediak-Higashi
						Type	
Name	Tyrosinase-negative	Yellow albinism	Tyrosinase-positive	Brown albinism	Nettleship-Falls		
Characteristics	No pigment VA around 20/200 Nystagmus Foveal hypoplasia Strabismus	Little or no pigment at birth—increases with age Phenotypic variability	Little pigment at birth—increases with age VA 20/60–20/400	Moderate hypopigmentation VA 20/60–20/200	Mild skin, iris, retinal hypopigmentation Iris transillumination defects	Lightly pigmented skin and iris Normal or decreased VA Bleeding diathesis Pulmonary fibrosis	Variable pigmentation Normal to moderately decreased VA Immune deficiency Decreased life span
Gene/gene map	Tyrosinase (TYR) 11p14–p21	Tyrosinase (TYR) 11p14–p21 (allelic with 1A)	P (pink eye dilution) 15q11.2–q12	Tyrosinase-related protein 1 9p22–p23	Melanosomal G protein-coupled receptor Xp22.3	Organelle structural membrane protein defect 12q12–q13	Intracellular protein transport defect 1q43
Inheritance	AR	AR	AR	AR	XR	AR	AR
Pathophysiology	Normal number of melanosomes with no melanin	Incomplete and decreased melanization	Abnormal transport of tyrosine across melanosome membrane	Defect in enzyme in melanin biosynthesis	Decreased number of melanosomes with normal melanin	Pheomelanosomes unevenly melanized melanosomes	Giant melanosomes Decreased number of melanosomes
Hairbulb melanosomes	Stage I and II premelanosomes	Stage I, II, and III premelanosomes	Stage II and III premelanosomes	Stage II and III premelanosomes with few stage IV melanosomes	Stage IV melanosomes Macromelanosomes	Stage I, II, and III premelanosomes	Stage II and II premelanosomes Stage IV melanosomes Macromelanosomes
Diagnostic tests	Hairbulb test negative Carriers: decreased TYR activity	Hairbulb test negative or weakly positive (positive with l-cysteine)	Hairbulb test positive Visual evoked potentials	Hairbulb test positive	Hairbulb test positive Macromelanosomes Carriers: tigroid fundus	Hairbulb test positive Prolonged bleeding time Ceroid accumulation	Hairbulb test positive Giant lysosomal granules Decreased natural killer cell activity

AR = autosomal recessive; XR = X-linked recessive; VA = visual acuity; XLOA = X-linked ocular albinism.

Source: Abrams LS, Traboulsi EI: Albinism. In: Traboulsi EI, ed: *Genetic Diseases of the Eye.* New York: Oxford University Press; 1998:697–721.

Female carriers of the X-linked ocular form have pathognomonic fundus findings. Mottled pigmentation at the posterior pole merges with peripheral linear streaks of hypopigmentation and normal pigmentation, giving the fundus a "mud-splattered" appearance.

THERAPEUTIC ASPECTS

Puerto Rican albinos or those with easy bruisability should be screened for a bleeding diathesis and Hermansky-Pudlak syndrome.

Patients with albinism and recurrent infections should be suspected of having Chediak-Higashi syndrome.

There is a predisposition to actinic-induced skin cancer. Patients are instructed to avoid direct prolonged sun exposure, use sunscreens, and have regular examinations for cutaneous neoplasms in sun-exposed areas. Tinted glasses are useful for patients with significant light sensitivity. Optimal correction of refractive errors should be attempted. Low-vision aids may be helpful.

Strabismus is common, and patients may require patching and/or surgery. Kestenbaum procedures can be used in patients who adopt a head posture to reduce the torticollis.

REFERENCES

Abrams LS, Traboulsi EI: Albinism. In: Traboulsi EI, ed: *Genetic Diseases of the Eye.* New York: Oxford University Press; 1998:697–721.

Riemann B, Traboulsi EI: Overview of human albinism. *Contemporary Ophthalmology* 2003:2(3).

RESOURCES

The National Organization for Albinism and Hypopigmentation
www.albinism.org
University of Minnesota Computational Biology Centers
www.cbc.umn.edu/tad/genes.htm

Alport Syndrome

OMIM NUMBERS

X-linked: 301050
Autosomal: 203780
Autosomal dominant: 104200

INHERITANCE

X-linked is the most frequent type (85% of patients), but the autosomal recessive type has also been documented. The existence of an autosomal dominant form is considered less clear.

GENE/GENE MAP

X-linked form at Xq22.3 (*COL4A5*)

Autosomal recessive form at 2q36–q37: mutation in either the *COL4A3* gene (collagen 4 alpha 3 polypeptide) (OMIM 120070) or the *COL4A4* gene (collagen 4 alpha 4 polypeptide) (OMIM 120131)

Fechtner syndrome (OMIM 153640) at 22q12.1–q13.2, 22q11.2

Epstein syndrome (OMIM 153650) at 22q11–q13

EPIDEMIOLOGY

1 in 5000

CLINICAL FINDINGS

The features are hereditary chronic nephritis, sensorineural hearing loss, and ocular abnormalities. All the following criteria are required for diagnosis:

1. Hematuria with or without proteinuria, hypertension, and renal failure
2. Proven renal disease in at least one affected relative
3. Neural hearing loss in the proband or in a relative

Nephritis usually presents as hematuria or proteinuria in childhood or early adult life and may persist without further deterioration of renal function or may progress to renal failure.

Males are more likely to have progressive kidney disease than are females.

Fechtner syndrome is Alport syndrome with leukocyte inclusions and macrothrombocytopenia.

Epstein syndrome is Alport syndrome with macrothrombocytopenia.

OCULAR FINDINGS

Dot-and-fleck retinopathy occurs in about 85% of affected adult males.

Anterior lenticonus occurs in about 25% of patients.

Rarely, patients have a posterior polymorphous corneal dystrophy.

The retinopathy and anterior lenticonus are not usually demonstrated in childhood, but worsen with time so that the retinal lesion is often present at the onset of renal failure and the anterior lenticonus later. The demonstration of dot-and-fleck retinopathy in any individual with a family history of Alport syndrome or with end-stage renal disease is diagnostic of Alport syndrome. The presence of anterior lenticonus or posterior polymorphous corneal dystrophy in any individual is highly suggestive of the diagnosis.

Additional ocular features described in X-linked Alport syndrome include other corneal

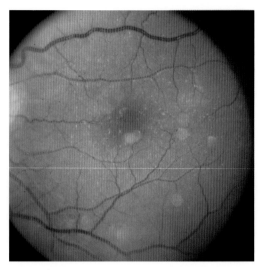

Alport syndrome Subretinal fine hard flecks in a patient with Alport syndrome.

dystrophies, microcornea, arcus, iris atrophy, cataracts, spontaneous lens rupture, spherophakia, posterior lenticonus, a poor macular reflex, fluorescein angiogram hyperfluorescence, electro-oculogram and electroretinogram abnormalities, and retinal pigmentation.

The ocular and other clinical features of autosomal recessive Alport syndrome are identical to those seen in X-linked disease, while retinopathy and cataracts are the only ocular abnormalities described in the rare autosomal dominant form.

THERAPEUTIC ASPECTS

Renal transplantation has been performed successfully in patients with advanced renal failure.

Generally, the anterior lenticonus does not require cataract surgery.

REFERENCES

Aubler M, Levy M, Broyer M, et al: Alport's syndrome: a report of 58 cases and a review of the literature. *Am J Med* 1981;70:493–505.

Colville DJ, Savige J: Alport syndrome: a review of the ocular manifestations. *Ophthalmic Genet* 1997;18:161–173.

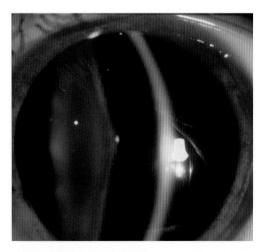

Alport syndrome Anterior lenticonus in a 14-year-old with Alport syndrome.

Pajari H, Setala K, Heiskari N, et al: Ocular findings in 34 patients with Alport syndrome: correlation of the findings to mutations in *COL4A5* gene. *Acta Ophthalmol Scand* 1999;77:214–217.

Patterson LA, Rao KV, Crosson JT, et al: Fechtner syndrome: a variant of Alport's syndrome with leukocyte inclusions and macrothrombocytopenia. *Blood* 1985;65:397–406.

Polak BC, Hogewind BL: Macular lesions in Alport's disease. *Am J Ophthalmol* 1977;84:532–535.

RESOURCES

Alport Syndrome Home Page
  alport.cjb.net
Hereditary Nephritis Foundation
  1390 W 6690 S, #202H
  Murray, UT 84123
  801-262-5901
  www.cc.utah.edu/~cla6202/HNF.htm

Alström Syndrome

OMIM NUMBER
203800

INHERITANCE
Autosomal recessive

GENE/GENE MAP
ALMS1 gene
2p13

EPIDEMIOLOGY
Frequent among French Acadians of Yarmouth County, Nova Scotia, and of Louisiana

CLINICAL FINDINGS
Patients have retinitis pigmentosa, deafness, obesity, and diabetes mellitus that results from resistance to insulin. Patients can develop a dilated cardiomyopathy even in infancy. In contrast to patients with Bardet-Biedl syndrome, there is no polydactyly, mental retardation, or hypogonadism.

Other less common clinical features include a slowly progressive chronic nephropathy, deafness, acanthosis nigricans, diabetes insipidus, and liver failure and cirrhosis.

OCULAR FINDINGS
Photophobia and nystagmus are present early in life. Electroretinography shows severe cone impairment, with mild or no rod involvement early in the disease and progression to more severe rod dysfunction as patients grow older.

Russell-Eggitt et al. found 37 cases of the syndrome in the world literature since 1959. Of 22 patients admitted to the Great Ormond Street Hospital for Children in London, 18 had infantile cardiomyopathy. These authors confirmed the severe and progressive infantile retinal dystrophy with better-preserved rod than cone function. Visual acuity decreased to less than 20/200 by 10 years of age and to no light perception by 20 years of age.

THERAPEUTIC ASPECTS
The syndrome should be considered in children and infants with obesity and a cone-rod dystrophy, especially in the presence of a dilated cardiomyopathy.

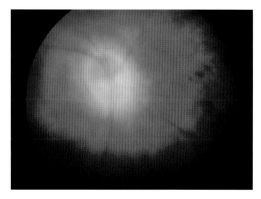

Alström syndrome Fundus photograph of a patient with Alström syndrome. (Courtesy of Alex Levin, M.D.)

REFERENCES

Collin GB, Marshall JD, Cardon LR, et al: Homozygosity mapping of Alström syndrome to chromosome 2p. *Hum Mol Genet* 1997;6:213–219.

Michaud JL, Heon E, Guilbert F, et al: Natural history of Alström syndrome in early childhood: onset with dilated cardiomyopathy. *J Pediatr* 1996; 128:225–229.

Millay RH, Weleber RG, Heckenlively JR: Ophthalmologic and systemic manifestations of Alström's disease. *Am J Ophthalmol* 1986;102:482–490.

Russell-Eggitt IM, Clayton PT, Coffey R, et al: Alström syndrome: report of 22 cases and literature review. *Ophthalmology* 1998;105:1274–1280.

RESOURCES

None listed

Angelman Syndrome

OMIM NUMBER

105830

INHERITANCE

The syndrome results from an absence of a maternal contribution to the imprinted 15q11–q13 region. This may arise from a de novo deletion in most cases or (rarely) from uniparental disomy. An absence of paternal genes from the 15q11–q13 segment results in Prader-Willi syndrome.

Most cases are sporadic and, less commonly, autosomal dominant that have been modified by imprinting with some nondeletion and some deletion cases.

GENE/GENE MAP

UBE3A gene, imprinting center *UPD* 15q11–q13

EPIDEMIOLOGY

1000 to 5000 cases in the United States and Canada

CLINICAL FINDINGS

The diagnosis is clinical and can be confirmed by laboratory testing in 80% of patients.

Table 10 lists the clinical findings that suggest the diagnosis.

Chromosome studies, as well as molecular analysis by fluorescent in situ hybridization (FISH), polymorphism analysis, or methylation testing to look for alterations in 15q11–q13, should be obtained in individuals in whom the diagnosis is highly probable. A positive genetic test confirms the diagnosis, but a normal result

TABLE 10. Diagnostic Criteria for Angelman Syndrome

Consistent (100%)
  Developmental delay, functionally severe
  Speech impairment, none or minimal use of words; receptive and nonverbal communication skills higher than verbal ones
  Movement or balance disorder, usually ataxia of gait and/or tremulous movement of limbs
  Behavioral uniqueness: any combination of frequent laughter/smiling, apparently happy demeanor

Frequent (more than 80%)
  Delayed, disproportionate growth in head circumference, usually resulting in microcephaly (absolute or relative) by age 2 years
  Seizures, onset usually <3 years of age
  Abnormal electroencephalogram, characteristic pattern with large-amplitude slow-spike waves (usually 2 to 3 seconds), facilitated by eye closure

Associated (20% to 80%)
  Flat occiput, occipital groove
  Protruding tongue, tongue thrusting, suck/swallowing disorders, feeding problems during infancy
  Strabismus
  Hypopigmented skin, light hair and eye color compared to family (seen only in deletion cases)
  Hyperactive lower limb deep tendon reflexes; uplifted, flexed arm position, especially during ambulation
  Increased sensitivity to heat
  Sleep disturbance
  Attraction to/fascination with water

Source: Williams CA, Angelman H, Clayton-Smith J, et al: Angelman syndrome: consensus for diagnostic criteria. Angelman Syndrome Foundation. *Am J Med Genet* 1995;56: 237–238.

does not exclude it. A positive genetic test is presumptive evidence for the presence of the syndrome even in individuals who do not have strong clinical evidence of the condition.

The diagnosis is usually not suspected during the first year of life but becomes a more frequent diagnostic consideration between 1 and 4 years of age. An abnormal electroencephalogram may be the first sign requiring diagnostic evaluation. During infancy, other clinical disorders can mimic the features of the syndrome. These include Rett syndrome, nonspecific cerebral palsy, Lennox-Gastaut syndrome, static encephalopathy with mental retardation, and infantile autism.

Patients with nondeletion Angelman syndrome have a less severe phenotype. These include patients with paternal uniparental disomy, imprinting mutations, and *UBE3A* mutations. The clinical severity is greatest in patients with deletions and less severe in those with *UBE3A* mutations, imprinting mutations, and uniparental disomy.

OCULAR FINDINGS
Ocular hypopigmentation
Optic atrophy (rare)
Strabismus

THERAPEUTIC ASPECTS
Most cases result from typical large de novo deletions of 15q11–q13 and are expected to have a low (less than 1%) risk of recurrence. Angelman syndrome due to paternal uniparental disomy, which occurs in the absence of a parental translocation, is likewise expected to have a recurrence risk of less than 1%.

In instances where there is no identifiable large deletion or uniparental disomy, the risk of recurrence may be as high as 50% as a result of either a maternally inherited imprinting center mutation or a mutation in the *UBE3A* gene. Individuals with the syndrome who have none of the above abnormalities comprise a significant proportion of cases, and some may have a 50% recurrence risk.

REFERENCES

Chan C-TJ, Clayton-Smith J, Cheng XJ, et al: Molecular mechanisms in Angelman syndrome: a survey of 93 patients. *J Med Genet* 1993;30:895–902.

Clayton-Smith J: Clinical research on Angelman syndrome in the United Kingdom: observations on 82 affected individuals. *Am J Med Genet* 1993;46:12–15.

Clayton-Smith J, Pembrey ME: Angelman syndrome. *J Med Genet* 1992;29:412–415.

Dickinson AJ, Fielder AR, Young ID, et al: Ocular findings in Angelman's (happy puppet) syndrome. *Ophthalmic Paediatr Genet* 1990;11:1–6.

Mah ML, Wallace DK, Powell CM: Ophthalmic manifestations of Angelman syndrome. *J Am Assoc Pediatr Ophthalmol Strabismus* 2000;4:248–249.

Williams CA, Angelman H, Clayton-Smith J, et al: Angelman syndrome: consensus for diagnostic criteria. Angelman Syndrome Foundation. *Am J Med Genet* 1995;56:237–238.

Zori RT, Hendrickson J, Woolven S, et al: Angelman syndrome: clinical profile. *J Child Neurol* 1992;7:270–280.

RESOURCE

Angelman Syndrome Foundation
www.angelman.org

Aniridia

OMIM NUMBERS
Aniridia: 106200
Gillespie syndrome: 206700

INHERITANCE
Autosomal dominant
Autosomal recessive in Gillespie syndrome
Sporadic in patients with 11p13 deletions

GENE/GENE MAP
Autosomal dominant: 11p13 with *PAX6* homeobox developmental gene mutations

Sporadic: chromosomal deletion at 11p13, location of *WT1* gene

EPIDEMIOLOGY

1.8 in 100,000 live births

CLINICAL FINDINGS

There are three recognized phenotypes:

1. Eighty-five percent are not associated with systemic abnormalities.
2. Thirteen percent have the WAGR association of Wilms' tumor (nephroblastoma), aniridia, genitourinary abnormalities, and mental retardation. Some of these patients have other malformations, such as hemihypertrophy. Ambiguous genitalia, mental and growth retardation, and multiple minor anomalies are part of this association (anomalies of the pinna, inguinal and umbilical hernias, microcephaly). Thirty-eight percent of WAGR patients develop nephropathy and renal failure in their lifetime.
3. Two percent have Gillespie syndrome of aniridia, developmental delay, and cerebellar ataxia.

OCULAR FINDINGS

There are congenital ocular findings of bilateral total or partial absence of the iris. *Aniridia* is a misnomer because careful examination of all patients reveals some iris tissue.

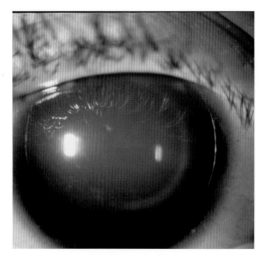

Aniridia Edge of the lens and cataract in aniridia.

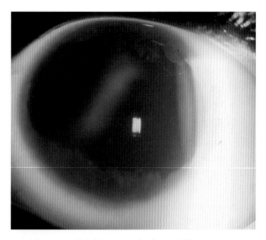

Aniridia Superficial keratopathy in aniridia.

Aniridia is a malformation of the whole eyeball, with abnormalities in most ocular tissues. Patients may have microcornea, corneal pannus, and opacification resulting from absence of limbal stem cells.

Isolated autosomal dominant keratitis is a variant of aniridia and results from mutations in the *PAX6* gene.

Cataracts are found in 85% of cases and dislocated lenses in 35%.

Secondary glaucoma occurs in up to 50% of patients; glaucoma is usually seen after the second decade of life as the peripheral iris stump adheres to the angle, occluding it. Goniodysgenesis is noted in some cases.

Foveal and optic nerve hypoplasia are seen frequently.

Nystagmus is present in the majority of cases, and photophobia is common.

Bilateral ptosis has been reported.

Visual acuity is less than 20/60 in all patients and less than 20/200 in more than 60%.

Rare families, with a very mild phenotype, have been reported in whom the incidence of cataracts and glaucoma is less than that of the classical, more common form of the disease and in whom visual acuity is better preserved.

Some patients with *PAX6* mutations may present with Peters anomaly or with isolated cataracts or foveal hypoplasia.

THERAPEUTIC ASPECTS

A karyotype should be obtained in all isolated cases to rule out a deletion at 11p13.

All patients with sporadic aniridia in whom mutation analysis of the *PAX6* gene has not been done or in whom no intragenic mutation has been demonstrated should have renal sonograms to rule out Wilms' tumor. Sonograms are started at age 6 months and are continued every 6 months until age 4. Sonograms are not necessary in familial cases since these are due to intragenic *PAX6* mutations, with no chance of deletions involving the neighboring Wilms' tumor gene.

Glaucoma and the complications of its surgical treatment are the main causes of blindness in patients with aniridia. Surgical treatment may be necessary if the glaucoma is not controlled by medications.

REFERENCES

Fraumeni JE Jr, Glass AG: Wilms' tumor and congenital aniridia. *JAMA* 1968;206:825–828.

Gillespie FD: Aniridia, cerebellar ataxia, and oligophrenia in siblings. *Arch Ophthalmol* 1965;73: 338–341.

Glaser T, Ton C, Mueller R, et al: Absence of *PAX6* gene mutations in Gillespie syndrome (partial aniridia cerebellar ataxia and mental retardation). *Genomics* 1994;19:145–148.

Glaser T, Walton D, Maas R: Genomic structure, evolutionary conservation and aniridia mutations in the human *PAX6* gene. *Nat Genet* 1992;2:232–239.

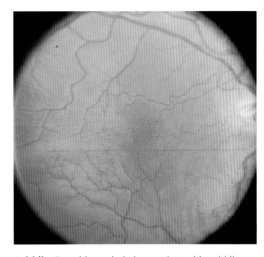

Aniridia Foveal hypoplasia in a patient with aniridia.

Hanson I, Fletcher J, Jordan T, et al: Mutations at the *PAX6* locus are found in heterogeneous anterior segment malformations including Peters' anomaly. *Nat Genet* 1994;6:168–173.

Miller RW, Fraumeni JF Jr, Manning MD: Association of Wilms' tumor with aniridia, hemihypertrophy and other congenital malformations. *N Engl J Med* 1964;270:922–927.

Mirzayans F, Pearce W, MacDonald I, et al: Mutation of the *PAX6* gene in patients with autosomal dominant keratitis. *Am J Hum Genet* 1995;57:539–548.

RESOURCE

The Human PAX6 Allele Variant Database Web Site
http://pax6.hgu.mrc.ac.uk/

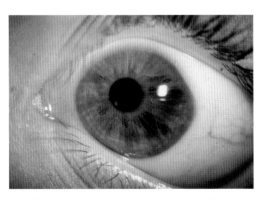

Aniridia Significant remnants of an iris resembling Rieger anomaly.

Anterior Segment Dysgenesis

See **Axenfeld-Rieger Syndrome**

Autosomal Dominant Vitreoretinochoroidopathy (ADVIRC)

OMIM NUMBER
193220

INHERITANCE
Autosomal dominant

GENE/GENE MAP
Not mapped

EPIDEMIOLOGY
Only three families have been reported.

CLINICAL FINDINGS
No systemic clinical findings

OCULAR FINDINGS
Vitreoretinochoroidopathy, with choroidal atrophy and diffuse vascular incompetence. Very slow progression of visual and electro-physiologic dysfunction. Patients do not complain of night blindness.

Presenile cataracts occur in all patients.

Less commonly, glaucoma, retinal detachment, and vitreous hemorrhage occur.

Ophthalmoscopy shows coarse pigmentary degeneration beyond vortex veins. Cystoid macular edema has been reported in one case. Preretinal white opacities, vitreous cells, and fibrillary changes can also occur.

THERAPEUTIC ASPECTS
Extraction of presenile cataracts

REFERENCES

Blair NP, Goldberg MF, Fishman GA, et al: Autosomal dominant vitreoretinochoroidopathy (ADVIRC). *Br J Ophthalmol* 1984;68:2–9.

Kaufman SJ, Goldberg MF, Orth DH, et al: Autosomal dominant vitreoretinochoroidopathy. *Arch Ophthalmol* 1982;100:272–278.

Traboulsi EI, Payne J: Autosomal dominant vitreoretinochoroidopathy and presenile cataracts: report of the third family. *Arch Ophthalmol* 1993; 111:194–196.

RESOURCES

None listed

Autosomal dominant vitreoretinochoroidopathy (ADVIRC) Peripheral pigmentary changes with well-delineated transition from normal retina in a 40-year-old female with ADVIRC.

Axenfeld-Rieger Syndrome

OMIM NUMBERS
See Table 11.

INHERITANCE
All variants are inherited in an autosomal dominant fashion.

GENE/GENE MAP
The genes for Axenfeld-Rieger syndrome and its variants, also known as *anterior segment dysgenesis*, are autosomal dominant, fully penetrant, and variable in expressivity. Clues to the location

TABLE 11. Anterior Segment Dysgenesis

Condition	OMIM Number	Gene (OMIM Number)/Gene Map
Anterior segment mesenchymal dysgenesis (ASMD) with autosomal dominant cataracts	107250	*PITX3* (602669)/10q25
Axenfeld-Rieger anomaly		*FOXC1* (601090)/6p25
Iridogoniodysgenesis anomaly	601631	6p25
Iridogoniodysgenesis syndrome (iris hypoplasia)	137600	*PITX2* (601542)/4q25
Peters anomaly	106210	*PAX6*/11p13 *PITX2* (601542)/4q25
Rieger syndrome type I	180500	*PITX2* (601542)/4q25
Rieger syndrome type II	601499	13q14

of these genes came from the reports of patients with anterior segment dysgenesis and chromosomal aberrations involving chromosomes 4, 6, 10, 13, 16, and 22. Using linkage analysis, Murray et al. mapped the gene for Rieger syndrome to 4q in one large family. Genetic heterogeneity was suggested by Mears et al., who mapped the gene of what they termed *iridogoniodysgenesis anomaly* (IGDA) to 6p25. Phillips et al. identified another locus for Rieger syndrome on chromosome 13q14. Semina et al. cloned the Rieger syndrome gene located at 4q25. This gene, now designated *PITX2*, is a *bicoid*-related homeobox transcription factor gene. Its murine homolog, *RIEG*, is expressed in periocular mesenchyme, maxillary and mandibular epithelia, the umbilicus, Rathke's pouch, vitelline vessels, and limb mesenchyme. Semina et al. identified six *RIEG* mutations in families with Rieger syndrome.

See also Table 11.

EPIDEMIOLOGY

Isolated Axenfeld anomaly (prominent and anteriorly displaced Schwalbe's line) is present in up to 15% of normal individuals.

Variants of Rieger anomaly and syndrome are rare. The exact incidence is not known.

CLINICAL FINDINGS

The Axenfeld-Rieger spectrum of ocular anomalies results from an abnormality of neural

crest development and/or resorption in the developing iris, anterior chamber angle, and cornea.

In Rieger syndrome, systemic anomalies are also due to abnormal neural crest differentiation in structures such as facial bones and cartilage, dental papillae, and the primitive periumbilical ring. This leads to a phenotype characterized by

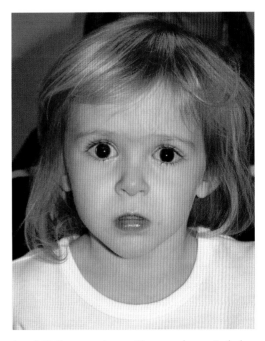

Axenfeld-Rieger syndrome: Rieger syndrome Typical facial appearance with malar hypoplasia and pointed chin. Red reflex from the right eye is due to extensive absence of iris tissue. This patient also has glaucoma.

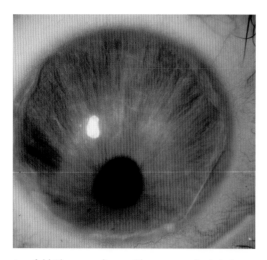

Axenfeld-Rieger syndrome: Rieger anomaly Anterior segment photograph showing a prominent Schwalbe's line, ectopic pupil, and iris hypoplasia.

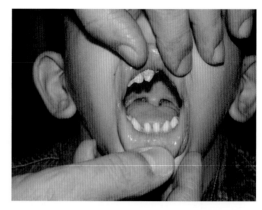

Axenfeld-Rieger syndrome: Rieger syndrome Dental abnormalities in a patient with Rieger syndrome.

facial dysmorphism, with maxillary hypoplasia and a receding chin, hypodontia and peg-shaped teeth, and redundant periumbilical skin. Less common abnormalities include congenital cardiac defects and hydrocephalus.

OCULAR FINDINGS

There is extreme variability in the appearance of the anterior segment of patients with Axenfeld-Rieger syndrome. Some family members of patients with classic iris, angle, and corneal changes have elevated intraocular pressure with a normal-appearing anterior segment, while rare others have a clinical picture compatible with Peters anomaly or aniridia. The most common clinical picture is characterized by a prominent and anteriorly displaced Schwalbe's line to which attach strands of peripheral iris; the pupil is displaced and the iris is so thin in some areas as to be absent, leading to the formation of atypical colobomas or polycoria. In families with predominant iris thinning and absence of an Axenfeld-type anomaly, Axenfeld-Rieger syndrome has been reported and later shown to result from mutation of *PITX2*.

Individuals with isolated Axenfeld anomaly are probably not at increased risk of glaucoma.

However, patients with any variant of Axenfeld-Rieger syndrome are extremely likely to have increased intraocular pressure, with a lifetime risk of glaucoma of 50%.

Cataracts are uncommon except in patients whose phenotype resembles Peters anomaly or those with mutations in *PITX3*.

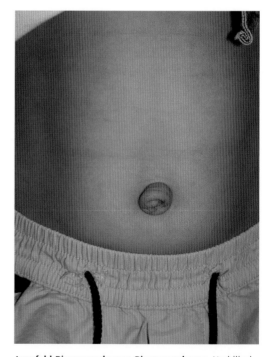

Axenfeld-Rieger syndrome: Rieger syndrome Umbilical protrusion because of absence of the umbilical ring derived from neural crest cells.

THERAPEUTIC ASPECTS

Monitoring for elevation of intraocular pressure is mandatory for these patients who have a 50% lifetime risk of glaucoma.

If glaucoma develops, medical therapy can be tried and may be effective, but most patients require surgical intervention. Tube surgery may be most effective.

REFERENCES

Alward WL: Axenfeld-Rieger syndrome in the age of molecular genetics. *Am J Ophthalmol* 2000;130: 107–115.

Lines MA, Kozlowski K, Walter MA: Molecular genetics of Axenfeld-Rieger malformations. *Hum Mol Genet* 2002;11:1177–1184.

Mears AJ, Mirzayans F, Gould DB, Pearce WG, Walter MA: Autosomal dominant iridogoniodysgenesis anomaly maps to 6p25. *Am J Hum Genet* 1996;59:1321–1327.

Murray J, Bennett S, Kwitek A, Small K, Schinzel A, Alward W, et al: Linkage of Rieger syndrome to the region of the epidermal growth factor gene on chromosome 4. *Nat Genet* 1992;2:46–49.

Phillips J, Del Bono E, Haines J, Pralea A, Cohen J, Greff L, et al: A second locus for Rieger syndrome maps to chromosome 13q14. *Am J Hum Genet* 1996;59:613–619.

Semina E, Reiter R, Leysens N, Alward W, Small K, Datson N, et al: Cloning and characterization of a novel *bicoid*-related homeobox transcription factor gene, *RIEG*, involved in Rieger syndrome. *Nat Genet* 1996;14:392–399.

Traboulsi EI: Malformations of the anterior segment of the eye. In: Traboulsi EI, ed: *Genetic Diseases of the Eye*. New York: Oxford University Press; 1998:81–98.

RESOURCES

None listed

Bardet-Biedl Syndrome (BBS)

OMIM NUMBERS
Type I: 209901
Type II: 209900
Type III: 600151
Type IV: 600374
Type V: 603650
Type VI: 605231
Type VII: 607590

INHERITANCE
Autosomal recessive

GENE/GENE MAP
There is genetic heterogeneity.
1. Type I: *BBS1* at 1q13
2. Type II: *BBS2* at 6q21
3. Type III: 3p13–p12
4. Type IV: *BBS4* at 5q22.3–q23
5. Type V: 2q31
6. Type VI: caused by mutations in *MKKS* on 20p12; the same recessive gene defect causes McKusick-Kaufman syndrome of hydrometrocolpos, polydactyly, and cardiac defects
7. Type VII: 4q27

There is now evidence that more than one of the BBS genes are involved in any one family with the syndrome.

EPIDEMIOLOGY
The prevalence in Newfoundland is about 10 times greater than in Switzerland (1 in 160,000) and is similar to the prevalence among the Bedouin of Kuwait (1 in 13,500).

CLINICAL FINDINGS
The modified diagnostic criteria according to Beales et al. (1999) require the presence of 4 of 6 major criteria or 3 of 6 major criteria plus 2 of 11 minor criteria.

Major diagnostic criteria:
1. Rod-cone or cone-rod dystrophy
2. Obesity
3. Polydactyly
4. Learning disabilities
5. Hypogonadism
6. Renal anomalies

Minor diagnostic criteria:
1. Speech disorder/delay
2. Strabismus, cataracts, astigmatism
3. Brachydactyly, syndactyly
4. Developmental delay
5. Polyuria, polydipsia (nephrogenic diabetes insipidus)
6. Ataxia, poor coordination, imbalance
7. Mild spasticity (lower limbs)
8. Diabetes mellitus
9. Dental crowding, hypodontia, high arched palate
10. Left ventricular hypertrophy, congenital heart disease
11. Hepatic fibrosis

The Laurence-Moon syndrome (OMIM 245800) is not characterized by obesity or polydactyly. Patients do, however, have spastic paraplegia or ataxia.

If iris coloboma is present instead of pigmentary retinopathy, patients have Biemond syndrome (OMIM 210350).

If diabetes mellitus, obesity, cardiomyoathy, and deafness are associated with other features of Bardet-Biedl syndrome, a diagnosis of Alström syndrome (OMIM 203800) should be considered.

Anosmia has recently been discovered in humans with BBS and results from a generalized defect in ciliated epithelia.

OCULAR FINDINGS

Pigmentary degeneration of the retina (80% of patients) has features of cone-rod dystrophy rather than typical retinitis pigmentosa. However, patients have been described with typical retinitis pigmentosa, retinitis pigmentosa sine pigmento, retinitis punctata albescens, congenital amaurosis of Leber, and optic atrophy.

Visual acuity deteriorates rapidly with age so that, by age 20, more than 75% of patients are legally blind (by age 30, more than 90%) from the retinal dystrophy.

Visual fields are markedly constricted, and severe abnormalities of color vision occur in the majority of patients.

The electroretinogram is nonrecordable or substantially reduced, with elevated dark-adaptation thresholds.

Nystagmus is present in 5% of patients.

THERAPEUTIC ASPECTS

There is no treatment to prevent deterioration of vision.

Surgical excision of the extra digit can be performed.

Obesity is a major source of stress for patients and parents. Early referral to a dietitian is important. A multidisciplinary approach to weight loss that includes a combination of dietary assessment, behavioral therapy, and exercise is recommended.

Educational needs and speech therapy for

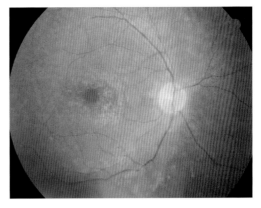

Bardet-Biedl syndrome (BBS) Peripheral fine pigmentary changes and macular atrophic changes in a patient with BBS.

these developmentally challenged patients should be addressed early.

The treatment of renal complications depends on the type of renal dysfunction. Antibiotics are prescribed for reflux. Monitoring for renal failure is essential. A minority of patients require dialysis. An occasional patient may need renal transplantation. Patients may die of renal failure in middle age.

Diabetes mellitus is usually of the non-insulin-dependent type, but some patients require insulin.

Endocrinologic issues include hypogonadism and short stature and may need to be treated with hormonal replacement.

REFERENCES

Beales PL, Badano JL, Ross AJ, Ansley SJ, Hoskins BE, Kirsten B, Mein CA, Froguel P, Scambler PJ, Lewis RA, Lupski JR, Katsanis N: Genetic interaction of *BBS1* mutations with alleles at other BBS loci can result in non-Mendelian Bardet-Biedl syndrome. *Am J Hum Genet* 2003;72:1187–1199.

Beales PL, Elcioglu N, Woolf AS, et al: New criteria for improved diagnosis of Bardet-Biedl syndrome: results of a population survey. *J Med Genet* 1999;36:437–446.

Beales PL, Katsanis N, Lewis RA, et al: Genetic and mutational analyses of a large multiethnic Bardet-Biedl cohort reveal a minor involvement of *BBS6* and delineate the critical intervals of other loci. *Am J Hum Genet* 2001;68:606–616.

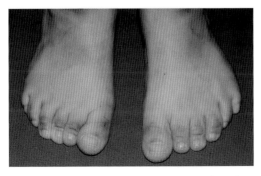

Bardet-Biedl syndrome (BBS) Postaxial (away from the vertical central axis of the body) polydactyly of both feet in a patient with BBS.

Green J, Parfrey P, Harnett J, et al: The cardinal manifestations of Bardet-Biedl syndrome, a form of Laurence-Moon-Biedl syndrome. *N Engl J Med* 1989;321:1002–1009.

Katsanis N, Ansley SJ, Badano JL, Eichers ER, Lewis RA, Hoskins BE, Scambler PJ, Davidson WS, Beales PL, Lupski JR: Triallelic inheritance in Bardet-Biedl syndrome, a Mendelian recessive disorder. *Science* 2001;293:2256–2259.

Katsanis N, Beales PL, Woods MO, et al: Mutations in *MKKS* cause obesity, retinal dystrophy and renal malformations associated with Bardet-Biedl syndrome. *Nat Genet* 2000;26:67–70.

Katsanis N, Lupski JR, Beales PL: Exploring the molecular basis of Bardet-Biedl syndrome. *Hum Mol Genet* 2001;10:2293–2299.

Klein D, Ammann F: The syndrome of Laurence-Moon, Bardet-Biedl and allied diseases in Switzerland: clinical, genetic and epidemiological studies. *J Neurol Sci* 1969;9:479–513.

Schachat AP, Maumenee IH: Bardet-Biedl syndrome and related disorders. *Arch Ophthalmol* 1982;100:285–288.

RESOURCE

Laurence-Moon-Bardet-Biedl Society
www.lmbbs.org.uk

Best Disease

See Vitelliform Dystrophy *under* Retinal Dystrophies and Degenerations

Blepharophimosis Syndrome (BPES)

OMIM NUMBERS

Blepharophimosis, ptosis, and epicanthus inversus 1 (BPES1): 110100

Blepharophimosis, ptosis, epicanthus inversus, and infertility (BPES2): 601649

INHERITANCE

Autosomal dominant with high penetrance

Sporadic cases may occur

GENE/GENE MAP

Forkhead transcription factor *FOXL2* gene mutations on 3q22–q23 cause BPES1 and BPES2.

Another gene is present on 7p21–p13.

EPIDEMIOLOGY

Incidence and prevalence unknown

CLINICAL FINDINGS

The main features of BPES1 are related to dysplasia of the lids (see Ocular Findings).

Some patients have low-set and simple ears.

The syndrome can be associated with primary amenorrhea and female infertility in some families (BPES2).

Blepharophimosis is a feature of several systemic syndromes and, in those instances, is inherited in the same fashion as the syndrome.

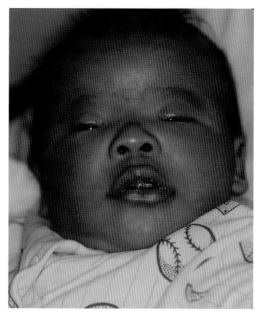

Blepharophimosis syndrome (BPES) Typical midfacial features of a baby with blepharophimosis syndrome. There is bilateral ptosis, epicanthus inversus, and telecanthus.

OCULAR FINDINGS

Dysplasia of lids (hypoplasia and fibrosis of the levator muscle and hypoplasia of the upper tarsi) featuring:

1. Bilateral ptosis
2. Lateral displacement of inner canthi (telecanthus)
3. Shortened horizontal palpebral fissure (lids are short)
4. Inverted epicanthal fold between upper and lower lids

Strabismus may be present.

Lacrimal system abnormalities may be present.

Severity of periocular findings may vary among affected family members.

Blepharophimosis is differentiated from simple congenital ptosis, in which there is no shortening of the palpebral fissure or telecanthus. It is also differentiated from congenital fibrosis of the extraocular muscles by the normal eye movements in blepharophimosis syndrome.

THERAPEUTIC ASPECTS

Ptosis repair is performed early in severe cases to prevent deprivation amblyopia.

Canthoplasty can be performed at a later stage.

REFERENCES

Crisponi L, Deiana M, Loi A, et al: The putative forkhead transcription factor *FOXL2* is mutated in blepharophimosis/ptosis/epicanthus inversus syndrome. *Nat Genet* 2001;27:159–166.

Fraser IS, Shearman RP, Smith A, et al: An association between blepharophimosis, resistant ovary syndrome and true premature menopause. *Fertil Steril* 1988;50:747–751.

Johnson CC: Surgical repair of the syndrome of epicanthus inversus, blepharophimosis, and ptosis. *Arch Ophthalmol* 1964;71:510–516.

Kohn R, Romano PE: Blepharoptosis, blepharophimosis, epicanthus inversus, and telecanthus: a syndrome with no name. *Am J Ophthalmol* 1971; 72:625–632.

Small KW, Stalvey M, Fisher L, et al: Blepharophimosis syndrome is linked to chromosome 3q. *Hum Mol Genet* 1995;4:443–448.

RESOURCE

Blepharophimosis, Ptosis, Epicanthus Inversus Family Network
SE 820 Meadow Vale Dr.
Pullman, WA 99163
509-332-6628
lschauble@wsu.edu
www.wsu.edu/~i0144069

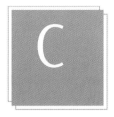

Cataract, Congenital

A discussion of all the clinical and therapeutic aspects of congenital cataracts is beyond the scope of this monograph. Table 12 summarizes the gene and gene-mapping information on a number of isolated inherited cataracts. Additional information can be obtained from OMIM.

CLINICAL FINDINGS

Most pediatric cataracts are genetic or secondary to an intrauterine infection. Unilateral cataracts are less likely to be genetically determined. Associated systemic or ocular anomalies are often present. Systemic anomalies may include:

1. Metabolic disease (galactosemia, galactokinase deficiency, glucose-6-phosphate dehydrogenase deficiency, mannosidosis, Fabry, Refsum, or Wilson disease)
2. Renal disease (Lowe or Alport syndrome)
3. Musculoskeletal disease (chondrodysplasia punctata, myotonic dystrophy, Stickler or Robert syndrome) or connective tissue disorders (Marfan or Ehlers-Danlos syndrome)
4. Central nervous system disorders (Marinesco-Sjogren or Meckel syndrome, neurofibromatosis type 2)
5. Dermatologic disorders (Cockayne or Rothmund-Thomson syndrome, incontinentia pigmenti, ichthyosis)
6. Craniofacial malformations (François, Rubinstein-Taybi, Smith-Lemli-Opitz, Marshall, or cerebro-facial-skeletal syndrome)
7. Several chromosomal disorders include cataract in their usual manifestations: trisomies 8, 13, 17, 21, and 22; monosomy 21; deletions 2q, 3q, 4p, 5p (cri du chat syndrome), 13q, 18p, and 18q; duplication 2p, 3q, 5p, 9p, 10q, 15q; and many others

OCULAR FINDINGS

Cataract may occur as an isolated finding or associated with other inherited ocular anomalies (Norrie disease, aniridia, colobomatous microphthalmos, microphthalmia without coloboma, or dominant or X-linked microcornea).

Noninherited cataracts may also have associated ocular findings, such as persistent hyperplasia of the primary vitreous, glaucoma in congenital rubella, or retinal scars in congenital toxoplasmosis.

Isolated cataracts are usually inherited as an autosomal dominant trait. They are usually bilateral, but asymmetry is not unusual. Depending on their location, size, and density, they may or may not require surgery. Anterior and posterior polar, stellate, cortical, nuclear, zonular, and total cataracts have been described. Nuclear and anterior polar cataracts are usually congenital. Lamellar cataracts can develop later in life, even though they are often inherited.

Anterior polar cataracts are nonprogressive and usually do not require surgery. Lamellar cataracts usually increase in opacity. Visual prognosis is good for anterior polar and lamellar cataracts but only fair for nuclear cataracts.

A genetic effect has also been found for cortical cataracts associated with age, even though well-known factors such as light exposure, nonwhite race, diabetes, or female gender are known to play a role.

X-linked cataracts are present in some families. Males have nuclear opacities and microcornea and are strongly predisposed to glaucoma. Carrier females have microcorneas and sutural opacities; they develop additional cataractous changes with advancing age.

Less commonly, cataracts can be inherited in an autosomal recessive pattern.

THERAPEUTIC ASPECTS

Table 13 summarizes the workup of patients with congenital cataract.

TABLE 12. Congenital Cataracts

Type	OMIM Number	Gene/Gene Map
Aculeiform	115700	2q33–q35
Anterior polar 1 (CTAA1)	115650	14q24–qter
Anterior polar 2 (CTAA2)	601202	17p13
Cerulean type I (CCA1)	115660	17q24
Cerulean type II (CCA2)	601547	CRYBB2/22q
Congenital total	302200	Xp
Autosomal dominant		CRYAA/21q22.3
Coppock-like (CCL)		CRYGA/2q33–q35
Marner type (CAM)	116800	16q22.1
Posterior polar (CPP)	116600	1pter–p36.1
Volkmann type	115665	1p36
Dominant, zonular pulverulent (CZP3)	601885	GJA3/13q11–q12
Lamellar, zonular pulverulent (CZP1), Coppock (CAE)	116200	GJA8/1q21.1
Zonular with sutural opacities (CCZS)	600881	17q11–q12

A familial history of cataracts should always be sought, and both parents should undergo slit-lamp examination for the presence of sub-clinical lenticular opacities.

Bilateral cataracts in the first weeks or months of life, in the absence of a family history, should arouse the suspicion of a metabolic disorder. Galactosemia and galactokinase deficiency can be detected by enzymatic analysis of erythrocytes. Galactose restriction in the diet can result in regression of cataracts in both disorders.

A complete ophthalmologic examination is necessary to detect associated ocular anomalies that may affect the visual prognosis.

Only visually significant cataracts need prompt surgery. The prognosis is improved if

TABLE 13. Workup of Patients with Congenital Cataract

Laterality of Cataract	Workup
Unilateral	Prenatal and family history
	Slit-lamp examination of both eyes through dilated pupils
	Dilated fundus examination
	Toxoplasmosis, rubella, cytomegalovirus, herpes (TORCH) titers, Venereal Disease Research Laboratory (VDRL) test
Bilateral	Prenatal and family history
	Systemic examination and review of systems
	Slit-lamp examination of both eyes through dilated pupils
	Dilated fundus examination
	Genetic evaluation
	Complete blood count (CBC), blood urea nitrogen level (BUN), TORCH titers, VDRL test, urine for reducing substances, red cell galactokinase, urine for amino acids, calcium, and phosphorus
	Consider computed tomography scan of head and hearing test as needed

surgery is performed within the first 6 to 8 weeks of life. Untreated visually significant cataracts will result in deep amblyopia. Later in childhood, the age of onset of significant opacities determines the visual prognosis.

For children younger than 2 years of age, there is no consensus about the indication of inserting an intraocular lens at the moment of surgery. Usually, cataracts are removed using a vitreous cutting instrument or a manual aspiration device. Phacoemulsification is not necessary. To prevent posterior capsule opacification, posterior capsulectomy and anterior vitrectomy are performed at the time of surgery. The peripheral posterior capsule is left to facilitate secondary posterior chamber intraocular lens implantation years later. Optical correction and amblyopia therapy should begin as soon as possible after surgery.

For children older than 2 years, posterior chamber intraocular lens implantation is preferred whenever possible. Some surgeons prefer to keep the posterior capsule intact if it is transparent, whereas others perform a posterior capsulectomy at the time of surgery, in some cases using a pars plana approach. In the former case, postoperative yttrium aluminum garnet (YAG) capsulotomy in cooperative children is almost inevitable due to the high rate of posterior capsule opacification.

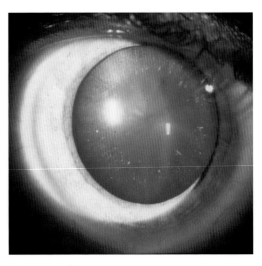

Cataract Cerulean cataract.

Postoperative control of inflammation is very important, and the frequent instillation of topical corticosteroids is necessary, slowly tapering the dose over several weeks.

Improvement in surgical techniques and cataract management has resulted in a better visual prognosis for both bilateral and unilateral cataracts, and visual acuity of 20/40 or better can be achieved in a significant proportion of properly managed cases. A recent study of unilateral pediatric cataracts found that 36.5% of

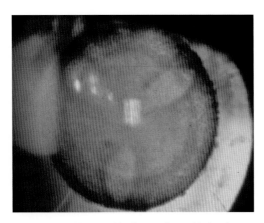

Cataract Lamellar opacities in a patient with dominant lamellar cataracts.

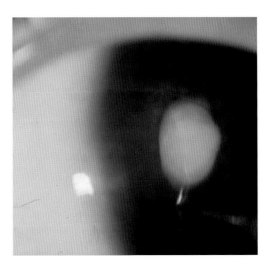

Cataract Anterior pyramidal cataract.

eyes achieved visual acuity of 20/40 or better. In 11 of 75 cases, good binocular vision (better than 100 sec arc) was obtained.

REFERENCES

Biglan AW, Cheng KP, Davis JS, et al: Secondary intraocular lens implantation after cataract surgery in children. *Am J Ophthalmol* 1997;123:224–234.

Brady KM, Atkinson CS, Kilty LA, et al: Cataract surgery and intraocular lens implantation in children. *Am J Ophthalmol* 1995;120:1–9.

Buckley E, Lambert SR, Wilson ME: IOLs in the first year of life. *J Pediatr Ophthalmol Strabismus* 1999;36:281–286.

Cassidy L, Taylor D: Congenital cataract and multisystem disorders. *Eye* 1999;13:464–473.

Cheng KP, Hiles DA, Biglan AW, et al: Management of posterior lenticonus. *J Pediatr Ophthalmol Strabismus* 1991;28:143–149.

Francis PJ, Berry V, Bhattacharya SS, Moore AT: The genetics of childhood cataract. *J Med Genet* 2000; 37(7):481–488.

Hosal BM, Biglan AW, Elhan AH: High levels of binocular function are achievable after removal of monocular cataracts in children before 8 years of age. *Ophthalmology* 2000;107:1647–1655.

Mori M, Keech RV, Scott WE: Glaucoma and ocular hypertension in pediatric patients with cataracts. *J Am Assoc Pediatr Ophthalmol Strabismus* 1997;1:98–101.

RESOURCES

None listed

Central Areolar Choroidal Dystrophy

See **Retinal Dystrophies and Degenerations**

CHARGE Association

OMIM NUMBER
214800

INHERITANCE
Most cases are isolated
Rare dominant inheritance

GENE/GENE MAP
Chromodomain helicase DNA-binding protein-7 (CHD7) on chromosome 8q12.1

EPIDEMIOLOGY
Probably the most common cause of microphthalmia with other systemic abnormalities and accounts for 15%–30% of patients with microphthalmia/coloboma.

CLINICAL AND OCULAR FINDINGS
The components of this association are Coloboma of the uvea, congenital *H*eart disease, *A*tresia of the choanae, *R*etardation of growth and mental development, *G*enital anomalies, and *E*ar malformations with hearing loss. Four of the six major findings are generally required for diagnosis. Additional abnormalities include seventh cranial nerve palsy in up to 45% of patients and facial clefts.

Russell-Eggitt and coworkers reviewed the ophthalmic features of 50 patients with the CHARGE association examined at the Hospital for Sick Children in London. Males and females were equally represented. Thirteen patients died in the first year of life. One of 48 karyotypes showed a balanced translocation between chromosomes 6 and 8. Eighty-eight percent of patients had ocular abnormalities that included a typical coloboma of the iris of varying severity in 82% of cases. Two patients had nasal iris colobomas. Posterior segment colobomatous defects were present in 38 of the 50 patients and varied from large chorioretinal colobomas to subtle optic nerve colobomas and inferior small retinal pigment epithelial defects. Eight patients had bilateral and 13 had unilateral microphthalmia. The reduction in the size of the globe was mild in all cases. Four patients had optic nerve hypoplasia. Persistent hyperplastic primary vitreous was present unilaterally

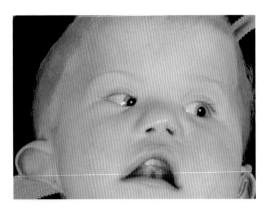

CHARGE association Patient with CHARGE association with bilateral colobomatous microphthalmia, simple ears, hearing loss, and choanal atresia.

in two patients. Two patients had congenital cataracts and 17 had strabismus. Facial palsy was bilateral in 2 patients and unilateral in 20. One patient had Marcus-Gunn jaw winking and ptosis. Four patients had delayed visual maturation.

The differential diagnosis of the CHARGE association includes the cat-eye syndrome (partial tetrasomy 22), Di George syndrome, and retinoic acid embryopathy

THERAPEUTIC ASPECTS

The management of these patients is quite complex and requires the collaborative efforts of ear, nose, and throat specialists, cardiologists, ophthalmologists, pediatricians, educators, and other health care specialists.

REFERENCE

Russell-Eggitt I, Blake K, Taylor D, Wyse R: The eye in the CHARGE association. *Br J Ophthalmol* 1990;421–426.

RESOURCES

None listed

Chondrodysplasia Punctata

Dominant type: **Conradi-Hunermann disease**
Recessive type: **rhizomelic type**

OMIM NUMBERS

Chondrodysplasia punctata I, X-linked recessive (CDPX1): 302950

Chondrodysplasia punctata II, X-linked dominant (CDPX2): 302960

Chondrodysplasia punctata syndrome: 215105

Chondrodysplasia punctata, autosomal dominant: 118650

Rhizomelic chondrodysplasia punctata type 1 (RCDP1): 215100

Rhizomelic chondrodysplasia punctata type 2 (RCDP2): 222765

Rhizomelic chondrodysplasia punctata type 3 (RCDP3): 600121

INHERITANCE

X-linked and autosomal recessive forms are the most common

GENE/GENE MAP

There is genetic heterogeneity.

X-linked forms

1. Conradi-Hunermann disease, an X-linked form affecting females only, is caused by mutations in the delta(8)-delta(7) sterol isomerase emopamil-binding protein (*EBP* 300205) at Xp11.23–p11.22.

2. X-linked recessive chondrodysplasia punctata is caused by mutations in the arylsulfatase E gene (*ARSE* 300180) at Xp22.3.

Rhizomelic dwarfism is a peroxisomal disorder; four peroxisomal abnormalities have been identified in the classic form of RCDP, all of which are transmitted as autosomal recessive traits:

1. RCDP1 is caused by mutations in the *PEX7* gene (OMIM 601757), which encodes the

peroxisomal type 2 targeting signal (PTS2) receptor at 6q22–q24.

2. RCDP2 is caused by a deficiency of the enzyme acyl-CoA:dihydroxyacetonephosphate acyltransferase (DHAPAT 602744) at chromosome 1.

3. RCDP3 is caused by mutations in the alkyldihydroxyacetonephosphate synthase (alkyl-DHAP synthase) gene (*AGPS* 603051) at 2q31.

Autosomal dominant chondrodysplasia punctata is a benign form of Conradi-Hunermann disease.

EPIDEMIOLOGY

Not applicable

CLINICAL FINDINGS

Skeletal dysplasia

Dominant form (Conradi-Hunermann disease):

1. Koala bear facial features, ichthyosiform skin changes, cataracts, and leg-length discrepancies are the primary clinical features.

2. At birth, the skin may be thick, red, and covered with cream-colored honey plaques. Some of the plaques may be peeled off without bleeding; others leave a raw, bleeding surface. The skin changes common at the neck, elbow, and groin (areas of flexion and moisture) are present in about 30% of patients. The eruption typically resolves during infancy and may be superseded by a follicular atrophoderma and patchy alopecia.

3. Intelligence is normal.

4. Scoliosis is a prominent feature. Stippled epiphyses (chondrodysplasia punctata) are the characteristic X-ray findings. This defect, which is seen in various settings and inherited disorders, often in association with peroxisomal deficiency, disappears by about age 3 to 4 years. Punctate calcifications are present in the ends of the long

bones, carpal and tarsal bones, vertebrae, and pelvis. Unilateral, and at times striking, shortening of the long tubular bones is seen.

Recessive form (rhizomelic type)

1. This form of chondrodysplasia punctata calcifans is usually more severe, and both legs are symmetrically short. There is marked proximal shortening of the extremities, with splaying of the long bones and abnormal ossification of epiphyses of both the humerus and the femur.

2. A depressed midface, saddle-nose deformity, frontal bossing, and high arched palate are constant findings.

3. Vertebral bodies have a coronal cleft filled by cartilage that is a result of an embryonic arrest.

4. Patients may have low birth weight and fail to thrive. Flexion contractures, dislocation of the hips, and microcephaly are common. The children are severely retarded mentally.

5. Skin changes such as those observed in ichthyosiform erythroderma are present in 25% of patients.

X-linked chondrodysplasia punctata is due to a contiguous gene deletion affecting the recessive X-linked ichthyosis locus. The scaling resembles that in X-linked ichthyosis; peroxisomal function is normal.

The differential diagnosis includes:

1. Symptomatic calcifications: cerebrohepatorenal syndrome of Zellweger, chromosomal abnormality, and prenatal infections

2. Multicentric epiphyseal ossification: in multiple epiphyseal dysplasia

3. Stippled epiphyses: in Zellweger syndrome, Smith-Lemli-Opitz syndrome, cretinism, and trisomy 18

OCULAR FINDINGS

Overall, cataracts occur in 20% of patients. They are seen in more than 70% of the patients with the more severe recessive form. The cataracts begin in early postnatal life in the dominant variety. It has been suggested that cataracts are consistently absent in the autosomal dominant form and present in two-thirds of the rhizomelic and X-linked 302950 forms. Lens opacities have been documented as early as days 22 and 66 in two patients. The early changes were vacuoles in the posterior lens cortex. Mature cataracts have been seen at age 11 weeks in the recessive variety.

There may be optic nerve hypoplasia and a reduced number of ganglion cells in the retina. The rods and cones are dysplastic. In one patient, the optic nerve was reported as normal.

Posterior embryotoxon, posterior lenticonus, and atrophy of the ciliary processes have been noted. The equatorial lens epithelium is replaced by vacuoles.

Strabismus and nystagmus are accompanying features.

Hypertelorism has been found.

THERAPEUTIC ASPECTS

In the dominant variety, cataract surgery should be considered routinely if the lens opacities are visually significant. However, in the recessive variety, no surgical intervention is indicated, because severe neurologic and ocular abnormalities indicate a poor prognosis for life and vision. Only an occasional patient with the recessive disease survives beyond age 2 years.

Life expectancy and mental development are normal in the dominant variety if the patient survives the first few weeks of life. Orthopedic problems are frequent due to asymmetric shortening of the limbs and/or scoliosis. Patients with the autosomal recessive variety usually die prior to age 2 years.

REFERENCES

Levine RE, Snyder AA, Sugarman GI: Ocular involvement in chondrodysplasia punctata. *Am J Ophthalmol* 1974;77:1–859.

Ryan H: Cataracts of dysplasia epiphysalis punctata. *Br J Ophthalmol* 1970;54:197–199.

Spranger JW, Opitz JM, Bidder U: Heterogeneity of chondrodysplasia punctata. *Humangenetik* 1971; 11:190–212.

RESOURCES

None listed

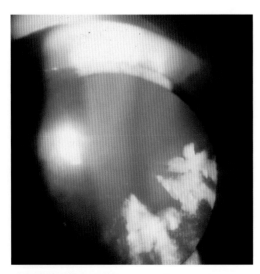

Chondrodysplasia punctata Sectoral cataract in Conradi-Hunermann disease.

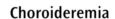

Choroideremia

See **Retinal Dystrophies and Degenerations**

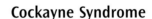

Cockayne Syndrome

OMIM NUMBERS
Type I: 216400
Type II: 133540
Type III: 216411

INHERITANCE
All forms are autosomal recessive.

GENE/GENE MAP

Type I: chromosome 5

Type II: 10q11

Type III: unmapped

Genetic heterogeneity has been demonstrated, and three complementation groups have been identified. Cultured fibroblasts from patients with the syndrome are very sensitive to the lethal effects of ultraviolet C light. There is defective recovery of DNA and RNA replication but no increase in chromosomal breakage or abnormalities in DNA repair, as in xeroderma pigmentosum or Bloom syndrome.

EPIDEMIOLOGY

Rare

Prevalence unknown

CLINICAL FINDINGS

This syndrome is characterized by early onset (type I) and sometimes congenital (type II) growth retardation, a progeroid facies with a small head, disproportionately long limbs, photodermatitis, and skeletal malformations with knee contractures resulting in a horseback-riding stance.

Sensorineural deafness and progressive neurodegeneration with mental deficiency, cerebellar ataxia, choreoathetosis, epilepsy, extrapyramidal tract signs, intracranial calcifications, and peripheral neuropathy become evident with time.

Photodermatopathy of sun-exposed areas, such as the cheeks, is a prominent feature.

Patients are not at increased risk for cancer.

Prenatal diagnosis is possible.

Patients may have hyperbetaglobulinemia, hyperinsulinemia, and hyperlipoproteinemia.

OCULAR FINDINGS

Enophthalmos is present in all patients and is due to loss of subcutaneous and orbital fat.

Visual acuity may be surprisingly preserved in most patients despite advanced optic atrophy and retinal dystrophic changes. Severe visual loss occurs late in the course of the disease.

Strabismus (exotropia or esotropia) is common. Nystagmus was present in 6 of 46 cases in one review.

A characteristic ocular finding is the poor pupillary response to dilating agents; this may be due to atrophy of the dilator iris muscle fibers, as evidenced by peripheral iris transillumination defects in some patients. Pigment dispersion in the anterior and posterior chambers has been documented in histopathologic studies by Levin et al.

Raised inferior corneal lesions, band keratopathy, and recurrent erosions have been described in some patients and are probably due to corneal exposure in neurologically impaired patients.

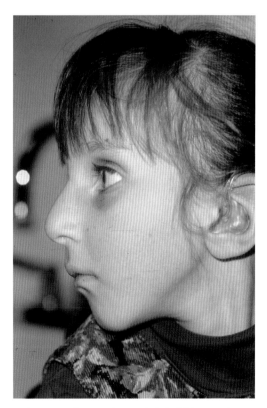

Cockayne syndrome Characteristic facial features in a patient with Cockayne syndrome.

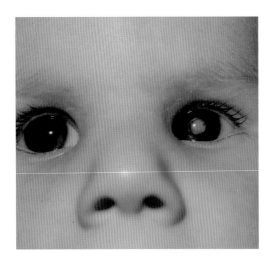

Cockayne syndrome Cataract in a baby who was later discovered to have Cockayne syndrome.

Cataracts have been described in 15% of patients and were present in both of Cockayne's original patients. They may be congenital or may develop with increasing age.

Hyperopic errors of refraction as high as +10.00 diopters are present in the majority of patients. Pigmentary retinopathy is one of the most consistent physical features.

The fundus has a salt-and-pepper appearance, with optic atrophy and arteriolar narrowing. Patients have been reported who lacked the typical salt-and-pepper appearance and exhibited denser black pigmentation at the posterior pole.

There is a variable degree of reduction of scotopic and photopic electroretinographic responses, which is most pronounced in older patients. Ocular histopathologic studies in one patient revealed degeneration of all retinal layers, pigment migration into the photoreceptor layer, thinning of the choriocapillaris, and moderate atrophy of the optic nerve with gliosis. The retinal pigment epithelium was intact, with excessive intracellular deposition of lipofuscin. Unusual pigmented cells were present in the retinal and subretinal space. There was widespread pigment dispersion in the anterior and posterior chambers and in the trabecular meshwork. The cornea was normal.

THERAPEUTIC ASPECTS

The skin should be shielded from ultraviolet light with sunscreen lotions.

Refractive errors and strabismus should be corrected, and cataracts should be extracted in infants and children in whom this is judged to be beneficial.

Death occurs in the second to fourth decades of life.

REFERENCES

Levin PS, Green WR, Victor DI, MacLean AL: Histopathology of the eye in Cockayne's syndrome. *Arch Ophthalmol* 1983;101:1093–1097.

Traboulsi EI, DeBecker I, Maumenee IH: Ocular findings in Cockayne syndrome. *Am J Ophthalmol* 1992;114:579–583.

RESOURCE

Share and Care Cockayne Syndrome Network
www.cockayne-syndrome.org

Cohen Syndrome

OMIM NUMBER
216550

INHERITANCE
Autosomal recessive

GENE/GENE MAP
COH1
8q22–q23

EPIDEMIOLOGY

Most reported patients are from Finland and Israel. Some patients have been reported from Lebanon, Palestine, and Japan. There is a high prevalence of Cohen syndrome among the Amish population of Ohio.

CLINICAL FINDINGS

The syndrome is characterized by congenital hypotonia, midchildhood truncal obesity, narrow hands and feet, and a typical facial appearance with a high nasal bridge, open mouth with prominent central incisors, short philtrum, and micrognathia.

Some patients have delayed puberty but no documentable endocrinologic abnormalities.

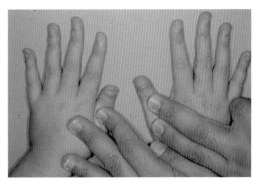

Cohen syndrome Elongated fingers.

Granulocytopenia may be present, and Warburg et al. postulated the existence of two types: type I (with granulocytopenia) and type II (without granulocytopenia).

The syndrome can be differentiated from Bardet-Biedl syndrome by the absence of polydactyly and hypogenitalism.

OCULAR FINDINGS

Progressive myopia is a hallmark of the disease and is present in the majority of patients.

Finnish patients have a progressive retinal dystrophy that is less severe than the one in Bardet-Biedl syndrome. Night blindness, with poor vision and constricted visual fields, is universal. Pigmentary retinopathy, with progressive chori-

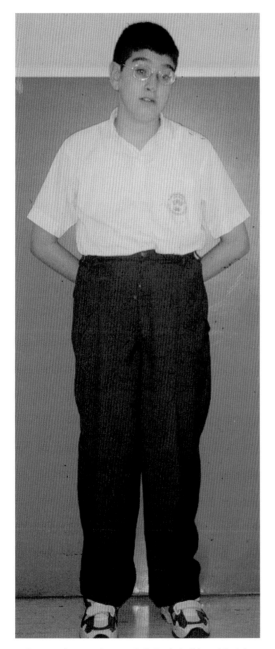

Cohen syndrome Characteristic body build and facial features.

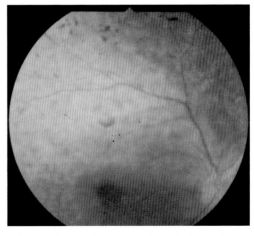

Cohen syndrome Pigmentary retinopathy in a patient with Cohen syndrome.

oretinal atrophy, develops as early as the first decade of life. The electroretinogram is non-recordable, and bony spicules are seen in the retinal periphery. Jewish patients appear not to have retinal involvement. Lebanese and Palestinian patients have a progressive retinal dystrophy.

Downslanting of the palpebral fissures occurs in all patients.

Cataracts develop in some patients in the fourth and fifth decades of life.

THERAPEUTIC ASPECTS

No specific treatment is available.

Despite the granulocytopenia, patients do not seem prone to infection.

REFERENCES

Beales PL, Elcioglu N, Woolf AS, et al: New criteria for improved diagnosis of Bardet-Biedl syndrome: results of a population survey. *J Med Genet* 1999; 36:437–446.

Cohen MM Jr, Hall BD, Smith DW: A new syndrome with hypotonia, obesity, mental deficiency, and oral, ocular and limb anomalies. *J Pediatr* 1973;83: 280–284.

Kivitie-Kallio S, Autti T, Salonen O, et al: MRI of the brain in the Cohen syndrome: a relatively large corpus callosum in patients with mental retardation and microcephaly. *Neuropediatrics* 1998;29: 298–330.

Kivitie-Kallio S, Eronen M, Lipsanen-Nyman M, et al: Cohen syndrome: evaluation of its cardiac, endocrine and radiological features. *Clin Genet* 1999;56:41–50.

Kivitie-Kallio S, Larsen S, Kajasto K, et al: Neurological and psychological findings in patients aged 11 months to 57 years. *Neuropediatrics* 1999;30: 181–189.

Kivitie-Kallio S, Summanen PS, Raitta C, et al: Ophthalmologic findings in Cohen syndrome: a long term follow-up. *Ophthalmology* 2000;107:1737–1745.

Kolehmainen J, Black GC, Saarinen A, et al: Cohen syndrome is caused by mutations in a novel gene, *COH1*, encoding a transmembrane protein with a presumed role in vesicle-mediated sorting and intracellular protein transport. *Am J Hum Genet* 2003;72:1359–1369.

Kondo I, Nagataki S, Miyagi N: The Cohen syndrome: does mottled retina separate a Finnish and a Jewish type? *Am J Med Genet* 1990;37:109–113.

Resnick K, Zuckerman J, Cotlier E: Cohen syndrome with bull's eye macular lesion. *Ophthalmic Genet* 1986;7:1–8.

Sack J, Friedman E: The Cohen syndrome in Israel. *Isr J Med Sci* 1986;22:766–770.

Tahvanainen E, Norio R, Karila E, et al: Cohen syndrome gene assigned to the long arm of chromosome 8 by linkage analysis. *Nat Genet* 1994;7; 201–204.

Warburg M, Pedersen SA, Horlyk H: The Cohen syndrome: retinal lesions and granulocytopenia. *Ophthalmic Paediatr Genet* 1990;11:7–13.

RESOURCE

Cohen Syndrome Support Group
  45 Compton Way
  Middleton Junction
  Manchester
  M24 2BU
  England
  0161-653-0876
  cohensyndrome@hotmail.com

Congenital Fibrosis of Extraocular Muscles (CFEOM)

OMIM NUMBERS
See Table 14.

INHERITANCE
See Table 14.

GENE/GENE MAP
See Table 14.

EPIDEMIOLOGY

The dominant CFEOM1 form is worldwide.

Recessive CFEOM2 has been reported from Saudi Arabia and from Iran.

A dominant CFEOM3 family has been reported from Turkey.

An unclassified recessive family, possibly mapping to 12q11, has been reported from Yemen.

TABLE 14. Types of Congenital Fibrosis Syndromes

Type	OMIM Number	Inheritance	Gene/Gene Map
CFEOM1	135700	Dominant	*KIF21A*/12q11–q12
CFEOM2	602078	Recessive	*ARIX*/11q13.2
CFEOM3	604361	Dominant	Not identified/16q24.2–q24.3
Unclassified	N/A	Recessive	Not identified/12q11–q12

CFEOM = congenital fibrosis of extraocular muscles.

CLINICAL FINDINGS

Patients with CFEOM have congenital bilateral ptosis and restrictive external ophthalmoplegia, with the eyes fixed in infraduction.

Initial reports of CFEOM1 showed that the trait is fully penetrant, with little variability in expression of the gene among or between families. Patients with CFEOM3, on the other hand, have a wide range of phenotypes, with some resembling those with CFEOM1 and others with no ptosis and only minimal abnormalities of vertical gaze. A more recent report of a Turkish family with chromosome 12–linked CFEOM, however, showed that some patients with this genotype can resemble those with CFEOM3.

Autosomal recessive CFEOM, which is much less common than the dominant form of the disease, has been described in three consanguineous Saudi Arabian families (CFEOM2) and in one Yemenite family (unclassified). Mutations in the *ARIX* developmental gene cause CFEOM2 through interference with the embryonic development of the cranial third nerve nucleus.

Neuropathologic studies have shown that chromosome 12–related CFEOM results from defects in the development of selective pools of brain stem alpha motoneurons and their corresponding axons. The superior division of the oculomotor nerve and its corresponding alpha motoneurons were absent in the midbrain of one individual with this condition.

OCULAR FINDINGS

See Clinical Findings.

Patients often have significant astigmatism.

THERAPEUTIC ASPECTS

Errors of refraction should be corrected.

Very large recessions (more than 10 mm) or free tenotomies of the inferior rectus muscles are necessary to bring the eyes up to midline.

Ptosis repair using frontalis suspension should be performed after or concurrent with inferior rectus surgery.

Amblyopia is treated as needed.

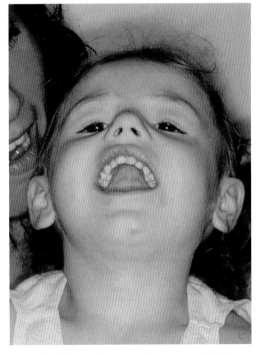

Congenital fibrosis of extraocular muscles (CFEOM)
Dominant CFEOM1. Characteristic facial features with bilateral ptosis and chin-up head position.

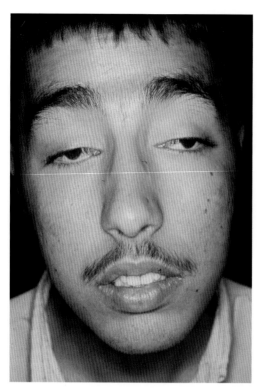

Congenital fibrosis of extraocular muscles (CFEOM) Recessive CFEOM2. Bilateral ptosis and bilateral exotropia.

REFERENCES

Brown HW: Congenital structural muscle anomalies. In: Allen JH, ed: *Strabismus Ophthalmic Symposium.* St Louis: CV Mosby Co; 1950:229.

Doherty E, Macy M, Sener SW, et al: CFEOM3: a new extraocular congenital fibrosis syndrome that maps to 16q24.2–q24.3. *Invest Ophthalmol Vis Sci* 1999;40:1687–1694.

Engle EC, Goumnerov BC, McKeown CA, et al: Oculomotor nerve and muscle abnormalities in congenital fibrosis of the extraocular muscles. *Ann Neurol* 1997;41:314–325.

Engle EC, Kunkel LM, Specht LA, et al: Mapping a gene for congenital fibrosis of the extraocular muscles to the centromeric region of chromosome 12. *Nat Genet* 1994;7:69–73.

Nakano M, Yamada K, Fain J, et al: Homozygous mutations in *ARIX* (*PHOX2A*) result in congenital fibrosis of the extraocular muscles type 2. *Nat Genet* 2001;29:315–320.

Sener EC, Lee BA, Turgut B, et al: A clinically variant fibrosis syndrome in a Turkish family maps to the CFEOM1 locus on chromosome 12. *Arch Ophthalmol* 2000;118:1090–1097.

Traboulsi EI, Jaafar MS, Kattan HM, et al: Congenital fibrosis of the extraocular muscles: report of 24 cases illustrating the clinical spectrum and surgical management. *Am Orthoptic J* 1993;43:45–53.

Traboulsi EI, Lee BA, Mousawi A, et al: Evidence of genetic heterogeneity in autosomal recessive congenital fibrosis of the extraocular muscles. *Am J Ophthalmol* 2000;129:658–662.

Wang SM, Zwaan J, Mullaney PB, et al: Congenital fibrosis of the extraocular muscles type 2, an inherited exotropic strabismus fixus, maps to distal 11q13. *Am J Hum Genet* 1998;63:517–525.

Yamada K, Andrews C, Chan WM, et al: Heterozygous mutations of the kinesin KIF21A in congenital fibrosis of the extraocular muscles type 1 (CFEOM1). *Nat Genet* 2003;35:318–321.

Yazdani A, Chung DC, Abbaszadegan MR, et al: A novel *PHOX2A/ARIX* mutation in an Iranian family with congenital fibrosis of extraocular muscles type 2 (CFEOM2). *Am J Ophthalmol* 2003;136:861–865.

RESOURCES

None listed

Congenital Stationary Night Blindness, X-Linked

See **X-Linked Congenital Stationary Night Blindness** *under* **Retinal Dystrophies and Degenerations**

Cornea Plana

OMIM NUMBERS
217300 for recessive form
121400 for dominant form

INHERITANCE

Eriksson et al. reported 34 Finnish sibships with 56 cases of cornea plana: 2 families consisting of 7 patients appeared to have a dominant form of the disease, while 26 patients from 13 sibships with the recessive form had common ancestors and lived in Lapland.

GENE/GENE MAP

The gene (*CNA2*) for the autosomal recessive form was mapped to 12q21 and was cloned by Pellegata et al., who found homozygosity for a founder missense mutation in the human *KERA* gene in 47 Finnish patients.

The dominant form of the disorder in Finland does not map to 12q21 but the gene in a dominant Cuban pedigree does, suggesting that mutations in the *KERA* gene may cause dominant as well as recessive cornea plana.

EPIDEMIOLOGY

Most patients have been reported from Finland, but the disorder has also been reported from the United States, Cuba, and Saudi Arabia.

CLINICAL FINDINGS

The radius of curvature of the cornea is larger than normal, resulting in apparent continuity of the sclera over the cornea.

Eriksson et al. list five clinical groups of signs in cornea plana. See Table 15.

The clinical findings were fairly consistent between the two eyes of one patient and among affected family members.

In mild cases, visual acuity is 20/25 to 20/30. In severe cases, other ocular abnormalities may be present, such as malformations of the iris, a slit-like pupil, or adhesions between the iris and the cornea.

Absence of the lens has been described.

Corneal curvature deviates from normal by 5 to 8 diopters only in dominant cases. In the recessive form, corneal refraction (K readings) may be as low as 23 diopters and most readings are below 34 diopters. Despite the expected decrease in refractive power of the cornea, based on keratometric readings, there is only modest hyperopia in most patients; this is probably due to the increased thickness of the central portion of the cornea. Patients with the milder dominant form do not exhibit the central opacity that is typical of the recessive form.

The average axial length of the eye is 24.1 mm (range: 21.4 to 27.4 mm). Some patients with long globes may even be myopic.

The parents of patients with the recessive form have a normal eye exam.

Some patients develop glaucoma later in life.

OCULAR FINDINGS

See Clinical Findings.

THERAPEUTIC ASPECTS

Management consists of correction of associated errors of refraction and the early detection and treatment of glaucoma.

TABLE 15. Cornea Plana Signs

Group of Signs	Description
1	Corneoscleral limbal area is widened, with superficial haziness of limbus and indistinct merge between sclera and cornea Clear-corneal diameter is small Arcus senilis occurs at early age
2	Round gray central corneal zone measuring 5 mm in diameter; corneal stroma is thin at the margin of this area and thicker in the middle; parenchyma of this disc-shaped central area is more opaque than the rest of the corneal stroma
3	Corneal radius is larger than normal; anterior portion of the eye is therefore less prominent or bulging than normal when visualized from the side
4	Cornea is thinner than normal
5	Mild ptosis in some patients

REFERENCES

Eriksson A, Lehmann W, Forsius H: Congenital cornea plana in Finland. *Clin Genet* 1973;4:301–310.

Pellegata NS, Dieguez-Lucena JL, Joensuu T, et al: Mutations in *KERA*, encoding keratocan, cause cornea plana. *Nat Genet* 2000;25:91–95.

Tahvanainen E, Forsius H, Karila E, et al: Cornea plana congenita gene assigned to the long arm of chromosome 12 by linkage analysis. *Genomics* 1995;26:290–293.

Tahvanainen E, Villanueva AS, Forsius H, et al: Dominantly and recessively inherited cornea plana congenita map to the same small region of chromosome 12. *Genome Res* 1996;6:249–254.

RESOURCE

Foundation Fighting Blindness
www.blindness.org

Corneal Dystrophies

OMIM NUMBERS

See Table 16.

INHERITANCE

Except for macular dystrophy, one form of congenital hereditary endothelial dystrophy, and one form of lattice dystrophy, which are autosomal recessive, all are inherited in an autosomal dominant fashion with variable expressivity.

GENE/GENE MAP

The genetic basis of corneal dystrophies is emerging, and specific genes are being identified for increasing types of dystrophies.

Molecular genetic studies of the corneal dystrophies suggest that genes on at least 10 human chromosomes are involved in the maintenance of corneal transparency (chromosomes 1, 5, 9, 10, 12, 16, 17, 20, 21, and X). Within the 10 chromosomes, specific genetic mutations in seven genes (*GSN*, *BIGH3*, *KRT3*, *KRT12*, *MSS1*, *GLA*, and *ARSC1*) have been identified in 15 corneal dystrophies.

Some corneal dystrophies that are considered distinct clinicopathologic entities are actually caused by different mutations in the same gene. For example, lattice dystrophy types I and IIIA,

TABLE 16. Corneal Dystrophies

Type	OMIM Number	Gene/Gene Map	Layer	Clinical and Ocular Findings
Epithelial basement membrane dystrophy (of Cogan; map-dot-fingerprint; microcystic)	121820	Not identified Not mapped	Epithelial basal membrane	Most common anterior segment dystrophy (6%–18% of population) Gray patches, microcysts, and/or fine lines in epithelium Recurrent epithelial erosions and transient blurry vision, especially in patients older than 30 years
Meesman corneal dystrophy	122100	*KRT3* (OMIM 148043) *KRT12* (OMIM 601687) 12q12–q13	Epithelial basal membrane	Rare Onset very early in life Tiny epithelial vesicles extending out to limbus Mild irritation and slight decrease in VA
Corneal dystrophy of Bowman's membrane, type II Thiel-Behnke	602802	*CDB2* 10q24	Epithelial basal membrane	Honeycomb deposits in Bowman's membrane Recurrent epithelial erosions and decreased VA

TABLE 16. Corneal Dystrophies (*Continued*)

Type	OMIM Number	Gene/Gene Map	Layer	Clinical and Ocular Findings
Reis-Bucklers corneal dystrophy (CDRB)	None	*BIGH3* (OMIM 601692): keratoepithelin gene 5q31	Bowman's membrane	Early onset Superficial reticular opacification in Bowman's membrane Recurrent epithelial erosions and decreased VA
Avellino corneal dystrophy (ACD)	None	*BIGH3* (OMIM 601692): keratoepithelin gene 5q31 (same mutation as lattice)	Stroma	Granular-lattice dystrophy deposits Decreased VA from haze in older patients
Granular corneal dystrophy (CDGG1)	121900	*BIGH3* (OMIM 601692): keratoepithelin gene 5q31	Stroma	Hyaline deposits Breadcrumb-like deposits with intervening clear cornea Type I (Groenow): most common, early onset, decreased VA Type II: milder form Type III: more superficial, recurrent erosions
Lattice corneal dystrophy (CDL1)	122200	*BIGH3* (OMIM 601692): keratoepithelin gene Type I: 5q31 Type II: 9q34	Stroma	Amyloid deposits Glass-like branching lines in stroma Type I (Biber-Haab-Dimer): classic form, early onset, decreased VA or erosions, recurrence in graft Type II (Meretoja): systemic amyloidosis Type III: late onset, recessive, variant IIIA is dominant, recurrent erosions
Macular corneal dystrophy	217800	*CHST6* sulfotransferase gene 16q22	Stroma	Early onset Glycosaminoglycan deposits Focal opacities with diffuse haze Decreased VA
Schnyder's crystalline corneal dystrophy	121800	Not identified	Stroma	Very early onset Lipid deposits Central opacities, corneal arcus, and diffuse stromal haze 50% systemic hypercholesterolemia Rarely, decreased VA
Central cloudy corneal dystrophy	None	Not identified Not mapped	Stroma	Multiple gray polygonal opacities separated by corneal dystrophy crack-like intervening clear zones

(*Continued*)

TABLE 16. Corneal Dystrophies (*Continued*)

Type	OMIM Number	Gene/Gene Map	Layer	Clinical and Ocular Findings
Gelatinous drop-like corneal dystrophy (primary familial amyloidosis)—AR	204870	Probably *M1S1* gene (OMIM 137290), tumor-associated antigen GA733-1 1p32–q12	Stroma	Multiple protruding mulberry-like subepithelial deposits
Posterior polymorphous corneal dystrophy	122000	*COL8A2* gene 20q11	Endothelium	Early onset Asymmetric Vesicles, geographic, or broad-band lesions in posterior corneal surface Stromal edema Anterior segment abnormalities 14% elevated intraocular pressure
Congenital hereditary endothelial corneal dystrophy—AD	121700	*CHED1* 20p13 (20p11.2–q11.2)	Endothelium	Corneal edema since the first or second year of life, progressive, pain, no nystagmus
Congenital hereditary endothelial corneal dystrophy—AR	217700	*CHED2* 20p13	Endothelium	More common Corneal edema from birth, stationary, nystagmus

AD = autosomal dominant; AR = autosomal recessive; VA = visual acuity.

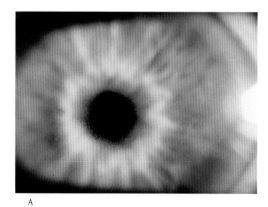

A

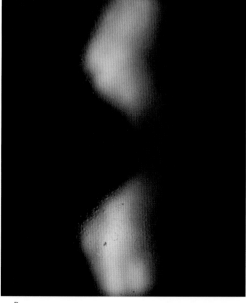

B

Meesman corneal dystrophy (A) Side illumination of the cornea in a patient with Meesman corneal dystrophy. Note the very fine vesicles in the superficial layers of the cornea. (B) shows a high-power view of the vesicles. (Courtesy of David Meisler, M.D.)

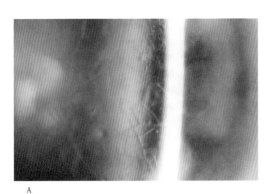 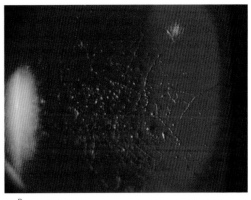

Lattice corneal dystrophy (A) High magnification slit-lamp view reveals characteristic lattice lines in the superficial and deeper layers of the stroma. (B) Retroillumination view of lattice lines and some "granular deposits." (Courtesy of David Meisler, M.D.)

granular corneal dystrophy types I, II (Avellino dystrophy), and III (Reis-Bucklers dystrophy), and Thiel-Behnke corneal dystrophy are the result of mutations in *BIGH3*.

Mutations in three genes (*GSN*, *BIGH3*, *MSS1*) are associated with amyloid deposition in the cornea.

EPIDEMIOLOGY

The most common anterior corneal dystrophy is map-dot-fingerprint (6% to 18% of the population).

The three most common stromal dystrophies are the lattice, granular, and macular types.

CLINICAL FINDINGS

Corneal dystrophies are hereditary disorders that affect both corneas.

Current and classical classifications of corneal dystrophies have been based on the layer of the cornea that is predominantly affected. It is now possible to classify these disorders on the basis of the genetic defects.

Table 16 summarizes the current status of knowledge of the genetics of corneal dystrophies and their most prominent clinical features. The reader is directed to more specialized texts for additional diagnostic and therapeutic aspects.

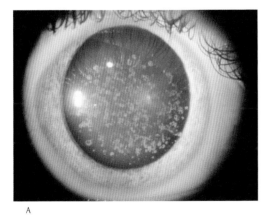 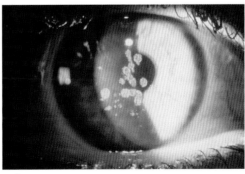

Granular corneal dystrophy (A) Diffuse fine granular stromal deposits. (B) Another patient with larger granular deposits.

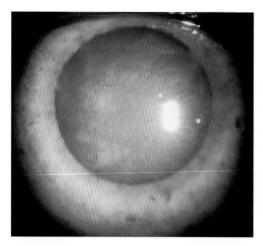

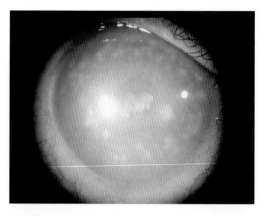

Macular corneal dystrophy There is diffuse corneal haze with numerous ill-defined opaque lesions. (Courtesy of David Meisler, M.D.)

Reis-Bucklers corneal dystrophy Central corneal opacification with orange-brown discoloration due to secondary siderosis. (Courtesy of David Meisler, M.D.)

OCULAR FINDINGS
See Table 16.

THERAPEUTIC ASPECTS
Treatment depends on the severity of symptoms. These include recurrent epithelial erosions in some patients and reduced vision in others.

Phototherapeutic, lamellar, or penetrating keratoplasty has been used in the various types. Discussion of the specific indications for each is beyond the scope of this book. The reader is referred to major cornea texts for that purpose.

Observation is often sufficient in patients with mild or even moderate symptoms.

REFERENCES

Afshari NA, Mullally JE, Afshari MA, et al: Survey of patients with granular, lattice, Avellino, and Reis-Bucklers corneal dystrophies for mutations in the *BIGH3* and gelsolin genes. *Arch Ophthalmol* 2001; 119:16–22.

Klintworth GK: Advances in the molecular genetics of corneal dystrophies. *Am J Ophthalmol* 1999; 128:747–754.

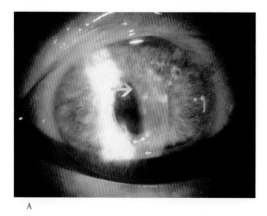

A

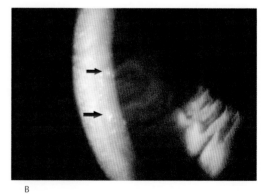

B

Posterior polymorphous corneal dystrophy (A) Slit-lamp view shows deep polymorphic opacities, best visualized in the light beam (*arrow*). (B) High-power view of polymorphic opacities at the level of the corneal endothelium (*arrows*).

Laibson PR: Anterior corneal dystrophies. In: Krachmer JH, Mannis MJ, Holland EJ, eds: *Cornea.* St Louis: CV Mosby Co; 1997;2:1033–1042.

Mannis MJ, DeSousa LB, Gross RH: The stromal dystrophies. In: Krachmer JH, Mannis MJ, Holland EJ, eds: *Cornea.* St Louis: CV Mosby Co; 1997;2: 1043–1062.

Munier FL, Korvatska E, Djemai A, et al: Keratoepithelin mutations in four 5q31-linked corneal dystrophies. *Nat Genet* 1997;15:247–251.

RESOURCES

None listed

Craniosynostosis Syndromes

OMIM NUMBERS

See Table 17.

INHERITANCE

See Table 17.

GENE/GENE MAP

Several of the craniosynostosis syndromes, such as Crouzon, Apert, Pfeiffer, and Jackson-Weiss syndromes, have been found to result from mutations in the family of fibroblast growth factor receptor (*FGFR*) genes. The proteins coded by these genes are membrane receptors that, when dimerized and bound to ligands (fibroblast growth factors), are activated to stimulate differentiation, chemotaxis, angiogenesis, mitogenesis, and cell survival. Hence, these receptors regulate key functions of growth and development.

All four of the craniosynostotic syndromes are allelic and result from mutations in the *FGFR2* gene located on 10q26. Furthermore, patients with different clinical types of craniosynostosis syndromes can have identical mu-

TABLE 17. Craniosynostosis Syndromes

Syndrome	OMIM Number	Gene/Gene Map	Digit Features	Ocular Features	Internal Organ Involvement
Crouzon	123500	*FGFR2/FGFR3* 10q26/4p16.3	None	Proptosis Exotropia Optic atrophy Extraocular muscle abnormalities	None
Apert	101200	*FGFR2* 10q26	Symmetric mitten-type syndactyly of hands and feet	Proptosis Hypertelorism Downslanting palpebral fissures Exotropia Extraocular muscle abnormalities	Cardiovascular (10%) Genitourinary (10%) Respiratory (1.5%) Gastrointestinal (1.5%) Intellectual impairment
Pfeiffer	101600	*FGFR1/FGFR2* 8p11.2–p11.1 10q26	Broad, medially deviated thumbs and great toes Brachydactyly	Proptosis Downslanting palpebral fissures Hypertelorism Strabismus	Various anomalies reported; more frequent in subtypes II and III

(Continued)

TABLE 17. Craniosynostosis Syndromes (*Continued*)

Syndrome	OMIM Number	Gene/Gene Map	Digit Features	Ocular Features	Internal Organ Involvement
Jackson-Weiss	123150	*FGFR2* 10q26 8p11.2–p11.1	Broad first metatarsal Abnormally shaped tarsal bones Calcaneocuboid fusion Hands unaffected	Proptosis Strabismus	None
Saethre-Chotzen	101400	*TWIST* *FGFR3* 7p21 4p16.3	Soft-tissue syndactyly (usually digits 2 and 3) of hands and feet	Ptosis Hypertelorism Strabismus	None
Boston type		*MSX2* 5q34–35	Single individual with triphalangeal thumb	Myopia Hyperopia Visual field defects	Single individual with cleft soft palate
Carpenter	201000	?	Brachydactyly Soft-tissue syndactyly Preaxial polydactyly of feet Decreased number of phalanges	Laterally displaced inner canthi Epicanthal folds	Cardiovascular (about 33%) Structural brain defects Intellectual impairment
Baller-Gerold	218600	?*TWIST*	Thumb aplasia or hypoplasia Radial aplasia or hypoplasia Shortened and bowed ulnae Lower limb anomalies in small percentage of patients	Downslanting palpebral fissures Epicanthal folds Exotropia Nystagmus Ectropion Severe myopia	Anal, renal, genital, cardiac, central nervous system defects Vertebral anomalies
Treacher Collins	154500	*TCOF1* 5q32–q33.1	None	Downslanting palpebral fissures Lower lid coloboma	None

Source: Lewanda AF, Traboulsi EI, Jabs EW: Syndromes with craniofacial anomalies. In: Traboulsi EI, ed: *Genetic Diseases of the Eye*. New York: Oxford University Press; 1998:777–796.

tations in *FGFR2*, suggesting the presence of modifying genes.

EPIDEMIOLOGY

Apert: 1 in 160,000

CLINICAL FINDINGS

Included in this category is a group of malformation syndromes that have in common the radiologic and clinical skull abnormalities associated with craniosynostosis or premature closure of one or more cranial sutures. Table 17 summarizes the clinical features of several of these syndromes and gives their genetic basis.

OCULAR FINDINGS

Many patients have associated ocular abnormalities. Ocular findings are secondary to the abnormal development of the orbits and the increased intracranial pressure.

Shallow orbits may be responsible for proptosis, which can be severe in some cases. Rarely, the eyes may be spontaneously subluxated.

True hypertelorism is present in 45% of patients.

Lids usually have an antimongoloid slant.

Strabismus occurs in 36.5% of patients. V-pattern exotropia, with overacting inferior obliques, is probably the most common pattern of strabismus in these patients. Diamond et al. reported the frequent absence of various extraocular muscles in patients with strabismus.

Disc swelling was present in 31% of Crouzon and 9.5% of Apert patients. Optic atrophy may

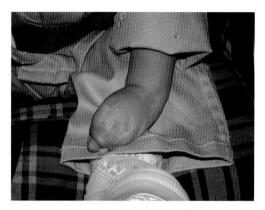

Craniosynostosis syndromes: Apert syndrome Polysyndactyly (mitten hand).

result from long-standing papilledema secondary to intracranial pressure.

Optic discs are pale or atrophic in 50% of Crouzon patients and 24% of Apert patients.

Intraocular abnormalities, such as iris coloboma, cataract, and ectopia lentis, are noted infrequently.

THERAPEUTIC ASPECTS

Care of these patients has advanced tremendously in the past few decades, and complex surgical procedures have allowed not only longer survival, but also a significant improvement in function and appearance.

These patients have a high incidence of strabismus because of their orbital anatomy and because of the congenital absence of the muscles, especially the superior oblique, in some. Special consideration should be given to strabismus surgery in these patients, keeping these facts in mind and allowing for recovery and planning for craniofacial reconstructive procedures.

REFERENCES

Diamond GR, Katowitz JA, Whitaker LH, et al: Ocular alignment after craniofacial reconstruction. *Am J Ophthalmol* 1980;90:248–250.

Diamond GR, Katowitz JA, Whitaker LA, et al: Variations in extraocular muscle number and structure in craniofacial dysostosis. *Am J Ophthalmol* 1980;90:416–418.

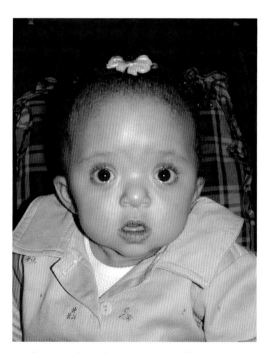

Craniosynostosis syndromes: Apert syndrome Facial features.

Dufier JL, Vinurel MC, Renier D, et al: Les complications ophtalmologiques des craniofaciostenoses: a propos de 244 observations. *J Fr Ophtalmol* 1986; 9:273–280.

RESOURCE

Birmingham Craniofacial Unit
www.craniofacial.org.uk.ukcf.htm

Cystinosis, Nephropathic

OMIM NUMBER
219800

INHERITANCE
Autosomal recessive

GENE/GENE MAP
CTNS encodes an integral membrane protein, designated *cystinosin*, that has features of a lysosomal membrane protein.

Forty-four percent of American patients are homozygous for a "European" 65 kb deletion.

The severity of the disease appears to be related to the type of mutation and the amount of residual function in cystinosin.

17p13

EPIDEMIOLOGY
1 in 180,000 worldwide

CLINICAL FINDINGS
The disease is characterized by widespread accumulation of intralysosomal cystine crystals.

There are three clinical types with variable degrees of severity: infantile (nephropathic), late onset (intermediate severity), and adult onset (benign).

1. Patients with the infantile form comprise more than 90% of cases. They are asymptomatic until 8 to 15 months of age, when they present with progressive renal failure, growth retardation, renal rickets, and hypothyroidism. There is hypopigmentation of skin and hair. If patients do not undergo renal transplantation, they will die in the first decade of life.
2. When the symptoms of cystinosis appear first in adolescence, mild renal failure may be present but growth is normal.
3. The adult type is a relatively benign condition characterized by deposition of cystine crystals in the cornea, polymorphonuclear leukocytes, and fibroblasts, but not in the kidney.

Crystals accumulate in the cornea, conjunctiva, and most ocular tissues in all three types.

The diagnosis is made on clinical grounds. Crystals are found in biopsy material, and there is an 80- to 100-fold increase in free cystine in peripheral leukocytes and cultured skin fibroblasts.

OCULAR FINDINGS
Corneal deposits cause severe photophobia and blepharospasm. The refractile, spindle-shaped crystals are present throughout the corneal stroma. Cystine crystals also deposit in the conjunctiva, causing injection and providing a source of tissue diagnosis. Decreased corneal sensitivity may also be present late in the course of the disease.

Cystine crystals accumulate in the cornea, conjunctiva, and most ocular tissues in all three types, but only patients with the nephropathic type develop the characteristic patchy depigmentation of the retinal pigment epithelium and fine pigment clumping. There is no significant visual disturbance. It is unclear whether the pigmentary retinopathy causes any reduction of vision.

Pupillary-block glaucoma has been reported.

THERAPEUTIC ASPECTS
Administration of topical cysteamine improves renal function and corneal clarity. The chemical reacts with lysosomal cystine to form a mixed disulfide that leaves the lysosome

through a transport system for cationic amino acids. This treatment, however, is available only at the National Institutes of Health.

Sunglasses are helpful in some patients.

REFERENCES

Kaiser-Kupfer MI, Caruso RC, Minckler DS, et al: Long-term ocular manifestations of nephropathic cystinosis. *Arch Ophthalmol* 1986;104:706–711.

Kaiser-Kupfer MI, Datiles MB, Gahl WA: Clear graft two years after keratoplasty in nephropathic cystinosis. *Am J Ophthalmol* 1988;105:318–319.

Kaiser-Kupfer MI, Fujikawa L, Kuwabara T, et al: Removal of corneal crystals by topical cysteamine in nephropathic cystinosis. *N Engl J Med* 1987;316:775–779.

Stenson SM, Siegel IM, Carr RE: Infantile cystinosis: ocular findings and pigment dilution of eye and skin. *Ophthalmic Paediatr Genet* 1983;3:169–180.

Wan WL, Minckler DS, Rao NA: Pupillary-block glaucoma associated with childhood cystinosis. *Am J Ophthalmol* 1986;101:700–705.

Wong VG, Schulman JD, Seegmiller JE: Conjunctival biopsy for the biochemical diagnosis of cystinosis. *Am J Ophthalmol* 1970;70:278.

Yamamoto GK, Schulman JD, Schneider JA, et al: Long term ocular changes in cystinosis: observations in renal transplant recipients. *J Pediatr Ophthalmol Strabismus* 1979;16:21.

RESOURCES

None listed

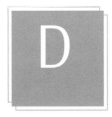

Distichiasis-Lymphedema Syndrome

Also called **Falls syndrome**

OMIM NUMBER
153400

INHERITANCE
Autosomal dominant with variable penetrance

GENE/GENE MAP
Caused by mutation in the forkhead family transcription factor gene *MFH1* (*FOXC2* 602402)
16q24.3

EPIDEMIOLOGY
Rare; incidence unknown

CLINICAL FINDINGS
This disorder consists of two unusual developmental anomalies:
1. Distichiasis, an extra row of lashes at the site of the meibomian gland openings.
2. Lymphedema, causing painless swelling of the extremities, predominantly below the knee. The lymphedema first becomes evident between 5 and 20 years of age, most commonly during adolescence. Mild pitting edema may be the earliest sign.

In some patients, distichiasis or lymphedema may occur alone.

Other features are epidural spinal cysts, vertebral anomalies, and pterygium colli (webbed neck).

The diagnosis is based on the physical findings and family history. Hypoplastic lymph channels can be demonstrated on lymphangiography.

Although rare, epidural cysts with secondary neurologic complications should always be looked for.

Distichiasis may be an isolated, dominantly inherited disorder unrelated to lymphedema. For this reason it is frequently confused with the distichiasis-lymphedema syndrome, especially before puberty, when the lymphedema usually first appears.

Lymphedema may also be an isolated hereditary disease.

OCULAR FINDINGS
The extra row of lashes may involve all four lids, but may be present only on the lower ones. The lashes may be fully developed or lanugo-like. Superficial punctate keratitis and photophobia are frequent findings if the lashes rub against the cornea.

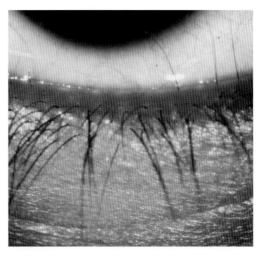

Distichiasis-lymphedema syndrome Lower lid with several extra lashes growing from the orifices of meibomian glands.

Partial ectropion of the lower lid has been described, causing a proptotic appearance of the eyes.

THERAPEUTIC ASPECTS

Early treatment of lymphedema with supportive stockings may be helpful, especially if instituted early.

Extra lashes that cause significant keratitis should be removed by plucking or electrolysis.

REFERENCES

Falls HF, Kertesz ED: A new syndrome combining pterygium colli with developmental anomalies of the eyelids and lymphatics of the lower extremities. *Trans Am Ophthalmol Soc* 1964;62:248–275.

Fang J, Dagenais SL, Erickson RP, et al: Mutations in *FOXC2* (*MFH-1*), a forkhead family transcription factor, are responsible for the hereditary lymphedema-distichiasis syndrome. *Am J Hum Genet* 2000;67:1382–1388.

Mangion J, Rahman N, Mansour S, et al: A gene for lymphedema-distichiasis maps to 16q24.3. *Am J Hum Genet* 1999;65:427–432.

Robinow M, Johnson GF, Verhagen AD: Distichiasis-lymphedema: a hereditary syndrome of multiple congenital defects. *Am J Dis Child* 1970;119:343–347.

Traboulsi EI, Al-Khayer K, Matsumoto M, et al: Lymphedema-distichiasis syndrome and *FOXC2* gene mutation. *Am J Ophthalmol* 2002;134:592–596.

RESOURCE

British Lymphology Society and Lymphoedema Support Network
www.lymphoedema.org

Dominant Cystoid Macular Dystrophy

See Retinal Dystrophies and Degenerations

Dominant Progressive Foveal Dystrophy

See Retinal Dystrophies and Degenerations

Down Syndrome

Also called trisomy 21

OMIM NUMBER

190685

INHERITANCE

Chromosomal trisomy 21 in 95% of cases
Translocation 21 in 5% of cases; critical interval is 21q22.2–22.3

GENE/GENE MAP

21q22.3

A region of 5 Mbp between D21S58 and D21S42 is associated with the mental retardation and most of the facial and other features of the syndrome.

DSCR1 (OMIM 602917) is highly expressed in brain and heart and is suggested as a candidate for involvement in the pathogenesis of the syndrome, in particular mental retardation and/or cardiac defects.

EPIDEMIOLOGY

The most common trisomy in live newborns; in the United States, the incidence is 1 in 700 newborns.

Incidence increases with maternal age: from 1 in 1550 live births in women under 20 years of age to 1 in 25 in women over 45.

CLINICAL FINDINGS

Various degrees of mental and growth retardation
Hypotonia

Brachycephaly

Flat face, large protruding tongue, small nose with small low bridge, high arched palate, small poorly defined ears, conductive hearing loss, and short, thick neck

Stubby hands with a single palmar crease (simian crease), clinodactyly of the fifth digit with hypoplasia of the middigital phalanges, short stubby feet with a wide gap between the first and second toes, and joint hypermobility

Dysplasia of pelvis, with hypoplastic iliac wings and a shallow acetabulum

Atlantoaxial instability, which may cause a variety of neurologic signs

Cardiac malformations occur in 40% to 50% of cases; most characteristic is closure defect of endocardial cushions. One-third of congenital heart defects are complex and a source of significant morbidity. Mitral valve prolapse is more frequent than in age- and gender-matched controls.

Intestinal atresia, imperforate anus, and Hirschsprung disease

Transient myelodysplasia of the newborn and a higher incidence of leukemia, especially the megakaryocytic subtype, acute myelogenous leukemia

Hypothyroidism

Males are usually sterile, although there is no evidence that they do not produce sperm, but females have borne offspring.

All patients over 40 years of age develop dementia.

OCULAR FINDINGS

Brushfield spots of iris (52%)

Lid abnormalities: epicanthus, upward-slanting palpebral fissures (82%), blepharitis, ectropion

Increased number of retinal vessels crossing the disc margin (frequent)

Nasolacrimal duct obstruction (30%)

Myopia, hypermetropia, and astigmatism (60%)

Strabismus (38%), esotropia more than exotropia

Nystagmus (18%)

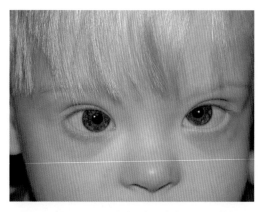

Down syndrome Upward slanting of the eyes, mild esotropia, Brushfield spots on the iris, and blepharitis in a young child with Down syndrome.

Congenital or acquired cataracts (13%)

Keratoconus (uncommon feature)

Infantile glaucoma (rare)

THERAPEUTIC ASPECTS

The most common causes of morbidity and mortality are congenital heart defects, malignant hematologic disease, and duodenal atresia. If these conditions are corrected, survival into the fifth decade and beyond is likely, but is complicated by progressive dementia of the Alzheimer type.

Functional prognosis has improved in recent decades with better supportive measures and periodic assessment and management of motor, language, social, and adaptive skills.

Because infants are prone to respiratory infections, immunization recommendations should be followed closely.

Screening for spine instability should be performed, and patients with myelopathy or marked instability without myelopathy are candidates for cervical spine fusion.

Early ophthalmologic evaluations are recommended, and correction of refractive errors, strabismus, and cataracts has a positive influence on vision and educational development.

The coexistence of congenital glaucoma, severe myopia, and cataracts strongly predisposes to the development of retinal detachment and a poor visual outcome.

Grafting in cases of keratoconus is associated with a higher incidence of complications.

REFERENCES

da Cunha RP, Moreira JB: Ocular findings in Down's syndrome. *Am J Ophthalmol* 1996;122:236–244.

Roizen NJ, Mets MB, Blondis TA: Ophthalmic disorders in children with Down syndrome. *Dev Med Child Neurol* 1994;36:594–600.

Traboulsi EI, Levine E, Mets MB, et al: Infantile glaucoma in Down's syndrome (trisomy 21). *Am J Ophthalmol* 1988;105:389–394.

RESOURCE

National Down Syndrome Society
www.ndss.org

Doyne Honeycomb Choroiditis

See **Familial Radial Drusen** *under* **Retinal Dystrophies and Degenerations**

Duchenne Muscular Dystrophy (DMD)

OMIM NUMBER
310200

INHERITANCE
X-linked

GENE/GENE MAP
Dystrophin
Xp21

EPIDEMIOLOGY
Duchenne muscular dystrophy (DMD) is the most common hereditary neuromuscular disease.

Duchenne muscular dystrophy affects males of all races and ethnic groups.

Incidence varies in different population groups: 21.7 in 100,000 live male births in Italy; 29.2 in 100,000 in Ontario, Canada; 1 in 4215 in the Netherlands.

CLINICAL FINDINGS
Duchenne muscular dystrophy is a progressive proximal muscular dystrophy with characteristic pseudohypertrophy of the calves.

A milder form of dystrophin-associated muscular dystrophy is called *Becker muscular dystrophy* (BMD).

Onset of DMD usually occurs before age 3 years. The patient is chair-ridden by age 12 and dead by age 20.

Myocardial involvement appears in a high percentage by 6 years of age, is present in 95% of patients in the last years of life, and causes heart failure.

Functional impairment of smooth muscle in the gastrointestinal tract can cause acute gastric dilation and intestinal pseudo-obstruction, which may be fatal.

High serum creatine kinase is present.

Skeletal abnormalities include increased lordosis, scoliosis, and flexion contractures in the joints.

Respiratory muscles are also affected, with pulmonary hypoventilation and eventual respiratory failure.

The diagnosis is based on clinical signs. Electromyography and muscle biopsy are confirmatory.

Inflammatory changes seen in biopsy sections taken early in the course of the disorder can erroneously suggest a diagnosis of polymyositis if careful note is not made of the histologic hallmarks of dystrophy.

OCULAR FINDINGS
Curiously, the extraocular muscles are usually spared.

Abnormal retinal neurotransmission as measured by electroretinography is observed;

however, there have been no reports of night blindness or other signs of visual dysfunction.

THERAPEUTIC ASPECTS

Management is largely symptomatic.

There have been experimental trials of myoblast transfer therapy in humans and gene replacement with dystrophin minigenes in animal models.

REFERENCE

Pillers DA, Bulman DE, Weleber RG, et al: Dystrophin expression in the human retina is required for normal function as defined by electroretinography. *Nat Genet* 1993;4:82–86.

RESOURCE

Muscular Dystrophy Association: Duchenne Muscular Dystrophy
www.mdausa.org/disease/dmd.html

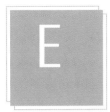

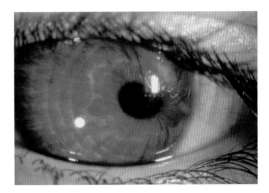

Ectopia lentis et pupillae The pupil is displaced nasally in this patient with ectopia lentis et pupillae. Remnants of the papillary membrane are present.

Ectopia Lentis

See **Marfan Syndrome**

Ectopia Lentis et Pupillae

OMIM NUMBER
225200

INHERITANCE
Autosomal recessive

GENE/GENE MAP
Unmapped

EPIDEMIOLOGY
Uncommon; incidence unknown

CLINICAL FINDINGS
Congenital and sometimes progressive subluxation of the crystalline lens is found.

Eccentric and sometimes miotic pupil is seen.

The lens and pupil are usually displaced in opposite directions.

Remnants of the pupillary membrane and subtle signs of anterior segment dysgenesis are characteristic and reveal the diagnosis.

Open-angle glaucoma and retinal detachment are not uncommon.

OCULAR FINDINGS
In a series of 16 patients, Goldberg found that 40% of eyes had visual acuity better than or equal to 20/40, and 90% had vision better than or equal to 20/400. Two eyes had very poor vision from failed retinal reattachment surgery, and one eye had very poor vision from amblyopia. Perimetry could not document glaucomatous damage in any eye.

THERAPEUTIC ASPECTS
Refraction is done either through the phakic or aphakic part of the pupil.

Lens extraction may be necessary if refraction is impossible, if the lens moves into and out of the visual axis, or if there is recurrent pupillary-block glaucoma. The vitreous is well formed, and the lens does not sink back toward the retina.

The patient should be monitored for intraocular pressure elevation.

Periodic ultrasonographic examination of the eye or visual field testing should be performed in patients with nondilating pupils.

REFERENCE

Goldberg M: Clinical manifestations of ectopia lentis et pupillae in 16 patients. *Ophthalmology* 1988;95: 1080–1087.

RESOURCES
None listed

Edwards Syndrome

Also called trisomy 18

OMIM NUMBERS
None

INHERITANCE
Chromosomal

GENE/GENE MAP
Trisomy 18

EPIDEMIOLOGY
Second most common autosomal trisomy: 1 in 6000 births

CLINICAL FINDINGS
Ninety percent of patients die in the first year of life

Low birth weight

Closed fists with index fingers overlapping the third digit, and the fifth digit overlapping the fourth

Narrow hips with limited abduction

Short sternum

Rocker-bottom feet

Microcephaly, prominent occiput, micrognathia

Complex cardiac malformations in 90% of patients

Renal malformations

Severe mental retardation

Advanced maternal age

OCULAR FINDINGS
Ptosis, short palpebral fissures, epicanthus, ankyloblepharon filiforme adnatum

Hypoplastic supraorbital ridges

Microphthalmia

Corneal opacities

Anisocoria

Cataracts

Uveoretinal and disc colobomas, retinal hypopigmentation

THERAPEUTIC ASPECTS
Prenatal detection of trisomies, followed by termination of pregnancy, is having a small but measurable impact on decreasing the incidence of Down, Edwards, and Patau syndromes.

Ten percent of patients live to 1 year and a few survive to adulthood, perhaps because of undetected mosaicism for a chromosomally normal cell line. However, central nervous system function is far less than in Down syndrome and leads to complex medical management and supportive care for long-term survivors.

Rarely should invasive diagnostic procedures or aggressive supportive measures be recommended.

REFERENCES

Bacal DA, Nelson LB, Zackai EH, et al: Ankyloblepharon filiforme adnatum in trisomy 18. *J Pediatr Ophthalmol Strabismus* 1993;30:337–339.

Holmes JM, Coates CM: Assessment of visual acuity in children with trisomy 18. *Ophthalmic Genet* 1994;15:115–120.

Velzeboer CM, van der Harten JJ, Koole FD: Ocular pathology in trisomy 18: a histopathological report of three cases. *Ophthalmic Paediatr Genet* 1989;10:263–269.

RESOURCE

Support Organization for Trisomy 18, 13, and Related Disorders
www.trisomy.org

Ehlers-Danlos Syndrome

OMIM NUMBERS
Ehlers-Danlos syndrome I: 130000
Ehlers-Danlos syndrome II: 130010
Ehlers-Danlos syndrome III: 130020
Ehlers-Danlos syndrome IV: 130050
Ehlers-Danlos syndrome V: 305200
Ehlers-Danlos syndrome VI: 225400

Ehlers-Danlos syndrome VII: 130060 autosomal dominant, 225410 autosomal recessive

Ehlers-Danlos syndrome VIII: 130080

INHERITANCE

Types I, II, III, IV, and VIIA and B are autosomal dominant.

Type V is X-linked recessive.

Types VI and VIIC are autosomal recessive.

GENE/GENE MAP

Ehlers-Danlos syndrome I and II: abnormal structure of type V collagen *COL5A1, COL5A2*

1. Ehlers-Danlos syndrome I: 2q31, 17q21.31–q22, 9q34.2–q34.3
2. Ehlers-Danlos syndrome II: 9q34.2–q34.3

Ehlers-Danlos syndrome III: 2q31

Ehlers-Danlos syndrome IV: abnormal structure of type III collagen *COL3A1*; 2q31

Ehlers-Danlos syndrome V: X-linked

Ehlers-Danlos syndrome VI: deficiency of lysyl hydroxylase; 1p36.3–p36.2

Ehlers-Danlos syndrome VIIA and B: no cleavage of N terminus of type I procollagen due to mutations in *COL1A1* or *COL1A2*; 17q21.31–q22, 7q22.1

Ehlers-Danlos syndrome VIIC: no cleavage of the N terminus of type I procollagen due to deficiency of peptidase; 5q23

Ehlers-Danlos syndrome VIII: unknown gene and locus

EPIDEMIOLOGY

1 in 5000 births

CLINICAL FINDINGS

The term *Ehlers-Danlos syndrome* is now known to encompass a heterogeneous group of connective tissue disorders that share hyperextensibility of the joints and skin due to an abnormality in collagen molecules.

At least eight distinct entities can be recognized on the basis of biochemical, genetic, and clinical findings.

1. Type I (gravis type) is the most commonly recognized.

   - Infants with the classic type are often born 4 to 8 weeks prematurely because of rupture of fetal membranes.
   - The skin is remarkably hyperextensible and bruises easily. Cigarette paper–like scarring is present over the forehead, chin, elbows, knees, and shins. Generalized tissue friability makes healing difficult. The lids are easily stretched on eversion.

2. Type II resembles type I but is a milder or *mitis* type.
3. Type III shows severe hypermobility of all joints without other musculoskeletal abnormalities. Skin changes are minimal.
4. Type IV (vascular type) manifests abnormalities of the large to medium-sized arterial vessels.

   - Spontaneous arterial rupture may occur at a young age.
   - Perforation of hollow organs, especially the colon and uterus, is a possible complication. Women with this type are especially at risk during pregnancy.
   - Because these events carry considerable morbidity, life expectancy is reduced, on average, by more than half.
   - The skin is very thin and transparent and may show elastosis perforans serpiginosa. Hyperextensibility of the joints and skin laxity are minimal.

5. Type V shows minimal joint hypermobility but marked hyperextensibility of the skin. A floppy mitral valve may be an associated feature.
6. Type VI (kyphoscoliotic or oculoscoliotic type) is primarily an ocular disease.

   - There is severe scoliosis with moderate joint and skin involvement. The hyperextensibility and joint laxity are not as severe as in type I (gravis type).

- Aortic root dilation and aortic regurgitation may occur.
- Rupture of the globe or retinal detachment may occur from minor trauma.
- This type results from a deficiency of lysyl hydroxylase, with the defect interfering in the cross-linking of collagen. However, spontaneous rupture of the globe has been observed in the absence of lysyl hydroxylase deficiency (Ia).
- Blue sclerae are a feature.
- Microcornea and myopia have been reported.

7. Type VII has some of the features of Marfan syndrome
8. Type VIII is characterized by short stature and extreme generalized joint hypermobility.

- Subluxation of the hips, knees, and feet is common.
- There is moderate skin stretchiness and bruisability.
- Hypertelorism and epicanthal folds are common.

The diagnosis is based on the clinical features. In the two autosomal recessive types (VI and VIC), biochemical documentation of the specific enzyme defect is possible.

Carrier detection is potentially possible in types V, VI, and VII, as is prenatal diagnosis.

The differential diagnosis includes cutis laxa, a disorder of reduced elastin fibers in which the skin hangs in loose folds. In Ehlers-Danlos syndrome, the skin shows increased stretchiness but resumes its normal position when not on stretch.

Larsen syndrome is a disorder of multiple congenital dislocations and skeletal abnormalities, but without hyperextensible skin.

In osteogenesis imperfecta, patients have blue sclerae, but globe rupture is rare.

OCULAR FINDINGS

Type VI
1. Epicanthus
2. Microcornea, keratoconus, and keratoglobus
3. Subluxation of the lens
4. Scleral fragility, with globe rupture caused by minor trauma
5. Myopia
6. Predisposition to retinal breaks

THERAPEUTIC ASPECTS

Management of skin and joint problems should be conservative and preventive.

The vascular type (IV) requires particular surgical care. The ruptured arteries are difficult to repair because of the pronounced vascular fragility. Rupture of the bowel is a surgical emergency. Because the risk of vascular rupture is especially high during pregnancy, women should be advised to avoid pregnancy. Patients should be advised to avoid contact sports and to treat blood pressure elevation aggressively.

The oculoscoliotic type (type VI) may improve with high doses of ascorbic acid (500 mg per day in children and up to 10 g per day in adults) because vitamin C is a cofactor for the enzyme that is deficient. No other metabolic or

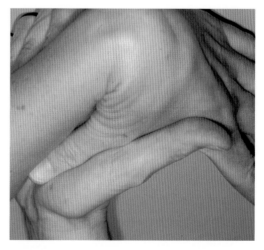

Ehlers-Danlos syndrome Hyperextensible wrist and thumb in a patient with Ehlers-Danlos syndrome.

genetic therapy is effective in other types of the syndrome.

Genetic counseling about inheritance patterns may be complicated.

REFERENCES

Judisch GF, Waziri M, Krachmer FH: Ocular Ehlers-Danlos syndrome with normal lysyl hydroxylase. *Arch Ophthalmol* 1976;94:1489–1491.

Macsai MS, Lemley HL, Schwartz T: Management of oculus fragilis in Ehlers-Danlos type VI. *Cornea* 2000;19:104–107.

Tilstra DJ, Byers PH: Molecular basis of hereditary disorders of connective tissue. *Annu Rev Med* 1994; 45:149–163.

RESOURCES

Ehlers-Danlos National Foundation
　www.ednf.org
Ehlers-Danlos Support Group
　www.atv.ndirect.co.uk

Enhanced S-Cone Syndrome

See **Retinal Dystrophies and Degenerations**

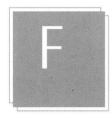

Fabry Disease

OMIM NUMBER
301500

INHERITANCE
X-linked

GENE/GENE MAP
Defect in alpha-galactosidase A
Xq22–q24

EPIDEMIOLOGY
1 in 40,000 males

CLINICAL FINDINGS
Affected males have extensive deposition of glycophospholipids in blood vessels, ganglion cells, the heart, kidneys, eyes, and most tissues.

Clinical sequelae include angiokeratomas in the skin and mucous membranes, paresthesias, and episodes of burning pain in the extremities.

Sweating defects and dependent edema may occur. Proteinuria develops in middle life, and kidney failure is a common cause of death.

Episodic severe pain in the extremities is usually the reason for initially seeking medical attention. Because the pain is rarely suspected as being caused by Fabry disease, the correct diagnosis is usually delayed until either an ophthalmologist sees the pathognomonic corneal or lens changes or kidney failure occurs.

Cardiovascular (left ventricular hypertrophy) and renal complications dominate the clinical course in the third and fourth decades of life.

Heterozygous females may have an attenuated form of the disease, but almost always have the whorl-like corneal epithelial dystrophy.

Prenatal diagnosis is possible by enzyme assay or urinalysis.

Most heterozygous females show skin and corneal lesions.

Some females may have renal or cardiac disease.

Both affected males and female carriers can be identified by decreased levels of alpha-galactosidase A activity in serum, leukocytes, tears, or cultured fibroblasts.

Maltese-cross figures in urinary sediment allow a presumptive clinical diagnosis.

Conjunctival, dermal, or gastrointestinal mucosal biopsy shows "zebra-like" electron-dense deposits in vascular endothelial and perithelial cells and in the cytoplasm of small unmyelinated neurons and perineural cells.

The episodes of pain in the extremities are often associated with fever and an elevated red blood cell sedimentation rate.

Corneal lesions similar to those in Fabry disease can be caused by chloroquine, indomethacin, and amiodarone, a cardiac antiarrhythmic drug.

Angiokeratomas are seen in some cases of fucosidosis.

The sutural cataracts resemble those in the mild phenotype of mannosidosis. The wedge-shaped cataracts are similar to hypocalcemic-induced lens opacities.

The pain in the extremities and other symptoms may be misdiagnosed as rheumatic fever, neurosis, erythromelalgia, or collagen vascular disease.

OCULAR FINDINGS
Ocular findings include conjunctival vascular tortuosity and aneurysmal dilations, a whorl-like corneal epithelial abnormality (cornea verticillata), lens opacities, and retinal vascular tortuosity.

The corneal epithelial swirl pattern (cornea verticillata) was found in 87% of affected males

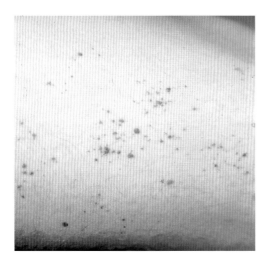

Fabry disease Characteristic skin lesions.

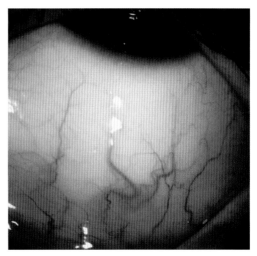

Fabry disease Tortuous conjunctival blood vessels.
(Courtesy of Maree Flaherty, M.D.)

and 76% of carrier females. The conjunctival vascular changes, which tend to appear in the second decade of life, are found in about half of affected males and carrier females.

The lens opacities, which may be evident before age 10 years, seem to be of two types:

1. The first type consists of triangles of white subcapsular granular opacities, with the base at the equator and the apex toward the center of the lens.
2. The second type consists of minute dots

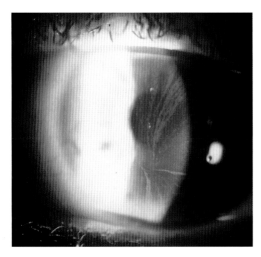

Fabry disease Corneal changes (cornea verticillata).
(Courtesy of Maree Flaherty, M.D.)

along the suture lines, best seen on retroillumination.

Impaired pupillary constriction with pilocarpine and reduced tear production are ocular signs of a generalized impaired autonomic nervous system.

Retinal vascular tortuosity may become apparent by the second decade of life.

Papilledema has been reported and is probably due to ischemic changes.

Central retinal artery occlusion has been reported in a 16-year-old boy.

Angiokeratomas of the lids are rare.

THERAPEUTIC ASPECTS

Neither the corneal lesion nor the cataract affects visual acuity.

Diphenylhydantoin or carbamazepine may provide some relief from the pain in the extremities.

Enzyme replacement therapy is available in Europe.

Renal insufficiency is progressive.

Mean survival is 42 years. Death usually results from renal failure, stroke, or cardiovascular disease.

REFERENCES

Brady RO, Schiffmann R: Clinical features of and recent advances in therapy for Fabry disease. *JAMA* 2000;284:2771–2775.

Sher NA, Reiff W, Letson RD, et al: Central retinal artery occlusion complicating Fabry's disease. *Arch Ophthalmol* 1978;96:815–817.

Spaeth GL, Frost P: Fabry's disease: its ocular manifestations. *Arch Ophthalmol* 1965;74:760–769.

RESOURCES

Fabry Community (Genzyme Therapeutics)
www.fabrycommunity.com
Fabry Support and Information Group (FSIG)
www.fabry.org
General Clinical Research Center: Fabry Disease
www.mssm.edu/crc/fabry

Familial Exudative Vitreoretinopathy (FEVR)

Also called **Criswick-Schepens syndrome**

OMIM NUMBERS
Autosomal dominant: 133780
X-linked: 305390

INHERITANCE
Autosomal dominant with 100% penetrance
X-linked

GENE/GENE MAP
Autosomal dominant forms: 11q13–q23 are caused by mutations in the frizzled-4 (*FZD4*) and the *LRP5* genes
X-linked form: Xp11.4; allelic with Norrie disease (OMIM 310600)

EPIDEMIOLOGY
Prevalence unknown

CLINICAL FINDINGS
Defective platelet function (rare); no other systemic associations reported

OCULAR FINDINGS
Extreme variability in expressivity: both eyes are affected, but asymmetry is common.

Retinopathy similar to retinopathy of prematurity is found. Most prominent is the abrupt cessation of peripheral retinal vessels in a scalloped pattern at the temporal equator. Dilated retinal vessels may result in peripheral neovascularization with adjacent preretinal hemorrhage that may evolve into a fibrovascular scar. Ectopia of the macula is present in 50% of patients. A positive angle kappa or strabismus is common.

Vitreous membranes, posterior vitreous detachment, and retinal traction may occur. The majority of retinal detachments occur in the first decade of life, with little progression after 10 years of age.

Other ocular findings include cataracts, neovascular glaucoma, vitreous hemorrhage, and subretinal exudates in 10% to 15% of eyes. The exudates can become massive, resembling those in Coats disease.

The results of electrophysiologic studies are normal to slightly decreased in amplitude.

Fluorescein angiography shows leakage from capillaries at the posterior pole, cessation of capillaries with leakage in the periphery, and fibrovascular masses.

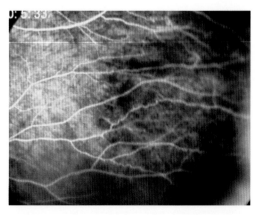

Familial exudative vitreoretinopathy (FEVR) Peripheral areas of vascular nonperfusion and avascular tortuosity in a patient with FEVR. (Courtesy of Johane Robitaille, M.D.)

THERAPEUTIC ASPECTS

Individuals at risk should be screened early to identify nonperfused peripheral retina and apply cryotherapy or laser photocoagulation as needed.

Scleral buckling, with or without vitrectomy, should be performed in patients with retinal detachment or vitreous hemorrhage.

REFERENCES

Chen ZY, Battinelli EM, Fielder A, et al: A mutation in the Norrie disease gene (*NDP*) associated with X-linked familial exudative vitreoretinopathy. *Nat Genet* 1993;5:180–183.

Downey LM, Keen TJ, Roberts E, et al: A new locus for autosomal dominant familial exudative vitreoretinopathy maps to chromosome 11p12–13. *Am J Hum Genet* 2001;68:778–781.

Li Y, Muller B, Fuhrmann C, et al: The autosomal dominant familial exudative vitreoretinopathy locus maps on 11q and is closely linked to D11S533. *Am J Hum Genet* 1992;51:749–754.

Robitaille J, MacDonald MLE, Kaykas A, et al: Mutant frizzled-4 disrupts retinal angiogenesis in familial exudative vitreoretinopathy *Nat Genet* 2002;32:326–330.

Tasman W, Augsburger JJ, Shields JA, et al: Familial exudative vitreoretinopathy. *Trans Am Ophthalmol Soc* 1981;79:211–226.

Toomes C, Bottomley HM, Jackson RM, et al: Mutations in LRP5 or FZD4 underlie the common familial exudative vitreoretinopathy locus on chromosome 119. *Am J Hum Genet* 2004;74:721–730.

RESOURCES

None listed

Familial Radial Drusen

See **Retinal Dystrophies and Degenerations**

Fetal Alcohol Syndrome (FAS)

OMIM NUMBERS

None

INHERITANCE

Not inherited

GENE/GENE MAP

Chromosomes are normal. However, genetic factors may modulate the expression of the teratogenic effects of alcohol. Polymorphisms in alcohol dehydrogenase genes (maternal or fetal) may be related to risk in this syndrome.

EPIDEMIOLOGY

0.4 to 3.1 in 1000 live births worldwide
1200 in the United States annually

CLINICAL FINDINGS

A constellation of physical abnormalities occurs in children of mothers who have abused alcohol during pregnancy. The three major diagnostic criteria are:

1. Specific craniofacial morphology, including short palpebral fissures, elongated midface, long and flat philtrum, thin upper vermilion, and flattened maxilla
2. Intrauterine growth retardation
3. Central nervous system dysfunction

The mechanism by which the abnormalities are produced is thought to be due to a direct teratogenic effect. To date, the syndrome has been described only in children of mothers who drank alcohol frequently during pregnancy. From 30% to 35% of the offspring of alcoholic mothers have the complete syndrome.

Abuse of crack cocaine or other agents during pregnancy may contribute to the syndrome in some infants.

The diagnosis is based on clinical findings.

OCULAR FINDINGS

Ptosis (20%), telecanthus, and epicanthus
Strabismus, including esotropia, Duane syndrome, and other types of ocular misalignment
Anterior segment malformations, especially Peters anomaly
Myopia
Occasional microphthalmos

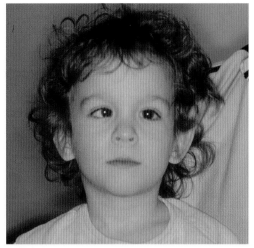

A

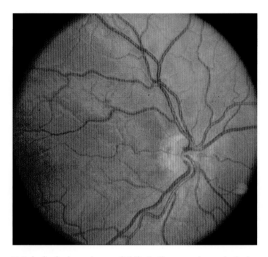

Fetal alcohol syndrome (FAS) Optic nerve hypoplasia in a patient with FAS.

Optic disc anomalies (48%), especially optic nerve hypoplasia, and increased tortuosity of retinal vessels, especially arteries (49%)

THERAPEUTIC ASPECTS

Maternal education regarding the toxic effects of alcohol is of paramount importance in preventing the syndrome. There is no safe minimum amount of alcohol consumption that can be guaranteed not to be toxic to a fetus, so mothers-to-be are urged to abstain entirely from alcohol throughout pregnancy.

There is no direct treatment for the effects of the syndrome.

One in six infants born with this syndrome die. Of the remainder, about half suffer permanent physical or mental handicaps.

REFERENCE

Johnson VP, Swayze VW II, Sato Y, et al: Fetal alcohol syndrome: craniofacial and central nervous system manifestations. *Am J Med Genet* 1996;61: 329–339.

RESOURCES

Fetal Alcohol Syndrome: Support, Training, Advocacy, and Resources (FASSTAR)
www.fasstar.com
National Organization on Fetal Alcohol Syndrome
www.nofas.org

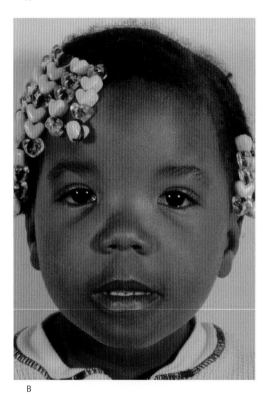

B

Fetal alcohol syndrome (FAS) Characteristic facial features of two patients with FAS. Note the esotropia in (A) and long philtrum, thin upper lip, and bilateral mild ptosis in (B).

Fragile X Syndrome

OMIM NUMBERS
FRAXA: 309550
FRAXE: 309548

INHERITANCE
X-linked

Expression of fragile X in females may depend in part on Lyonization and/or a parental source of abnormal X (imprinting)

GENE/GENE MAP
Four fragile sites are known on the X chromosome: FRAXA, FRAXD, FRAXE, and FRAXF. Only FRAXA and FRAXE are associated with clinical manifestations.

Each site is caused by a hypermethylated expansion of either a CCG or a CGG repeat, the size of which determines the range from normality to carrier to affected. Hypermethylation switches off transcription of the gene. The same effect may result from a deletion of the gene or a mutation within the gene.

FRAXA: Xq27; mutations in the *FMR1* gene
FRAXE: Xq28

EPIDEMIOLOGY
Fragile X is the most common cause of hereditary mental retardation. The incidence is between 1 in 1200 and 1 in 4000, depending on the population studied.

Because males have only one X chromosome, they are more susceptible to the effects of fragile X. However, 20% of males carry the gene without any apparent deleterious effects.

CLINICAL FINDINGS
The syndrome has very variable expressivity.
1. Mental retardation is the most common feature. Ten percent of prepubertal boys may have IQs in the borderline to low-normal range. However, some children have IQs below 20. Mean IQ in females is 80, with 25% functioning in the mentally retarded range. Almost one-third may function as normal or borderline normal. Affected females also tend to have more stable IQs and better outcomes than affected males.
2. Physical characteristics: Boys have large ears, a broad nasal bridge, a long prominent chin, and a narrow face. Dental anomalies (47%) and flat occiput (61%) are also common. Patients characteristically have joint hypermobility (89%) and large testes. Various heights have been observed. In girls, only prominent ears and a long face are common.

The diagnosis should be suspected in all mentally retarded boys.

OCULAR FINDINGS
Delayed visual motor integration
Poor eye contact
No consistent ocular malformations reported
Strabismus in up to one-third of patients

THERAPEUTIC ASPECTS
Special education, speech and language therapy, occupational therapy, and behavioral therapies are helpful in addressing many of the physical, behavioral, and cognitive impacts of fragile X syndrome.

Medical intervention can be helpful for aggression, anxiety, hyperactivity, and poor attention span.

Strabismus is treated as necessary.

REFERENCES

Hatton DD, Buckley E, Lachiewicz A, et al: Ocular status of boys with fragile X syndrome: a prospective study. *J Am Assoc Pediatr Ophthalmol Strabismus* 1998;2:298–302.

Storm RL, PeBenito R, Ferretti C: Ophthalmologic findings in the fragile X syndrome. *Arch Ophthalmol* 1987;105:1099–1102.

RESOURCE

The National Fragile X Foundation
www.nfxf.org

Fraser Syndrome

Also called cryptophthalmos-syndactyly syndrome

OMIM NUMBER
219000

INHERITANCE
Autosomal recessive

GENE/GENE MAP
Can be caused by mutations in the *FRAS1* gene on chromosome 4q21. The gene encodes a putative extracellular matrix protein.

EPIDEMIOLOGY
Minimal incidence is 0.43 in 100,000 live births and 11.06 in 100,000 stillbirths in Spain

Frequency among liveborn gypsy infants is about 130 times greater than in the nongypsy population

CLINICAL FINDINGS
Mental retardation

Dyscephaly with skull malformations mostly in the region of the temples and forehead; hair growth on temples extends to the lateral eyebrow

Meningomyelocele, encephalocele

Congenital heart disease

Anomalies of the auricles, ear canal, or inner ear

Anomalies of the nose and mouth: cleft lip and palate, crowding of teeth

Laryngeal atresia

Total or partial syndactyly of toes and/or fingers

Diastasis of the symphysis pubis

Renal malformations (85%): renal agenesis or dysplasia may occur, resulting in spontaneous abortion, stillbirth, or neonatal death

Malformations of genital organs, especially in females

Other less common malformations: anal atresia and umbilical hernia or low-set umbilicus

The diagnosis should be considered in the absence of cryptophthalmos if the other abnormalities are present. Suggested criteria for diagnosis of this condition include at least two major criteria (cryptophthalmos, syndactyly, abnormal genitalia, or a sibling with cryptophthalmos) and one minor criterion, or one major criterion and four minor criteria.

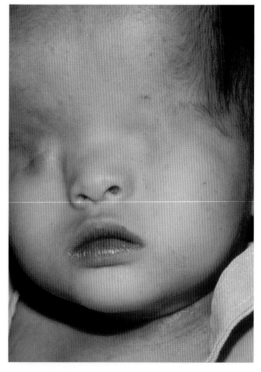

Fraser syndrome Face of a patient with cryptophthalmos. The forehead skin extends over the orbit and continues as the skin of the cheek.

Prenatal diagnosis of the severe forms of the syndrome should be possible using ultrasonography.

OCULAR FINDINGS

Cryptophthalmos: hidden eye, fused lids—absence of a palpebral fissure

Sometimes symblepharon occurs: adhesion of lid to globe

Microphthalmos in some cases

Absent or malformed lacrimal ducts

Hypertelorism

Flat supraorbital ridge

THERAPEUTIC ASPECTS

A lid fissure can be created, but the surgeon has to anticipate the possibility of finding an abnormal globe or penetrating the anterior chamber if the lids are fused to the cornea.

Imaging studies (ultrasonography, computed tomography, magnetic resonance imaging) should be performed prior to surgery to outline the anatomy of the globe and intraocular contents. Surgical options are then discussed based on findings in individual cases.

Twenty percent of patients die before age 1, usually secondary to renal or laryngeal defects.

REFERENCES

Boyd PA, Keeling JW, Lindenbaum RH: Fraser syndrome (cryptophthalmos-syndactyly syndrome): a review of eleven cases with postmortem findings. *Am J Med Genet* 1988;31:159–168.

Dibben K, Rabinowitz YS, Shorr N, et al: Surgical correction of incomplete cryptophthalmos in Fraser syndrome. *Am J Ophthalmol* 1997;124:107–109.

Martinez-Frias ML: Fraser syndrome: frequency in our environment and clinical-epidemiological aspects of a consecutive series of cases. *Ann Esp Pediatr* 1998;48:634–638.

McGregor L, Makela V, Darling SM, et al: Fraser syndrome and mouse blebbed phenotype caused by mutations in FRAS1/Fras1 encoding a putative extracellular matrix protein. *Nat Genet* 2003;34:203–208.

Thomas IT, Frias JL, Felix V, et al: Isolated and syndromic cryptophthalmos. *Am J Med Genet* 1986;25:85–98.

RESOURCE

National Organization for Rare Disorders
www.rarediseases.org

▦

Fucosidosis

OMIM NUMBER

230000

INHERITANCE

Autosomal recessive

GENE/GENE MAP

Deficiency of plasma and leukocyte enzyme alpha-L-fucosidase

FUCA1 on 1p34

EPIDEMIOLOGY

Carrier rate for fucosidosis mutations is high in persons of Italian descent

CLINICAL FINDINGS

This is a lysosomal storage disease with accumulation of fucose in tissues.

There are two forms: a severe form with death in early childhood and a milder form with survival into the third decade.

1. Severe phenotype: hepatosplenomegaly, cardiomegaly, mild dysostosis multiplex, thick skin, and resemblance to Hurler syndrome. Psychomotor retardation begins early in the first year of life.

2. Mild phenotype: later onset of psychomotor retardation. Features may be so mild that the diagnosis is unsuspected until the third or fourth decade of life. A characteristic feature is the presence of angiokeratomas on the face and upper body starting at age 4 years. Angiokeratomas are prominent in the groin, on the lower abdomen, and on the buttocks. They are clin-

ically indistinguishable from those in Fabry disease.

The diagnosis is based on the demonstration of low levels of alpha-L-fucosidase in plasma and leukocytes.

In the presence of angiokeratomas, normal levels of alpha-galactosidase should be documented to rule out Fabry disease.

The severe form must be differentiated from the mucopolysaccharidoses, generalized gangliosidosis, the mucolipidoses, the Austin variant of metachromatic leukodystrophy, and Farber lipogranulomatosis.

The mild form with angiokeratomas must be differentiated from Fabry disease.

OCULAR FINDINGS

In the severe phenotype, no ocular abnormalities have been described.

In the mild form:

1. Tortuous retinal vessels with beading or sausaging of retinal veins
2. Dilated and tortuous conjunctival vessels with local fusiform and saccular microaneurysms
3. Superficial diffuse central corneal opacities
4. Conjunctival biopsies reveal pathognomonic inclusion bodies

THERAPEUTIC ASPECTS

No treatment is known. Management is supportive.

REFERENCES

Libert J, van Hoff F, Tondeur M: Fucosidosis: ultrastructural study of conjunctiva and skin and enzyme analysis of tears. *Invest Ophthalmol* 1976; 15:626–639.

Snyder RD, Carlow TJ, Ledman J, et al: Ocular findings in fucosidosis. In: Bergsma D, Bron AJ, Cotlier E, eds: *The Eye in the Inborn Errors of Metabolism.* Birth Defects Original Articles Series 12(3). New York: Alan R. Liss; 1976:241–251.

RESOURCE

Lysosomal Diseases Australia
   www.lda.org.au/text.html

Fundus Albipunctatus

See **Retinal Dystrophies and Degenerations**

Fundus Flavimaculatus

See **Retinal Dystrophies and Degenerations**

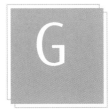

G

Glaucoma, Congenital

OMIM NUMBERS
231300
600975
137750

INHERITANCE
Autosomal recessive

Autosomal dominant in rare families and in the context of anterior segment dysgenesis

In the setting of a number of chromosomal defects

GENE/GENE MAP
Autosomal recessive
1. GLC3A (*CYP1B1*) on 2p21; codes for cytochrome P4501B1
2. GLC3B on 1p36

Autosomal dominant
1. GLC1A on 1q24.3–q25.2, 9q34.1

EPIDEMIOLOGY
1 in 10,000 patients seen for ophthalmologic care

Much more common in the Middle East than in Western ethnicities, with an incidence of 1 in 2500 births

CLINICAL AND OCULAR FINDINGS
Progressive enlargement of the cornea and globe (buphthalmos)

Corneal edema and breaks in Descemet's membrane (Haab striae), especially in early or

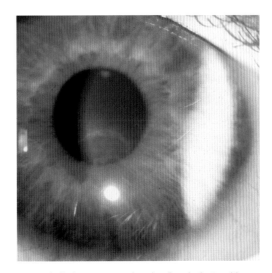

Congenital glaucoma Haab striae (breaks in Bruch's membrane) and corneal edema in a patient with congenital glaucoma.

intrauterine onset of intraocular pressure elevation

Increasing myopia and optic nerve head cupping with uncontrolled intraocular pressure

Symptoms are highly variable, but increased light sensitivity, squinting, and epiphora with exposure to even normal levels of light are typical. Some children may be completely asymptomatic, especially during the first few months of life.

Amblyopia from uncorrected high errors of refraction

THERAPEUTIC ASPECTS
Topical beta-blocker drops and topical or oral carbonic anhydrase inhibitors will decrease the intraocular pressure.

Surgical procedures, such as goniotomy, trabeculotomy, filtration surgery, and implant surgery, are indicated for long-term control of intraocular pressure.

Occlusion therapy and correction of high refractive errors are important to prevent amblyopia.

REFERENCES
Akarsu AN, Turacli ME, Aktan SG, et al: A second locus (GLC3B) for primary congenital glaucoma

(buphthalmos) maps to the 1p36 region. *Hum Mol Genet* 1996;5:1199–1203.

Stoilov I, Akarsu AN, Sarfarazi M: Identification of three different truncating mutations in cytochrome P4501B1 (*CYP1B1*) as the principal cause of primary congenital glaucoma (buphthalmos) in families linked to the GLC3A locus on chromosome 2p21. *Hum Mol Genet* 1997;6:641–647.

RESOURCES

Children's Glaucoma Foundation
www.childrensglaucoma.com

The Pediatric Glaucoma Cataract Family Association: Facts about Pediatric Glaucoma
www.pgcfa.org/glaucoma.htm

GM₂ Gangliosidoses

Includes Tay-Sachs disease *and* Sandhoff disease

OMIM NUMBERS

Tay-Sachs disease: 272800
Sandhoff disease: 268800

INHERITANCE

Autosomal recessive

GENE/GENE MAP

The GM₂ gangliosidoses are characterized by excessive intralysosomal accumulation of GM₂ ganglioside and related glycolipids. They result from the deficiency of β-hexosaminidase A (on 15q23–q24) in Tay-Sachs disease or β-hexosaminidases A and B (on 5q13) in Sandhoff disease. There is massive accumulation of GM₂ ganglioside in neurons, where they form characteristic inclusions.

EPIDEMIOLOGY

The infantile and adult forms of Tay-Sachs disease occur most frequently in descendants of Central and Eastern European (Ashkenazi) Jews. One in 30 American Jews carries the gene.

Non-Jewish individuals of French-Canadian ancestry, including the Cajun population in Louisiana, are at similarly increased risk. Both groups have 100 times the rate of occurrence of other ethnic groups. The juvenile form, however, is not increased in these groups.

CLINICAL FINDINGS

Observant parents notice an increased startle reaction to sound and hypotonia at 2 to 3 months of age.

There is progressive blindness, paralysis, and decreased awareness of the surroundings.

Death occurs by age 5.

There are four forms of the disease.

1. The classic infantile type is by far the most common, and its signs and symptoms are described above.
2. Children with the juvenile form develop symptoms between the ages of 2 and 5 years that closely resemble the symptoms of the classic infantile form. The course of the disease is slower, and death generally occurs by age 15.
3. Symptoms of chronic hexosaminidase A deficiency also may begin by age 5 but are far milder than those in the infantile and juvenile forms. Mental function, vision, and hearing remain intact, but affected individuals develop slurred speech, muscle weakness, muscle cramps, tremors, unsteady gait, and sometimes mental illness.
4. Individuals with adult-onset Tay-Sachs disease experience many of the same variable symptoms as individuals with the chronic form, but later in life.

Sandhoff disease is characterized by neuronal and visceral deposition of GM₂ gangliosides. Clinical and neurologic features are indistinguishable from those of classic Tay-Sachs disease, except for the presence of moderate hepatosplenomegaly and mild skeletal dysostosis in some patients. Death occurs before 10 years of age.

OCULAR FINDINGS

A macular cherry-red spot is one of the major diagnostic criteria. It results from the accumulation of gangliosides in retinal ganglion cells that surround the fovea, leading to their opacification. The central red spot represents normal choroidal background.

The cherry-red spot can be observed as early as 2 months of age. With time, ganglion cells die and optic atrophy ensues. The macular lesion disappears.

Visual evoked responses are absent, but the electroretinogram remains intact.

The macular cherry-red spot in Sandhoff disease is identical to that in Tay-Sachs disease. Both blindness and optic atrophy occur.

The diagnosis of Tay-Sachs disease should be entertained in the blind and neurologically impaired infant even in the absence of a cherry-red spot.

Hexosaminidase A activity can be measured in serum and in skin fibroblasts.

Absence of hexosaminidase A and B in serum and leukocytes confirms the diagnosis of Sandhoff disease.

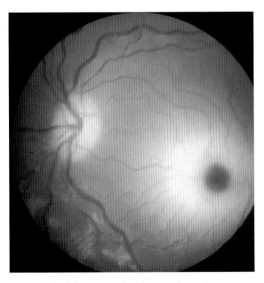

GM₂ gangliosidoses Macular cherry-red spot in a patient with Tay-Sachs disease. (Courtesy of Selwa Al-Hazzaa, M.D.)

THERAPEUTIC ASPECTS

There is no specific therapy; treatment is supportive.

REFERENCE

Kaback M et al: Tay-Sachs disease: carrier screening, prenatal diagnosis, and the molecular era. *JAMA* 1993;270:2307–2315.

RESOURCE

National Tay-Sachs and Allied Diseases Association www.ntsad.org

Goldenhar Syndrome

Also called oculoauriculovertebral dysplasia

OMIM NUMBER

164210

INHERITANCE

Most cases are isolated.

Autosomal dominant and presumed autosomal recessive inheritance have been reported.

GENE/GENE MAP

Not mapped

Goldenhar syndrome with ipsilateral radial defect has been mapped to chromosome 7p, but it may be a distinct entity.

EPIDEMIOLOGY

Over 70% of patients are males.

CLINICAL FINDINGS

Goldenhar syndrome is one of a group of disorders referred to as *hemifacial microsomia*. The term *Goldenhar syndrome* should be used only for those patients who have epibulbar dermoids associated with hemifacial microsomia.

Seventy percent of cases have unilateral involvement, the right side being affected more often.

Characteristic features
1. Malformations of the external ear with preauricular skin tags and pits
2. Vertebral hypoplasia
3. Micrognathia
4. Epibulbar dermoids

The cluster of developmental anomalies is the result of errors in morphogenesis of the first and second branchial arches.

Hypoplasia of the maxillary region and, in some cases, the mandibular region is frequent. The mouth may be large as a result of a lateral cleft-like extension (macrostomia). There is diminished to absent parotid secretion. Malfunction of the soft palate is common. Cleft lip and cleft palate are occasionally present, as are various abnormalities of the heart.

Occasional abnormalities include renal, limb, and rib anomalies.

Most patients have normal intelligence.

Hearing should be tested at an early age.

The diagnosis is made on the basis of the clinical findings.

If there are no epibulbar dermoids, a diagnosis of hemifacial microsomia should be made.

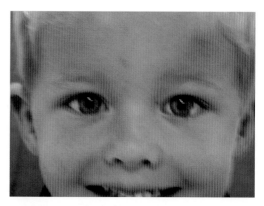

Goldenhar syndrome Bilateral limbal dermoids in a patient who also had preauricular tags.

Colobomas of the upper lid are associated with Goldenhar syndrome, whereas those of the lower lid are characteristic of Treacher Collins syndrome.

OCULAR FINDINGS

The characteristic feature is the epibulbar dermoid, almost invariably located at the limbus inferotemporally in one or both eyes. There may be irregular astigmatism and anisometropic amblyopia.

Subconjunctival lipodermoids (or dermolipomas) are not infrequent. They are most commonly present in the superotemporal quadrant of the globe.

Colobomas of the upper lid are estimated to be present in one-fourth of patients.

The association of Goldenhar syndrome with Duane syndrome has been reported on numerous occasions.

An occasional patient may have colobomatous microphthalmia.

THERAPEUTIC ASPECTS

Indications for the removal of epibulbar dermoids include continued growth, persistent irritation, and desired improvement in ocular appearance.

Excision of a lipodermoid may be complicated by its adherence to the conjunctiva and its extension posteriorly around the globe.

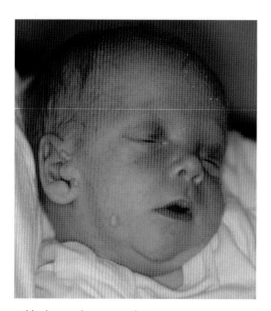

Goldenhar syndrome Hemifacial microsomia and preauricular tags in a baby with Goldenhar syndrome.

REFERENCES

Baum JL, Feingold M: Ocular aspects of Goldenhar's syndrome. *Am J Ophthalmol* 1973;75:250–257.

Pieroni D: Goldenhar's syndrome associated with bilateral Duane's retraction syndrome. *J Pediatr Ophthalmol* 1969;6:16–18.

RESOURCE

Goldenhar Syndrome Support Network
www.goldenharsyndrome.org

Goldmann-Favre Syndrome

See also **Enhanced S-Cone Syndrome** *under* **Retinal Dystrophies and Degenerations** *Includes* **clumped pigmentary retinal degeneration**

OMIM NUMBER
268100

INHERITANCE
Autosomal recessive with variable expressivity

GENE/GENE MAP
Caused by mutations in nuclear receptor gene *NR2E3* (OMIM 604485)
15q23

EPIDEMIOLOGY
1 in 56,000 to 1 in 164,000

CLINICAL FINDINGS
No known systemic associations

OCULAR FINDINGS
Unlike other retinal degenerations, this condition is characterized by an increased sensitivity of photoreceptors (cones) to blue light only.

Visual loss and night blindness are present early in the course of the disease.

The severe form of enhanced S-cone syndrome is called *Goldmann-Favre syndrome.*

Frequent associated ocular findings
1. Cataracts
2. Peripheral pigmentary retinopathy, some of which is in round "clumps" along the vascular arcades
3. Peripheral and macular retinoschisis
4. Opaque and nonperfused retinal vessels
5. Vitreoretinal degeneration with abnormal preretinal bands (veils) and posterior vitreous detachment
6. Retinal holes

Fluorescein angiography demonstrates cystoid macular edema.

Histopathology shows photoreceptor atrophy.

The electroretinogram is variably decreased.

The electro-oculogram is severely abnormal.

Dark adaptometry is abnormal.

Color vision is abnormal.

The differential diagnosis includes X-linked retinoschisis and autosomal dominant hyaloideoretinal degeneration.

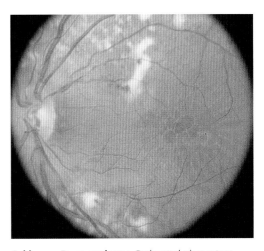

Goldmann-Favre syndrome Pericentral pigmentary changes and macular schisis in a young man with Goldmann-Favre syndrome.

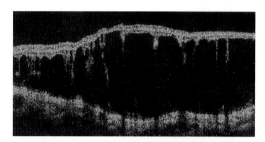

Goldmann-Favre syndrome Ocular coherence tomography demonstrating schisis in the patient with Goldmann-Favre syndrome in figure on page 77.

THERAPEUTIC ASPECTS

No specific therapy is available.

REFERENCES

Haider NB, Jacobson SG, Cideciyan AV, et al: Mutation of a nuclear receptor gene, *NR2E3*, causes enhanced S cone syndrome, a disorder of retinal cell fate. *Nat Genet* 2000;24:127–131.

Sharon D, Sandberg MA, Caruso RC, Berson EL, Dryja TP: Shared mutations in *NR2E3* in enhanced S-cone syndrome, Goldmann-Favre syndrome and many cases of clumped pigmentary retinal degeneration. *Arch Ophthalmol* 2003;121: 1316–1323.

RESOURCE

Foundation Fighting Blindness
www.blindness.org/index.html

Gorlin Syndrome

Also called basal cell nevus syndrome *or* nevoid basal cell carcinoma syndrome

OMIM NUMBER
109400

INHERITANCE
Autosomal dominant

GENE/GENE MAP
PTCH (601309) or *PTCH2* (603673)
9q22.3–q31

EPIDEMIOLOGY
1 in 55,600 people in northwestern England

CLINICAL FINDINGS
There are five major components:

1. Multiple nevoid basal cell carcinomas of the face, neck, and upper torso: basal cell nevi usually appear between the 15th and 35th year of life but have been observed as early as age 2 years; they are present in 90% of patients.

2. Jaw cysts (odontogenic keratocysts) occur in 65% to 75% of patients and are frequently associated with pain, tenderness, and swelling; they may be the initial presenting symptom.

3. Congenital vertebral and rib anomalies: short metacarpals, bifid ribs, partial bulging of the sella turcica, vertebral fusion, and scoliosis. Lamellar calcifications of the falx cerebri, tentorium cerebelli, or petroclinoid ligaments occur in more than 80% of patients. Head circumference may be 60 cm or more due to frontal and biparietal bossing.

4. Dyskeratotic pits on the palms and soles develop in the teenage or early adult years in over 60% of patients and are pathognomonic.

5. Neurologic abnormalities include defects of the corpus callosum, hydrocephalus, nerve deafness, seizures, and mental retardation.

There is sensitivity to ionizing radiation. Basal cell carcinomas develop in an irradiated region within 3 years. Susceptibility to other malignancies is also increased.

The differential diagnosis includes leopard syndrome, a disorder characterized by increasing numbers of pigmented spots on the face and body; Waardenburg syndrome, which exhibits telecanthus and mandibular prognathism; and pseudohypoparathyroidism, which is suggested by the shortened metacarpals and the calcification.

OCULAR FINDINGS

The basal cell nevi around the face tend to cluster on or around the lids and to undergo papillomatous and carcinomatous changes.

Forty percent of patients have true hypertelorism.

Other findings include strabismus, coloboma of the iris, cataract, glaucoma, and telecanthus in one-fourth of patients.

Four patients with extensive medullation of the nerve fibers have been reported, as well as one patient with a combined hamartoma of the retina and retinal pigment epithelium.

THERAPEUTIC ASPECTS

Families should be offered regular screening; see guidelines in *J Med Genet* 1993;30:460–464.

DNA testing is feasible using linkage or mutation analysis.

A large head circumference at birth is suggestive of the condition.

Rarely, infants can have fibromas in the heart. An echocardiogram is best performed before 3 months of age.

Routine scanning with computed tomography (which uses X-rays) is not recommended because of concerns about inducing skin malignancies.

Annual dental screening should start at age 8 years.

At least an annual examination of the skin should start at puberty. Early treatment for lesions of the lids, nose, ears, and scalp should be offered. Patients are advised to inspect all areas of the body; basal cell carcinomas have been reported on the vulva and the mucosa of the anal sphincter.

Basic sunscreening precautions should be taken.

REFERENCES

De Jong PT, Bistervels B, Cosgrove J, et al: Medullated nerve fibers: a sign of multiple basal cell nevi (Gorlin's) syndrome. *Arch Ophthalmol* 1985;103:1833–1836.

De Potter P, Stanescu D, Caspers-Velu L, et al: Photo essay: combined hamartoma of the retina and retinal pigment epithelium in Gorlin syndrome. *Arch Ophthalmol* 2000;118:1004–1005.

Kimonis VE, Goldstein AM, Pastakia B, et al: Clinical manifestations in 105 persons with nevoid basal cell carcinoma syndrome. *Am J Med Genet* 1997;69:299–308.

RESOURCES

The Gorlin-Syndrome Group
www.gorlin-group.pwp.blueyonder.co.uk

Neuroid Basal Cell Carcinoma/Gorlin Syndrome
hometown.aol.com/budcaruso/skinindex.html

Gyrate Atrophy of Choroid and Retina

Also called ornithine aminotransferase (OAT) deficiency

OMIM NUMBER

258870

INHERITANCE

Autosomal recessive

GENE/GENE MAP

Decreased activity of the enzyme OAT

10q26

EPIDEMIOLOGY

Rare

CLINICAL FINDINGS

There are no systemic abnormalities, except for mild proximal muscle weakness and fine, sparse hair in a minority of patients.

One-third of patients have slow waves on electroencephalography.

OCULAR FINDINGS

There are characteristic and progressive areas of geographic atrophy of the retinal pigment epithelium, choroid, and retina that appear first in the periphery and spread toward the posterior pole. The discrete round, atrophic patches coalesce to form well-defined diagnostic scalloped lesions. The macular area is spared until late in the disease. In some cases, peripapillary atrophy is also present, but the optic disc remains pink and healthy.

A ring scotoma may correspond to the areas of atrophy.

Retinal vessels become progressively narrow. In patients who have not been placed on the arginine-deficient diet early in life, the entire retina is atrophic by age 40 to 50 years.

Myopia appears in the first decade of life.

Night blindness begins in early childhood.

Cataracts develop and surgery is consistently needed prior to age 20 years.

The scotopic electroretinogram is nonrecordable.

The diagnosis is based on finding increased levels of ornithine in the plasma and urine. Plasma levels are 10 to 20 times normal.

Prenatal diagnosis is possible.

In the end stages, the differential diagnosis includes a fundus picture similar to that in choroideremia.

The characteristic patterned atrophy differentiates this disease from retinitis pigmentosa.

THERAPEUTIC ASPECTS

Ornithine aminotransferase uses pyridoxine (vitamin B_6) as a cofactor. Some patients' elevated plasma ornithine levels respond with a 50% reduction to pharmacologic dietary supplementation with vitamin B_6. Plasma ornithine levels should be tested before and after administration of oral doses of 300 to 500 mg vitamin B_6 per day in all patients to determine their biochemical response. Only those who show a significant reduction in plasma ornithine should take supplementary vitamin B_6.

An arginine-deficient diet (less than 15 g protein per day) is effective in lowering plasma ornithine levels and has halted progression of the

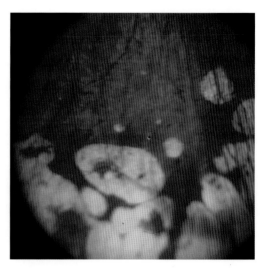

Gyrate atrophy of choroid and retina Peripheral gyriform and round areas of chorioretinal atrophy in a patient with gyrate atrophy.

disease in some patients. However, patients adopting this low-protein diet need to be monitored by a metabolic specialist to avoid a negative nitrogen balance or a deficiency of essential amino acids.

REFERENCES

O'Donnell JJ, Sipila I, Vannas A, et al: Gyrate atrophy of the retina and choroid: two methods for prenatal diagnosis. *Int Ophthalmol* 1981;4:33–36.

Simell O, Takki K: Raised plasma ornithine and gyrate atrophy of the choroid and retina. *Lancet* 1973;1:1031–1033.

Valle D, Walser M, Brusilow SW, et al: Gyrate atrophy of the choroid and retina: amino acid metabolism and correction of hyperornithinemia with an arginine-deficient diet. *J Clin Invest* 1980;65: 371–378.

Weleber RG, Kennaway NG, Buist NR: Vitamin B_6 in the management of gyrate atrophy of the choroid and retina. *Lancet* 1978;2:1213.

RESOURCE

Foundation Fighting Blindness
www.blindness.org/index.html

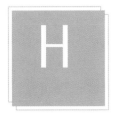

Hemangioma, Cavernous Familial

Also called cerebral capillary malformations, Cotlier syndrome

OMIM NUMBER
116680

INHERITANCE
Autosomal dominant with high penetrance and variable expressivity

GENE/GENE MAP
CCM1 on 7q11.2–q21, encoding for protein Krev interaction trapped-1 (*KRIT1*)
  CCM2 on 7p15–p13
  CCM3 on 3q25.2–q27

EPIDEMIOLOGY
0.39% to 0.9% worldwide

CLINICAL FINDINGS
Cavernous vascular malformations can involve any part of the central nervous system. They can be asymptomatic or cause seizures, mostly from hemorrhage, progressive or focal neurologic deficit, and headache. Intracranial hemorrhage occurs in 12% to 48% of patients.

Tumors can be detected by magnetic resonance imaging studies. Because of their venous nature, they are difficult to detect angiographically.

Skin lesions are the least common component and may be absent in certain families.

OCULAR FINDINGS
Ocular tumors are usually single at the disc or in the periphery and have the appearance of a cluster of grapes with overlying fibrosis. They do not enlarge with time.

Patients may present with vitreous hemorrhage.

Fluorescein angiography is diagnostic and shows a red blood cell fluid level in each saccule without evidence of leaking.

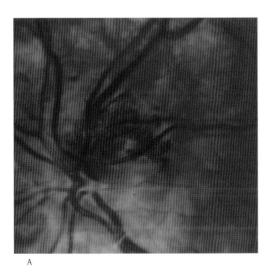

A

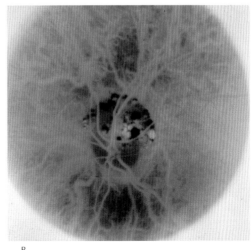

B

Cavernous familial hemangioma Fundus photograph (A) and corresponding angiogram (B) of cavernous hemangioma of the retina, here located at the optic nerve head; note the typical grape-like cluster of aneurysms and fluid levels in each. The patient had a brain hemangioma. (Courtesy of John F. Gillis, M.D.)

THERAPEUTIC ASPECTS

Early diagnosis of central nervous system lesions allows surgical excision or embolization.

No treatment is necessary for the retinal angiomas in the vast majority of patients. Laser photocoagulation may be used if vitreous hemorrhage ensues.

REFERENCES

Dobyns WB et al: Familial cavernous malformations of the central nervous system and retina. *Ann Neurol* 1987;21:578–583.

Dubovsky J, Zabramski JM, Kurth J, et al: A gene responsible for cavernous malformations of the brain maps to chromosome 7q. *Hum Mol Genet* 1995;4:453–458.

Laberge-le Couteulx S, Jung HH, Labauge P, et al: Truncating mutations in *CCM1*, encoding *KRIT1*, cause hereditary cavernous angiomas. *Nat Genet* 1999;23:189–193.

Lewis RA et al: Cavernous haemangioma of the retina and optic disc: a report of three cases and a review of the literature. *Br J Ophthalmol* 1975;59:422–434.

Rigamonti D, Hadley MN, Drayer BP, et al: Cerebral cavernous malformations: incidence and familial occurrence. *N Engl J Med* 1988;319:343–347.

RESOURCES

None listed

Homocystinuria

OMIM NUMBER

236200

INHERITANCE

Autosomal recessive

GENE/GENE MAP

Cystathionine β-synthetase
21q22.3

EPIDEMIOLOGY

Incidence in Europe has been estimated at 1 in 40,000 newborns, which corresponds to a carrier (heterozygote) frequency of about 1%.

In Ireland, where neonatal screening for homocystinuria is mandatory, the incidence is 1 in 52,544 births.

Incidence varies in different populations between 1 in 30,000 and 1 in 60,000 live births.

CLINICAL FINDINGS

Mental retardation

Coarse, fair hair

Connective tissue abnormalities causing skeletal findings similar to those of Marfan syndrome and ocular defects like ectopia lentis and myopia

Homocystine effects on vascular endothelium, platelets, and coagulation factors that predispose to repeated thromboembolic episodes

Malar flush

The diagnosis is based on elevated homocystine levels on serum and urine amino acid quantitation.

The urine nitroprusside test may be falsely negative in mildly affected adult patients. The sensitivity of testing can be improved by methionine loading.

OCULAR FINDINGS

Thirty-eight percent of 5-year-old patients with untreated homocystinuria have lens subluxation, and almost all patients have it by age 25. The zonules are absent, compared to the stretched zonules in Marfan syndrome.

The lenses move down and nasally in 50% of patients, posteriorly in 20%, and anteriorly in 10%. Pupillary block occurs in some patients with anterior lens subluxation and leads to elevation of intraocular pressure and to corneal decompensation from lens–endothelial contact.

THERAPEUTIC ASPECTS

Supplementation with pyridoxine (50 to 1000 mg/day) results in clinical and biochemical improvement in 50% of patients.

Vitamin B_6 nonresponders may benefit from a diet low in methionine and supplementation with cystine.

Early detection and treatment using dietary restriction and vitamin supplementation in an

Irish study of 14 patients by Burke et al. resulted in the prevention of ectopia lentis after a mean follow-up of 8.2 years compared with a 70% dislocation rate in untreated patients with a similar follow-up period. Ectopia lentis developed and progressed in five patients diagnosed later in life despite tight biochemical control.

In a study of 45 patients from Saudi Arabia, 84 surgical procedures were performed on 40 patients: 82 were done with general anesthesia and 2 with local anesthesia. Medical therapy was attempted initially in all patients with lens dislocation and was the sole therapy used for five patients. All patients had a history of lens subluxation or dislocation. Of the 45 patients, 14 (31%) were receiving dietary treatment at the time of presentation and 29 (64%) were mentally retarded. There were two surgical complications and one postsurgical complication. Lens dislocation into the anterior chamber was the most frequent indication for surgery (50%), followed by pupillary-block glaucoma (12%). Prophylactic peripheral iridectomy was not successful in preventing lens dislocation into the anterior chamber in five patients. Anesthetic precautions, such as stockings to prevent deep venous thrombosis, preoperative hydration, or aspirin, were taken in 85% of cases. Other common ophthalmic complications included optic atrophy (23%), iris atrophy (21%), anterior staphylomas (13%), lenticular opacities (9%), and corneal opacities (9%). Laser iridectomy was unsuccessful in preventing lens dislocation into the anterior chamber. With appropriate anesthetic precautions and modern microsurgical techniques, the risks associated with the surgical management of ocular complications are reduced. Surgical treatment should be considered, especially for cases of repeated lens dislocation into the anterior chamber or pupillary-block glaucoma. If a conservative nonsurgical approach is undertaken, these patients must be observed carefully for recurrent episodes of lens dislocation.

If the lens is in the anterior chamber, dilation of the pupil and gentle pressure over the

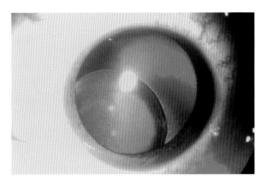

Homocystinuria Totally dislocated lens in a patient with homocystinuria.

cornea can lead to repositioning of the lens behind the pupil. Patients are then administered pilocarpine, and a laser peripheral iridotomy is performed to prevent pupillary-block glaucoma. In the case of recurrent dislocations into the anterior chamber, a lensectomy should be performed.

Prophylaxis of thromboembolic phenomena should be considered whenever these patients need general anesthesia. This should include a few weeks of supplementation with vitamin B_6 before surgery, good intravenous hydration before and during surgery, and dipyridamole or acetylsalicylic acid daily before and after surgery is performed.

REFERENCES

Burke JP, O'Keefe M, Bowell R, et al: Ocular complications in homocystinuria: early and late treated. *Br J Ophthalmol* 1989;73:427–431.

Cross HE, Jensen AD: Ocular manifestations in the Marfan syndrome and homocystinuria. *Am J Ophthalmol* 1973;75:405–419.

Harrison DA, Mullaney PB, Mesfer SA, et al: Management of ophthalmic complications of homocystinuria. *Ophthalmology* 1998;105:1886–1890.

Ramsey MS, Dickson DH: Lens fringe in homocystinuria. *Br J Ophthalmol* 1975;59:338–342.

RESOURCE

Homocystinuria Support
www.hcusupport.com

Hunter Syndrome

See also **Mucopolysaccharidoses**

OMIM NUMBER
309900

INHERITANCE
X-linked; the only mucopolysaccharidosis that is not autosomal recessive

GENE/GENE MAP
β-Iduronate-2-sulfatase
Xq28

EPIDEMIOLOGY
Incidence unknown

CLINICAL FINDINGS
Two phenotypes, severe and mild, are now accepted, and further heterogeneity is likely to be defined. Both types are due to different mutations at the X-chromosomal locus for the enzyme iduronate-2-sulfatase and are, therefore, allelic.

1. Severe phenotype: Death occurs prior to age 20 years. Many of the same features seen in Hurler syndrome are present. In general, skeletal and mental changes in Hunter syndrome are less severe than those in Hurler syndrome.

2. Mild phenotype: Patients may survive past age 50. Intelligence is normal and skeletal involvement is moderate. A characteristic clinical finding is pebbling of the skin over the scapula, neck, chest, or thigh.

The diagnosis is based on the demonstration of the deficient activity of alpha-L-sulfoiduronate sulfatase. As a screening test, the mucopolysaccharide spot test is useful.

Dermatan and heparan sulfate are present in the urine. The enzyme assay is available in only a few laboratories.

Conjunctival biopsy reveals typical lysosomal inclusions characteristic of mucopolysaccha-ride disorders but not specific for Hunter syndrome.

Hurler syndrome is differentiated because of its more severe phenotype and because of the absence of corneal clouding in Hunter patients early in the first decade of life.

Sanfilippo patients have no corneal clouding, but they have less dysmorphic features than do Hunter patients.

OCULAR FINDINGS
The absence of corneal clouding is a conspicuous feature.

Pigmentary retinopathy with an extinguished electroretinogram may lead to severe visual impairment in older patients with the severe phenotype or may be more benign in the mild phenotype.

Elevated and blurred disc margins have led to the diagnosis of chronic papilledema. This is presumed to be due to compression of the optic nerve by a posterior sclera that is thickened by the accumulation of mucopolysaccharides. Long-standing optic nerve swelling results in optic atrophy and loss of vision even in the mild phenotype. In other patients, vision may remain 20/20 and the electroretinogram may show only mild reduction of the b-wave in patients over 20 years of age.

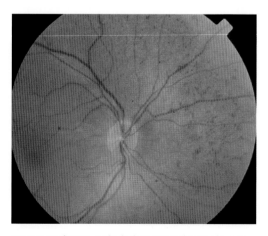

Hunter syndrome Retinal pigmentary changes in a patient with Hunter syndrome.

THERAPEUTIC ASPECTS

There is no specific therapy for the optic nerve and retinal disease.

The prognosis depends on the clinical severity. Survival to late adulthood has been observed.

REFERENCES

See **Mucopolysaccharidoses**

RESOURCES

National MPS Society, Inc.
17 Kraemer St.
Hicksville, NY 11801
516-432-1797
Fax: 410-538-4964
www.mpssociety.org
NYU Medical Center resource site
mcrcr2.med.nyu.edu/murphp01/lysosome/hgd.htm

Hurler Syndrome

See also **Mucopolysaccharidoses**

OMIM NUMBER
252800

INHERITANCE
Autosomal recessive

GENE/GENE MAP
Lysosomal alpha-L-iduronidase (*IDUA*)
4p16.3

EPIDEMIOLOGY
1 in 100,000 worldwide
30 new patients born annually in the United States

CLINICAL FINDINGS
The disease is not apparent at birth and development is normal in the first few months, followed by progressive mental and physical deterioration.

Photophobia, corneal clouding, coarse facial appearance, stiff joints, chest deformity, rhinitis, or visceromegaly prompts the initial medical consultation. Dwarfism and typical skeletal changes become apparent by 2 to 3 years of age. Hepatosplenomegaly follows.

Mental deterioration is evident after 1 year of age, and hydrocephalus is a frequent finding.

Other features include deafness, short neck, and wide-spaced teeth with hypertrophy of the gums. The reduced range of joint motion is especially striking in the fingers, resulting in the claw-hand deformity.

The absence of activity of lysosomal alpha-L-iduronidase renders cells incapable of cleaving iduronic acid residues in polysaccharide chains. Both heparan sulfate and dermatan sulfate contain the residue and cannot be degraded. As a result of the enzyme deficiency, both heparan sulfate and dermatan sulfate are excreted in the urine and stored in the tissues.

The diagnosis is based on clinical signs, excess mucopolysacchariduria (heparan sulfate and dermatan sulfate), and demonstration of deficient alpha-L-iduronidase in leukocytes or fibroblasts.

Carriers, or heterozygotes, have 50% normal alpha-L-iduronidase activity in cultured fibroblasts. A rapid new electrophoretic screening test for the presence of pathologic amounts of glycosaminoglycans (GAG) in urine has been reported. A sensitive assay for iduronidase, which allows unequivocal separation of normal individuals, carriers, and affected individuals using cultured amniotic fibroblasts, makes prenatal diagnosis possible. Two-dimensional electrophoresis of amniotic fluid for the presence of abnormal amounts of GAG is faster and may be more sensitive than the enzyme assay for prenatal diagnosis.

Patients with I-cell disease or mucolipidosis II have abnormalities at birth, whereas the clinical features of Hurler syndrome develop concurrently with the progressive accumulation of storage material and the child appears normal at birth.

Differentiation from Hunter syndrome is by the absence of corneal clouding in the latter.

Mannosidosis, multiple sulfatase deficiency, fucosidosis, aspartylglycosaminuria, and the GM_1 gangliosidoses must all be considered in the differential diagnosis because of their clinical similarities.

OCULAR FINDINGS

Corneal clouding appears early in life and is slowly progressive. It results from the accumulation of cytoplasmic and extracellular mucopolysaccharides.

Papilledema and/or optic atrophy occurs, along with pigmentary retinopathy. It has been demonstrated that the optic atrophy is due to both descending degeneration from hydrocephalus and accumulation of storage material in the ganglion cells.

The electroretinogram is abolished by age 5 or 6 years.

The orbits are shallow from premature closure of cranial sutures, resulting in proptosis.

THERAPEUTIC ASPECTS

Bone marrow transplantation has been tried and was effective in some patients, reversing the evidence of storage disease and clearing the corneal clouding.

Corneal transplant is not recommended because of the limited life span of the patient, the concurrent retinal degeneration, the difficulty of maintaining a clear graft in a child, and the severe anesthetic problems due to upper airway obstruction and excessive secretions.

Counseling, prenatal diagnosis, and abortion are available as primary prevention.

Death usually occurs before age 10 years and may be the result of respiratory infection or cardiac failure secondary to mucopolysaccharide deposition in the aortic or mitral valves, the intima of the coronary arteries, or the myocardium.

REFERENCES

See **Mucopolysaccharidoses**

RESOURCES

National MPS Society, Inc.
   17 Kraemer St.
   Hicksville, NY 11801
   516-432-1797
   Fax: 410-538-4964
   www.mpssociety.org
NYU Medical Center resource site
   mcrcr2.med.nyu.edu/murphp01/lysosome/hgd.htm

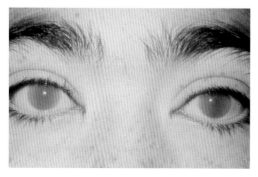

Hurler syndrome Corneal clouding in a patient with Hurler syndrome.

Hyperoxaluria

OMIM NUMBERS
   Type I: 259900
   Type II: 260000

INHERITANCE
   Each genetic type is inherited as an autosomal recessive trait.

GENE/GENE MAP
   Type I is caused by a defect in the peroxisomal enzyme alanine:glyoxylate aminotransferase: locus 2q36–q37. It involves a defect of the cytoplasmic enzyme N-ketoglutarate glyoxalate carboligase.

   Type II is a defect of cytosolic glyoxalate reductase located on 9cen.

EPIDEMIOLOGY
Unknown

CLINICAL FINDINGS
Primary hyperoxaluria comprises at least two types of heritable disorders of glyoxylate metabolism characterized by recurrent calcium oxalate nephrolithiasis, chronic renal failure, and death from uremia. Type II is a milder disorder, with urolithiasis as the only clinical feature. Initial symptoms of oxalate nephrolithiasis appear in the first decade of life.

Classification
1. Genetic: primary hyperoxaluria, type I (glycolic aciduria); primary hyperoxaluria, type II (glyceric aciduria), is milder and less frequent.
2. Acquired: increased ingestion of oxalate; increased intake of oxalate precursors: methoxyflurane, ethylene glycol, ascorbic acid, and xylitol; pyridoxine deficiency; hyperabsorption of oxalate (enteric hyperoxaluria).

The diagnosis is often not made until adulthood. Night blindness may be an early symptom.

The diagnosis is based on measurement of urinary oxalate excretion in the absence of pyridoxine deficiency, excessive oxalate ingestion, or bowel disease with excessive absorption. Plasma levels of phytanic acid are elevated. Enzyme assays are reported, but are difficult to standardize and reproduce.

The differential diagnosis includes fundus albipunctatus, Bietti crystalline fundus dystrophy, and crystalline retinopathy; systemic diseases with crystalline retinopathy such as cystinosis; and toxic retinopathies such as methoxyflurane oxalosis, tamoxifen, canthaxanthine, and talc embolism.

OCULAR FINDINGS
In most instances, ocular involvement has appeared in infants and children only in the retina. There are innumerable discrete white refractile lesions diffusely scattered throughout the posterior neural retina, with earlier development of well-circumscribed, semitransparent, yellowish, dome-shaped lesions at the level of the retinal pigment epithelium that may stain in late phases of fluorescein angiography. Some lesions develop a cuff of hyperpigmentation that may coalesce to involve the macular area in a large black lesion.

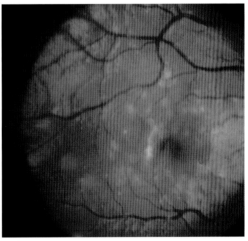

A

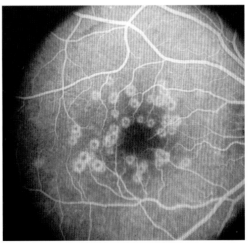

B

Hyperoxaluria Typical early macular lesions (A) and angiographic findings (B) in a 4-year-old boy with oxalosis.

THERAPEUTIC ASPECTS

Medical management has been directed at either symptomatic relief of associated conditions (polyarthritis, pericarditis) or supportive management of uremia (dialysis).

Renal transplantation has been uniformly unsuccessful due to rapid reaccumulation of oxalate crystals in the graft. Although oxalate is dialyzable, dialysis does not remove sufficient oxalate to control production rates in vivo.

Death within 10 years of symptom presentation occurs in more than 90% of patients with type I. Renal insufficiency does not occur in the rarer and milder type II variant.

REFERENCES

Small KW, Letson R, Scheinman J: Ocular findings in primary hyperoxaluria. *Arch Ophthalmol* 1990; 108:89–93.

Traboulsi EI, El-Baba FZ, Barakat A, et al: The retinopathy of primary hyperoxaluria. *Retina* 1985;5:151–153.

RESOURCE

The Oxalosis and Hyperoxaluria Foundation
www.ohf.org

Incontinentia Pigmenti (IP)

Also called **Bloch-Sulzberger syndrome**

OMIM NUMBER
308300

INHERITANCE
X-linked lethal

GENE/GENE MAP
The disease is caused by mutations in the *NEMO* (NF-Kappa-B Essential Modulator) gene and is referred to as IP2, or "classical" incontinentia pigmenti. Sporadic incontinentia pigmenti, originally called IP1, maps to Xp11 and is categorized as similar to hypomelanosis of Ito.

An 870 bp region of identity corresponding to an *MER67B* repeat exists in the *NEMO* gene both in intron 3 and in intron 3′ to exon 10; recombinations between the regions of identity delete exons 4 though 10 of *NEMO*. Accounting for 80% of new mutations, this rearrangement would result in a truncated molecule carrying the 133 N-terminal amino acids of *NEMO* plus at least 26 novel amino acids. It was predicted that this molecule would contain part of the first coiled-coil domain and may still interact with IKK2, but would be unlikely to respond to upstream signals.

EPIDEMIOLOGY
Unknown

CLINICAL FINDINGS
This genodermatosis is lethal prenatally in males, with rare exceptions.

In affected females, it causes highly variable abnormalities of the skin, hair, nails, teeth, eyes, and central nervous system. The prominent skin signs occur in four classic cutaneous stages: perinatal inflammatory vesicles, verrucous patches, a distinctive pattern of hyperpigmentation, and dermal scarring. The erythematous eruption with linear vesiculation in the newborn period is followed by a verrucous stage. After a few months, the verrucous growth is replaced by hyperpigmented areas, which disappear at age 20 years.

Twenty percent of patients have skeletal abnormalities, including hemivertebrae, kyphoscoliosis, syndactyly, and leg length discrepancies.

Hypodontia, delayed tooth eruption, and conical teeth are frequent.

Fifteen percent of patients show central nervous system involvement, developing mental deficiency, microcephaly, spasticity, or seizures.

The diagnosis is based on clinical features and family history.

Gene testing is possible.

OCULAR FINDINGS
Thirty-five percent of patients have significant ocular abnormalities, which are generally unilateral or markedly asymmetric.

Twenty percent of patients have significant visual loss, mostly from retinal disease.

The development of a retrolental mass of glial tissue may lead to confusion with retinoblastoma or retinopathy of prematurity.

Abnormal vascular anastomoses with peripheral zones of decreased perfusion and preretinal fibrosis are frequently present.

Less common ocular findings include cataracts (4%, and only if there is a retinal detachment), uveitis (2%), and blue sclerae (2%). Other abnormalities include nystagmus, strabismus, microphthalmos, pigmentation of the conjunctiva, corneal scarring, absence of the anterior chamber, optic atrophy, persistence of the hyaloid artery, and myopia.

Goldberg reported on the nature of the ocular complications of incontinentia pigmenti.

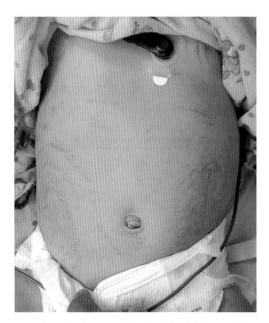

Incontinentia pigmenti (IP) Whorly healed linear skin lesions.

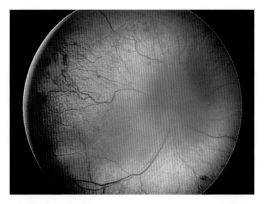

Incontinentia pigmenti (IP) Peripheral areas of avascular retina in a patient with IP. Also note the few scattered hemorrhages close to the avascular areas.

He emphasized that the ocular and cerebral abnormalities associated with this disease are far worse than the name would indicate. Although some patients have normal vision, total blindness or permanent visual deficiency may occur. Retinal vascular abnormalities, involving the periphery as well as the macula, appear to represent the primary disease process in the eye. Retinal detachment may ensue due to mechanisms that seem analogous to those of retinopathy of prematurity. Optic nerve atrophy and occipital lobe infarction are additional causes of severe visual dysfunction in some patients. Goldberg reported, for the first time, neonatal infarction of the macula in this disease.

When the eye is involved, retinopathy of prematurity and retinoblastoma are frequent misdiagnoses.

THERAPEUTIC ASPECTS

There is no specific therapy for the skin disorder.

Cryotherapy and laser photocoagulation have been used with some success in patients in whom the retinal disease was detected early.

REFERENCES

Goldberg MF: The blinding mechanisms of incontinentia pigmenti. *Ophthal Genet* 1994;15:69–76.
International Incontinentia Pigmenti Consortium: Genomic rearrangement in *NEMO* impairs NF-kappa-B activation and is a cause of incontinentia pigmenti. *Nature* 2000;405:466–472.

RESOURCE

Incontinentia Pigmenti International Foundation imgen.bcm.tmc.edu/NIPF

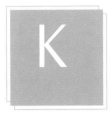

Kearns Syndrome

Formerly **Kearns-Sayre syndrome**

OMIM NUMBER

530000

INHERITANCE

Most cases are sporadic; however, familial cases with probable maternal transmission and several affected siblings have been reported.

Deletions of mitochondrial DNA are present in the majority of cases.

The mitochondrial DNA abnormality probably occurs in the oocyte or zygote and not in the mother. It is, however, likely that most severely affected ova are nonviable; thus, extensive pedigrees of the syndrome are not seen.

GENE/GENE MAP

Large deletions of mtDNA ranging from 1 to 8 kbp were found in muscle biopsies.

The exact site and size of the deletion, as well as the proportion of normal to abnormal mitochondria, vary among patients. This explains the variable clinical presentation.

EPIDEMIOLOGY

Incidence unknown

CLINICAL FINDINGS

In Kearns syndrome, mutant mitochondria are localized to muscle and the central nervous system; in chronic progressive external ophthalmoplegia, they are localized to muscle; and in Pearson syndrome, they are localized to blood.

The syndrome belongs to the group of disorders called *mitochondrial myopathies* and is characterized by onset before age 20 years, pigmentary degeneration of the retina, progressive external ophthalmoplegia, and at least one of the following abnormalities: heart block, cerebellar ataxia, and cerebrospinal fluid protein greater than 1 g/L.

Growth retardation, delayed sexual maturation, and mental deterioration are often present.

Less frequent features include pharyngeal and facial weakness, skeletal muscle weakness, and deafness.

Electrocardiographic abnormalities include complete heart block; thus, electrocardiograms must be performed on all patients suspected of having the syndrome.

Computed tomography may reveal diffuse leukoencephalopathy or cerebellar and brainstem atrophy with calcification of the basal ganglia.

Biochemical studies show abnormal pyruvate and lactate metabolism. Biopsy of skeletal mus-

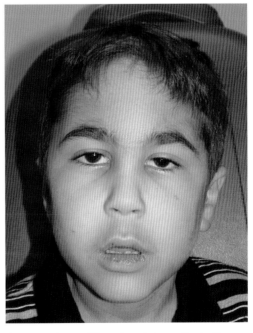

Kearns syndrome Bilateral ptosis in a patient with Kearns syndrome

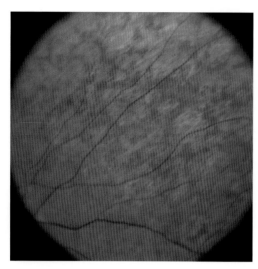

Kearns syndrome Pigmentary retinopathy in a patient with Kearns syndrome.

cle shows aggregates of abnormal mitochondria or ragged red fibers.

OCULAR FINDINGS

Progressive external ophthalmoplegia occurs with gradual loss of all extraocular movements and bilateral ptosis.

There is diffuse pigmentary retinopathy with a decreased electroretinogram; pigmentary changes are most evident in the macula; peripapillary atrophy has also been described.

THERAPEUTIC ASPECTS

Administration of coenzyme Q has been shown to improve the atrioventricular block, eye movements, and fatigue.

Patients usually die by the third or fourth decade of life from heart disease.

REFERENCES

Holt IJ, Harding AE, Morgan-Hughes JA: Deletions of muscle mitochondrial DNA in patients with mitochondrial myopathies. *Nature* 1988;331:717–719.

Kearns TP, Sayre GP: Retinitis pigmentosa, external ophthalmoplegia, and complete heart block: unusual syndrome with histologic study in one of two cases. *Arch Ophthalmol* 1958;60:280–289.

RESOURCES

United Mitochondrial Disease Foundation
www.umdf.org
Washington University: Mitochondrial Disorders resource site
www.neuro.wustl.edu/neuromuscular/mitosyn.html

Kjer Dominant Optic Atrophy

Also called juvenile optic atrophy

OMIM NUMBERS
Not applicable

INHERITANCE
Autosomal dominant

GENE/GENE MAP
OPA1 at 3q28–q29 codes for a polypeptide with homology to dynamin-related guanosine triphosphatases
OPA4 at 18q12.2–q12.3

EPIDEMIOLOGY
Incidence and prevalence unknown; probably the most common type of inherited optic atrophy after Leber's hereditary optic neuropathy

CLINICAL FINDINGS
Slowly progressive decrease in vision; patients lose about 1 line of Snellen acuity per decade of life
Color vision defect
Cecocentral scotomas
Wide intrafamilial and interfamilial variability in severity of visual loss
No neurologic or systemic abnormalities

OCULAR FINDINGS
A mild degree of temporal or diffuse pallor of the optic disc and minimal color vision defects, in the context of a family history of dominant optic atrophy, is highly suggestive of the diagnosis even if visual acuity is normal.

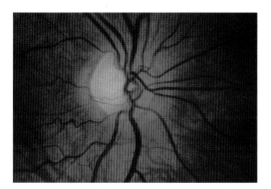

Kjer dominant optic atrophy Temporal pallor of the optic nerve head in a patient with dominant optic atrophy.

Only 58% of patients have visual loss before age 10.

Temporal pallor and "excavation" of the optic nerve head are characteristic.

Histopathologic studies reveal loss of ganglion cells and optic atrophy.

THERAPEUTIC ASPECTS
There is no specific therapy.

REFERENCES

Alexander C, Votruba M, Pesch UE, et al: *OPA1*, encoding a dynamin-related GTPase, is mutated in autosomal dominant optic atrophy linked to chromosome 3q28. *Nat Genet* 2000;26:211–215.

Delettre C, Lenaers G, Griffoin JM, et al: Nuclear gene *OPA1*, encoding a mitochondrial dynamin-related protein, is mutated in dominant optic atrophy. *Nat Genet* 2000;26:207–210.

Eliott D, Traboulsi EI, Maumenee IH: Visual prognosis in Kjer type autosomal dominant optic atrophy. *Am J Ophthalmol* 1993;115:360–367.

Johnston PB, Gaster RN, Smith VC, et al: A clinicopathologic study of autosomal dominant optic atrophy. *Am J Ophthalmol* 1979;88:868–875.

Johnston RL, Seller MJ, Behnam JT, et al: Dominant optic atrophy: refining the clinical diagnostic criteria in light of genetic linkage studies. *Ophthalmology* 1999;106:123–128.

Kerrison JB, Arnould VJ, Ferraz Sallum JM, et al: Genetic heterogeneity of dominant optic atrophy, Kjer type: identification of a second locus on chromosome 18q12.2–12.3. *Arch Ophthalmol* 1999;117:805–810.

Votruba M, Fitzke FW, Holder GE, et al: Clinical features in affected individuals from 21 pedigrees with dominant optic atrophy. *Arch Ophthalmol* 1998;116:351–358.

RESOURCES
None listed

Kniest Syndrome
Also called metatrophic dwarfism type II

OMIM NUMBER
156550

INHERITANCE
Autosomal dominant
Most cases are presumably caused by new mutations

GENE/GENE MAP
COL2A1
12q13.11–q13.2

EPIDEMIOLOGY
200 patients worldwide

CLINICAL FINDINGS
Clinical manifestations are present at birth.

Skeletal features include short stature in most patients, prominent knobby joints, scoliosis, a flat midface with a depressed nasal bridge, and a short trunk with a broad thorax and protrusion of the sternum. Diffuse atrophy of the interosseous muscles of the hands is invariably present, with flaring of epiphyses and metaphyses.

In a series of eight patients from Johns Hopkins Hospital, all had the skeletal features described above. Cleft palate or one of its variations (submucous cleft or bifid uvula) was present in three of these patients. Hearing loss was present in six.

Generalized osteoporosis and widening of the metaphyses are present. The epiphyses are translucent, and the joint spaces narrowed. The growth plate is abnormal on light microscopy, with a "Swiss cheese" appearance of the cartilage.

Facial features are similar to those in Stickler syndrome, but the bone dysplasia is more severe.

Metatrophic dwarfism is differentiated clinically from Kniest syndrome by the absence of a broad thorax and radiographically by the lack of radiolucency at the ends of the long bones. No myopia is present.

Spondyloepiphyseal dysplasia congenita is a dwarfing syndrome associated with myopia, but these patients have a near-normal facial profile and usually are more severely dwarfed than Kniest patients.

Patients with Marshall syndrome are short but not dwarfed. They have a facial appearance similar to that in Kniest and Stickler syndromes.

OCULAR FINDINGS

Patients have severe vitreoretinal degeneration.

Retinal detachment occurred in six eyes of five patients in the Johns Hopkins series.

Cataracts and bilateral subluxated lenses have also been reported.

THERAPEUTIC ASPECTS

Retinal examination, photographs, and fundus drawings should be made at regular intervals.

Prophylactic cryotherapy or vitrectomy may be considered if extensive lattice degeneration is found.

The indications for cataract surgery should be thoroughly weighed, considering the propensity to retinal detachments, the axial myopia, fluid vitreous, and the likelihood of encountering a hard nucleus.

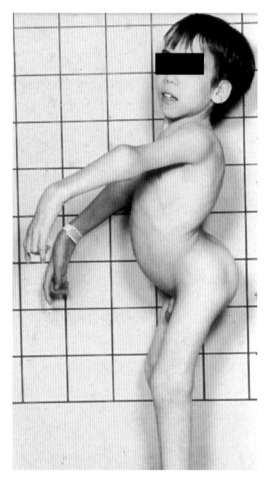

Kniest syndrome Note the short trunk dwarfism, severe kyphoscoliosis, and wide wrists, elbows, and knees.

REFERENCES

Maumenee IH: Vitreoretinal degeneration as a sign of generalized connective tissue diseases. *Am J Ophthalmol* 1979;88:432–449.

Maumenee IH, Traboulsi EI: The ocular findings in Kniest dysplasia. *Am J Ophthalmol* 1985;100:155–160.

RESOURCE

Little People of America, Inc.
www.lpaonline.org

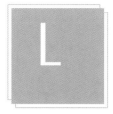

Leber Congenital Amaurosis

See **Retinal Dystrophies and Degenerations**

Leber Hereditary Optic Neuropathy (LHON)

Also called **Leber optic neuritis**

OMIM NUMBER

535000

INHERITANCE

Mitochondrial

Many cases are sporadic. The proportion of familial cases depends on the mutation and ranges between 43% for the 11778 mutation and 78% for the 3460 mutation.

Fifteen percent of families are heteroplasmic; that is, both mutant and wild-type mtDNA coexist within an individual. The level of heteroplasmy among different tissues can vary markedly. Mitochondrial DNA mutations alone are not sufficient to cause visual loss in LHON, since not all individuals harboring a pathogenic LHON mutation express the disease.

GENE/GENE MAP

Although more than 18 mutations in mtDNA have been identified in LHON, 3 mutations are considered definitely pathogenic:

1. Mutation at position 11778 (Wallace mutation) results in the substitution of histi-

dine for arginine at position 340 in subunit 4 of reduced nicotinamide adenine dinucleotide (NADH). This mutation accounts for 65% of European and American patients.
2. Mutation at position 14484 in subunit 6 of NADH accounts for 25% of patients.
3. Mutation at position 3460 in subunit 1 of NADH is present in 10% of patients.

Some families have no detectable mutations of mtDNA.

EPIDEMIOLOGY

Males are affected more often than females. This ratio is as high as 5 to 1, except in Asia, where only 68% of patients are male.

CLINICAL FINDINGS

Subacute (1 day to several months; average, 2 weeks), progressive, painless visual loss affects both eyes sequentially (average, 2 months) or, less commonly, at the same time.

Age of onset is between the late teens and mid-30s, although the neuropathy may occur at any age. Women have a slightly older age of onset.

Most patients have isolated optic neuropathy. Associated systemic findings have been reported in some families and include abnormal electrocardiographic findings, such as a prolonged QT interval and Wolff-Parkinson-White conduction anomaly, and a variety of minor or progressive, severe neurodegenerative disease and dystonia in other families. The 11778 mutation has also been associated with multiple sclerosis in some families.

Two of 12 patients with tobacco-alcohol amblyopia had LHON mutations: 1 had the 11778 mutation and 1 the 3460 mutation. It is believed that the mutations increase the patient's susceptibility to optic neuropathy from alcohol and tobacco abuse.

OCULAR FINDINGS

Central vision is lost almost completely, while the peripheral field is variably spared.

Color vision is profoundly affected, mainly in the red-green axis. Visual acuity ranges from 20/50 to no light perception and depends on the nature of the mutation. Vision is most severely impaired in 11778 mutation patients, followed in order of decreasing severity by those with 3460, 15257, and 14484 mutations.

Partial recovery of vision is possible in a small percentage of patients but does not start until 6 months or several years after disease onset. Visual recovery depends on the type of mutation, being more likely in patients with the 14484 mutation, in whom recovery occurs in up to 37%. Visual recovery is also noted in 22% of patients with the 3460 mutation and 28% with the 15257 mutation. Only 4% of patients with the 11778 mutation recover some vision.

The appearance of the disc in the acute stage is diagnostic. There is subtle disc elevation, with peripapillary telangiectasia and absence of leakage on fluorescein angiography. The peripapillary telangiectasias disappear within months, leaving nonspecific optic atrophy.

Light and electron microscopic studies in two patients revealed preferential loss of axons from P-cells, the smaller retinal ganglion cells. This explains the clinical features and preservation of the pupillary light response in LHON patients.

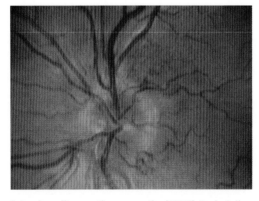

Leber hereditary optic neuropathy (LHON) Typical dilated small vessels at and around the optic nerve head in a patient in the acute phase of LHON.

THERAPEUTIC ASPECTS

There is no effective treatment.

Patients should avoid alcohol and smoking.

Vitamin supplements have been advocated but have not proven to be of value.

Management of the psychosocial aspects of the disease is essential.

Low-vision aids and visual rehabilitation may be needed.

REFERENCES

Cullom ME, Heher KL, Miller NR, et al: Leber's hereditary optic neuropathy masquerading as tobacco-alcohol amblyopia. *Arch Ophthalmol* 1993; 111:1482–1485.

Huoponen K: Leber hereditary optic neuropathy: clinical and molecular genetic findings. *Neurogenetics* 2001;3:119–125.

Leber T: Ueber hereditaere und congenital angelegte Sehnervenleiden. *Graefes Arch Clin Ophthalmol* 1871;17:249–291.

Mackey DA, Buttery RG: Leber hereditary optic neuropathy in Australia. *Aust N Z J Ophthalmol* 1992;20:177–184.

Mackey DA, Oostra RJ, Rosenberg T, et al: Primary pathogenic mtDNA mutations in multigeneration pedigrees with Leber hereditary optic neuropathy. *Am J Hum Genet* 1996;59:481–485.

Sadun AA, Win PH, Ross-Cisneros FN, et al: Leber's hereditary optic neuropathy differentially affects smaller axons in the optic nerve. *Trans Am Ophthalmol Soc* 2000;98:223–235.

Wallace DC: A new manifestation of Leber's disease and a new explanation for the agency responsible for its unusual pattern of inheritance. *Brain* 1970;93:121–132.

Wallace DC, Singh G, Lott MT, et al: Mitochondrial DNA mutation associated with Leber's hereditary optic neuropathy. *Science* 1988;242:1427–1430.

RESOURCES

International Foundation for Optic Nerve Disease: LHON resource site
www.ifond.org/lhon.php3
Leber's Optic Neuropathy resource site
www.leeder.demon.co.uk/pages/1honhome.htm
For testing, check www.genetests.org and search for LHON

Lowe Syndrome

OMIM NUMBER
309000

INHERITANCE
X-linked recessive

GENE/GENE MAP
OCRL1 gene mutations that lead to deficiency

Oculocerebrorenal syndrome results from a lipid phosphatase that may control cellular levels of a critical metabolite, phosphatidylinositol 4,5-bisphosphate. This phosphatase appears to be important in the transport of vesicles within the Golgi apparatus, and its deficiency causes the protean manifestations of Lowe syndrome.

Xq26.1

EPIDEMIOLOGY
In the United States, between 1 and 10 boys per million people are affected, or 250 to 2500 cases.

CLINICAL FINDINGS
There is a diagnostic association of renal tubular dysfunction with congenital cataract, congenital glaucoma, mental retardation, and hypotonia.

Patients present with failure to thrive. There is severe mental deficiency with moderate to severe diffuse electroencephalographic abnormalities.

Renal tubular dysfunction is manifested by decreased ammonia production and metabolic acidosis with hyperphosphaturia, as well as a generalized aminoaciduria.

There is moderate to severe osteoporosis, and occasionally vitamin D–resistant rickets develops.

The joints are hypermobile, and there is generalized hypotonia characterized by absent deep tendon reflexes and muscle hypoplasia.

The diagnosis is based on finding decreased ammonia production, hyperphosphaturia, hypophosphatemia, and generalized aminoaciduria.

Slit-lamp examination is a very sensitive and specific test for the detection of carriers.

Mutation analysis of the gene is possible.

Prenatal diagnosis by molecular analysis is limited to families in whom the mutation is already known or in whom linkage is informative.

Suchy et al. performed prenatal diagnosis by measuring phosphatidylinositol 4,5-bisphosphate 5-phosphatase activity in cultured amniocytes.

Other causes of congenital cataract and systemic illness should be ruled out. They include, among others, congenital rubella syndrome, recessive renal-retinal dystrophy, and Alport syndrome.

OCULAR FINDINGS
Congenital cataracts are present in all patients. The lenses are small, and may be membranous and thick.

Concurrent or sequential infantile glaucoma is present in 60% of patients.

Virtually all carrier females have characteristic and diagnostic cortical lens opacities with radial bands or wedges of "snowflecks" in the anterior cortex, and 15% have central posterior cortical opacities.

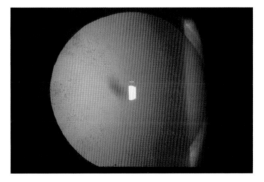

Lowe syndrome Characteristic lens opacities in a female carrier of Lowe syndrome.

THERAPEUTIC ASPECTS

In the absence of severe congenital glaucoma, cataract surgery may be successful in restoring vision. Surgical difficulties should be anticipated because of the membranous nature of the cataracts. Intraocular scissors and vitrectomy instruments may be needed.

REFERENCES

Duden R, Griffiths G, Frank R, et al: Beta-COP, a 110 kd protein associated with non-clathrin-coated vesicles and the Golgi complex, shows homology to beta-adaptin. *Cell* 1991;64:649–665.

Lin T, Lewis RA, Nussbaum RL: Molecular confirmation of carriers for Lowe syndrome. *Ophthalmology* 1999;106:119–122.

Lowe CU, Terrey M, MacLachland EA: Organic-aciduria, decreased renal ammonia production, hydrophthalmos, and mental retardation. *Am J Dis Child* 1952;83:164–184.

Suchy SF, Lin T, Horwitz JA, et al: First report of prenatal biochemical diagnosis of Lowe syndrome. *Prenat Diag* 1998;18:1117–1121.

RESOURCE

Lowe Syndrome Association
www.lowesyndrome.org

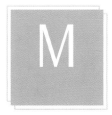

Malattia Leventinese

See **Familial Radial Drusen** *under* **Retinal Dystrophies and Degenerations**

Marfan Syndrome

Also includes **AD simple ectopia lentis**

OMIM NUMBER
154700

INHERITANCE
Autosomal dominant with variable expression and high penetrance

GENE/GENE MAP
Fibrillin 1, a microfibrillar glycoprotein component of the extracellular matrix, is the defective gene product.
15q21.1

EPIDEMIOLOGY
1 in 3000 to 1 in 10,000 worldwide
A paternal age effect in sporadic cases has been described.

CLINICAL FINDINGS
The syndrome is characterized by abnormalities of the eye (ectopia lentis), aorta (dilation of the aortic root and aneurysm of the ascending aorta and aortic aneurysm), and skeleton (dolichostenomelia, upper segment/lower segment ratio two standard deviations below the mean for age, pectus excavatum, and kyphoscoliosis).

In addition to these three major criteria, auxiliary signs may be present, such as myopia, mitral valve prolapse, arachnodactyly, joint laxity, tall stature, pes planus, striae distensae, pneumothorax, and dural ectasia.

About 35% of patients do not develop lens subluxation. There is a large family with Marfan syndrome without ectopia lentis in whom the disease gene was mapped to 3p24.2–p25.

The clinical diagnosis may be difficult in mild cases, and the spectrum of patients with connective tissue abnormalities simulating Marfan syndrome is wide.

OCULAR FINDINGS
Ocular abnormalities are present in at least 60% of patients. The most characteristic and usually diagnostic ocular abnormality is lens subluxation, which varies from mild superior and posterior displacement to significant subluxation with the equator of the lens in the pupillary axis. Inferior, nasal, or lateral subluxation also occurs. Subluxation is slowly progressive in some patients and is most noticeable in the first few years of life or in the late teens and early 20s. Total dislocation into the vitreous cavity has been documented in older patients, in whom it may rarely be complicated by phacolytic glaucoma. Lens dislocation into the pupil or anterior chamber is characteristic of untreated homocystinuria.

Microspherophakia is present in about 15% of patients and results in high myopia. The cornea is flat, with keratometric readings in the high 30s in about 20% of patients. Megalocornea (corneal diameter measuring more than 13.5 mm) may be present in some patients. The iris has a thin velvety texture, and the pupil is difficult to dilate in the more severely affected patients in whom there is atrophy of the dilator muscle fibers. Iridodonesis results from lens subluxation.

Wheatley et al. found fibrillin to be ubiquitous in the eye and a major component of the cornea, sclera, anterior chamber angle, uvea, zonules, lens capsule, and optic nerve septae. The authors concluded that ocular abnormalities could be correlated to the distribution pattern of fibrillin in the eye. The normal lens capsule has three distinct and adjacent zones in the equatorial and periequatorial regions that contain fibrillin. Fibrillin fibers are abnormal and disrupted in all three zones in Marfan patients.

Exotropia occurs in 10% of patients and esotropia in 2%. Strabismic and/or anisometropic or ametropic amblyopia should be suspected in all patients with reduced visual acuity.

Open-angle glaucoma is significantly more common in Marfan patients in all age groups compared to the general population and becomes more prevalent with increasing age. Pupillary block is unusual but has been documented. Phacolytic glaucoma has been noted in older patients with mature dislocated lenses.

Retinal detachment may occur spontaneously in eyes with axial myopia or following cataract extraction, especially in longer eyes. Loewenstein et al. identified and retrospectively reviewed the charts of one cohort of 12 patients (15 eyes) with retinal detachment who were operated on at the Wilmer Institute and a second cohort of 16 such patients (24 eyes) who were operated on several years earlier and elsewhere. They concluded that the results of retinal detachment surgery in the past were worse when the eye was aphakic. In most patients operated on more recently, the prognosis for successful repair was good regardless of whether the eye was phakic. In another study, Abboud found bilateral retinal detachment in 9 of 13 (69%) patients. The lens was ectopic in all eyes. Retinal breaks were small horseshoe tears or holes located anterior to the equator in 11 of 16 (69%) eyes. The retina of 12 of 16 (75%) eyes remained successfully reattached after a follow-up period ranging from 4 to 132 months. All 12 eyes had a visual acuity of 20/300 or better (range: 20/30 to 20/300); 8 had a visual acuity of 20/125 or better; and the cause of failure in the remaining 4 eyes was proliferative vitreoretinopathy.

Cataracts develop earlier than in the general population.

THERAPEUTIC ASPECTS

Periodic echocardiography should be performed to assess aortic dilation. Oral beta blockers reduce the incidence of aortic rupture. Aortic replacement may be necessary when aortic root measurements reach 50 to 55 mm in the adult. The average age of death has been delayed from the 40s to the 60s.

Careful refractions at regular intervals are necessary to achieve the best possible vision. The necessity of lensectomy in patients with significant subluxation and astigmatism continues to be debated. With the advent of vitrectomy instrumentation, small-incision lensectomy has become safer. Before lens extraction is contemplated, patients should have a prolonged trial of aphakic or phakic correction, as well as patching if amblyopia is suspected.

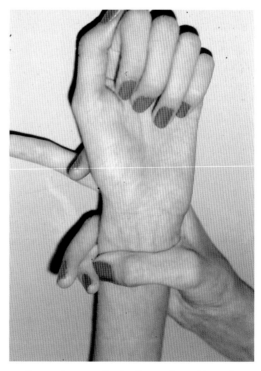

Marfan syndrome Wrist sign in a patient with Marfan syndrome

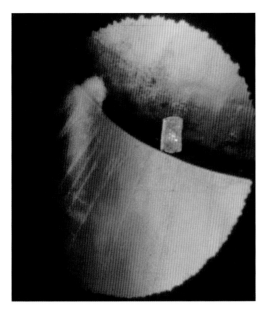

Marfan syndrome Superotemporal lens subluxation in a patient with Marfan syndrome; note the stretched zonules.

The prognosis for vision is good if the diagnosis is made early, errors of refraction are corrected, and amblyopia is managed properly.

REFERENCES

Abboud EB: Retinal detachment surgery in Marfan's syndrome. *Retina* 1998;18:405–409.

Izquierdo NJ, Traboulsi EI, Enger C, et al: Glaucoma in the Marfan syndrome. *Trans Am Ophthalmol Soc* 1992;90:111–117; discussion 118–122.

Izquierdo NJ, Traboulsi EI, Enger C, et al: Strabismus in the Marfan syndrome. *Am J Ophthalmol* 1994;117:632–635.

Loewenstein A, Barequet IS, De Juan E, et al: Retinal detachment in Marfan syndrome. *Retina* 2000;20:358–363.

Maumenee IH: The eye in the Marfan syndrome. *J Am Ophthalmol Soc* 1981;79:684–733.

Mir S, Wheatley HM, Hussels IE, et al: A comparative histologic study of the fibrillin microfibrillar system in the lens capsule of normal subjects and subjects with Marfan syndrome. *Invest Ophthalmol Vis Sci* 1998;39:84–93.

Traboulsi EI, Whittum-Hudson JA, Mir SH, et al: Microfibril abnormalities of the lens capsule in patients with Marfan syndrome and ectopia lentis. *Ophthalmic Genet* 2000;21:9–15.

Wheatley HM, Traboulsi EI, Flowers BE, et al: Immunohistochemical localization of fibrillin in human ocular tissues: relevance to the Marfan syndrome. *Arch Ophthalmol* 1995;113:103–109.

RESOURCES

The Canadian Marfan Association
www.marfan.ca
The National Marfan Foundation
www.marfan.org

Megalocornea

OMIM NUMBER
309300

INHERITANCE
X-linked
Possible rare autosomal recessive form

GENE/GENE MAP
MGCN
Xq21.3–q22

EPIDEMIOLOGY
Rare; prevalence unknown

CLINICAL FINDINGS
There are no systemic abnormalities in most patients.

An autosomal recessive syndrome of macrocephaly, megalocornea, and mental retardation (OMIM 249310; Neuhauser syndrome) exists.

A large corneal diameter may be present in patients with Marfan syndrome, Soto syndrome, and some craniofacial dysotosis syndromes.

OCULAR FINDINGS
Corneal diameter of more than 12 mm
Myopia frequently present
Annulus juvenilis
Posterior crocodile shagreen
Presenile cataracts

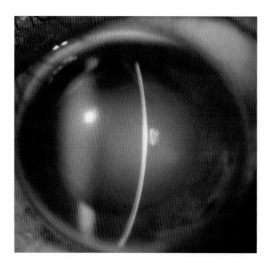

Megalocornea Peripheral arcus juvenilis and central crocodile shagreen in a patient with meglocornea. (Courtesy of David Mackey, M.D.)

THERAPEUTIC ASPECTS

Differentiation from congenital glaucoma in infants

Cataract extraction as needed

REFERENCES

Mackey DA, Buttery RG, Wise GM, et al: Description of X-linked megalocornea with identification of the gene locus. *Arch Ophthalmol* 1991;109:829–833.
Verloes A, Journel H, Elmer C, et al: Heterogeneity versus variability in megalocornea-mental retardation (MMR) syndromes: report of new cases and delineation of 4 probable types. *Am J Med Genet* 1993;46:132–137.

RESOURCES

None listed

Mitochondrial Encephalopathy, Lactic Acid, and Stroke-Like Episodes

Also called MELAS syndrome

OMIM NUMBER

540000

INHERITANCE

Mitochondrial

Family history consistent with maternal inheritance in 25% of cases

GENE/GENE MAP

Mitochondrial tRNA (*Leu-UUR*) gene encoded by nucleotides 3230–3304

Eighty percent of patients have a heteroplastic A-to-G point mutation in the dihydrouridine loop of this gene at position 3243.

EPIDEMIOLOGY

Very rare

CLINICAL FINDINGS

This progressive neurodegenerative disease has an onset before 20 years of age (80% between 5 and 15 years).

The most frequent symptom is episodic sudden headache with vomiting and convulsion.

There are recurrent cerebral insults resembling strokes and causing hemiplegia, aphasia, hemianopsia, or cortical blindness. The cerebral infarcts are nonvascular, caused by a transient dysfunction of oxidative phosphorylation within parenchyma. In imaging studies, infarcted areas do not respect vascular territories.

Seizures are common.

Mitochondrial myopathy and angiopathy, cardiomyopathy, and cardiac conduction defects are typical.

Proximal renal tubule dysfunction and lactic acidosis occur.

Diabetes mellitus type 2 may be present.

Deafness is not uncommon.

The diagnosis is suspected on clinical grounds. Elevated resting lactic acidosis that increases on exercise is found. Ragged red fibers are discovered on biopsy. Abnormalities are seen on magnetic resonance imaging.

The diagnosis can be confirmed by analysis of mtDNA for known point mutations in blood cells and muscle.

The differential diagnosis includes other mitochondrial disorders, such as myoclonic epilepsy with ragged red fibers (MERRF), chronic progressive external ophthalmoplegia, and the Kearns syndrome.

In adults, demyelinating diseases should be ruled out.

OCULAR FINDINGS

Ophthalmoplegia and ptosis are common.

Cortical visual impairment results from the stroke-like episodes.

Slowly progressive geographic macular atrophy occurs in some patients. Atrophic and retinal pigmentary changes in the macula and fundus periphery exist in at least 50% of patients. No optic atrophy is found.

Ocular histologic examination was performed in one patient by Rummelt et al. and in two patients by Chang et al. Abnormal mitochondria were present in the retinal pigment epithelium and in corneal endothelial and muscle cells.

THERAPEUTIC ASPECTS

Coenzyme Q10

Corticosteroids and a novel quinone, idebenone, have reduced the neurologic symptoms.

REFERENCES

Chang TS, Johns DR, Walker D, et al: Ocular clinicopathologic study of the mitochondrial encephalomyopathy overlap syndromes. *Arch Ophthalmol* 1993;111:1254–1262.

Hirano M, Pavlakis SG: Mitochondrial myopathy, encephalopathy, lactic acidosis and strokelike episodes (MELAS): current concepts. *J Child Neurol* 1994;9:4–13.

Latkany P, Ciulla TA, Cacchillo PF, et al: Mitochondrial maculopathy: geographic atrophy of the macula in the MELAS-associated A to G 3243 mitochondrial DNA point mutation. *Am J Ophthalmol* 1999;128:112–114.

Rummelt V, Folberg R, Ionasescu V, et al: Ocular pathology of MELAS syndrome with mitochondrial DNA nucleotide 3243 point mutation. *Ophthalmology* 1993;100:1757–1766.

Sue CM, Mitchell P, Crimmins DS, et al: Pigmentary retinopathy associated with the mitochondrial DNA 3243 point mutation. *Neurology* 1997;49: 1013–1017.

RESOURCE

United Mitochondrial Disease Foundation
www.umdf.org

Morning-Glory Disc Anomaly (MGDA)

OMIM NUMBER

Not listed

INHERITANCE

No documented familial cases

GENE/GENE MAP

No gene identified or mapped

EPIDEMIOLOGY

Rare congenital malformation of the optic nerve head and peripapillary region

CLINICAL FINDINGS

The anomaly is characterized by an enlarged, excavated, funnel-shaped optic disc with a central white glial tuft and a raised annulus of pigmentary chorioretinal changes at its edge. The term *morning-glory disc anomaly* was coined because of its resemblance to the flower of the same name.

There is an association between the anomaly and basal encephaloceles of the transsphenoidal or transethmoidal type. Hypopituitarism can also be present. Patients may also have a flat midface and midline clefts of the lip and palate.

A significant number of patients with the anomaly and stenotic lesions of the internal carotid system with Moyamoya disease have been reported. These patients can develop strokes. Agenesis of the corpus callosum and an absent chiasm are other intracranial anomalies that have been reported. Congenital renal abnormalities and orbital hemangiomas are other associated defects.

Neuroimaging or ultrasonographic studies outline the funnel-shaped junction of the optic nerve with the posterior aspect of the globe. The neuroimaging studies also uncover associated brain malformations, such as encephaloceles and agenesis of the corpus callosum.

OCULAR FINDINGS

The appearance varies, depending on the size of the posterior scleral opening, the degree of surrounding chorioretinal pigmentation, the vascular pattern, and the amount of gliosis and remnants of the hyaloid system at the center of the disc. The macula is usually dragged nasally to the edge of the disc, and the yellow macular xanthophyll pigment is frequently noticeable at that location. The retinal arterioles and venules emerge in a radial pattern from the enlarged scleral canal and are frequently bridged by vascular arcades close to the optic nerve head. Other straight arterio-arterial bridging vessels can be seen more peripherally.

The majority of cases are unilateral, with no left or right eye predominance.

Males and females are affected equally.

Fifty percent of patients present with strabismus, but patients may be detected because of leukocoria or poor vision or during routine examinations.

Total retinal detachment occurs in up to 30% of cases and may be present in infancy or early childhood. The detachment is usually nonrhegmatogenous and may result from communication between the subarachnoid and subretinal spaces. Spontaneous retinal reattachment has been reported.

Contractile movements of the peripapillary area have been observed and are presumably due to the presence of heterotopic smooth muscle fibers.

Visual impairment is variable but may be generally substantial, with visual acuity ranging from 20/30 to poor light perception.

Some cases are probably misdiagnosed as

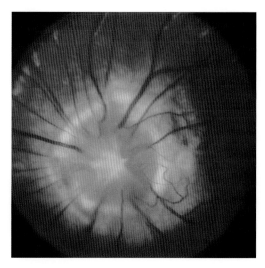

Morning-glory disc anomaly (MGDA) Typical large excavated disc with a central tuft of glial tissue.

typical uveal colobomas at the optic disc. Slusher et al. reported a large kindred in which cavitary optic disc anomalies ranging from optic pits to large, anomalous discs and typical

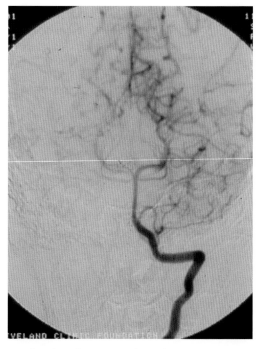

Morning-glory disc anomaly (MGDA) Moyamoya disease in a patient with MGDA. Note the narrowing of the internal carotid artery and distal collateral blood vessels.

colobomas were inherited in an autosomal dominant fashion. The great majority of cases with the anomaly and optic pits, however, are isolated, and the recurrence risk in siblings is negligible.

THERAPEUTIC ASPECTS

Careful refraction and treatment of associated strabismic or anisometropic amblyopia should be performed.

The retinal detachment is treated as needed.

Magnetic resonance imaging and magnetic resonance angiography should be performed in all patients, and the scans should be scrutinized for the presence of midline brain abnormalities and stenotic lesions of the internal carotid circulation.

REFERENCES

Bakri S, Siker D, Masaryk T, et al: Moyamoya disease, ocular malformations and midline cranial defects: a distinct syndrome. *Am J Ophthalmol* 1999;127:356–357.

Slusher MM, Weaver RG Jr, Creven CM, Mundorf TK, Cashwell LF: The spectrum of cavitary optic disc anomalies in a family. *Ophthalmology* 1989; 96:342–347.

Traboulsi EI, O'Neill JF: The spectrum in the morphology of the so-called morning glory disc anomaly. *J Pediatr Ophthalmol Strabismus* 1988; 25:93–98.

RESOURCES

None listed

Mucolipidoses

The mucolipidoses have clinical features characteristic of both the mucopolysaccharidoses (such as Hurler-like face, hepatosplenomegaly, and dysostosis multiplex) and the neurodegeneration of the sphingolipidoses.

OMIM NUMBERS

See Table 18.

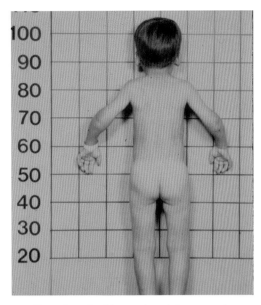

Mucolipopolysaccharidase III (MLIII) Posture and contractures of hands in patient with MLIII. (Reproduced with permission from *Am J Ophthalmol*)

INHERITANCE

Autosomal dominant for all types

GENE/GENE MAP

See Table 18.

EPIDEMIOLOGY

See Table 18.

CLINICAL FINDINGS

See Table 18.

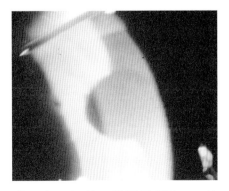

Mucolipopolysaccharidase III (MLIII) Mild corneal haze in patient with MLIII. (Reproduced with permission from *Am J Ophthalmol*)

TABLE 18. Mucolipidoses

Type	OMIM Number	Gene/Gene Map	Clinical Findings	Ocular Findings
MLI—severe	256550	α-N-acetyl neuraminidase deficiency 6p21.3	Excess sialic acid (sialidosis) Onset before age 2 years Hurler-like face Hepatosplenomegaly Delayed development Hearing deficiency Small stature Progressive neurodegeneration	Cherry-red spot that may disappear, leaving gray macular area Optic atrophy Cataracts (rare) Fine corneal opacities
MLI—late-onset type		β-galactosidase with or without α-N-acetyl neuraminidase deficiency	Myoclonic seizures (myoclonus syndrome)	Same as MLI—severe
MLII 1/M I-cell disease	2525000	N-acetylglucosamine-1-phosphotransferase deficiency Fibroblasts able to pinocytose normal exogenous lysosomal hydrolases, but cannot readmit hydrolases they themselves excrete into extracellular space because of lack of phosphate recognition marker 6-Phosphomannose residue as hydrolase recognition marker preventing excretion from cell, causing excessive intracellular depletion and extracellular excess of I-cell hydrolase 4q21–q23	Inclusions in cultured fibroblasts At birth, wizened little-old-man face, bulbous nose, and doughy skin Psychomotor retardation since birth Hurler-like facial appearance Gingival hypertrophy	Lid swelling Mild late corneal clouding Congenital glaucoma (rare)
MLIII	252600	Same as MLII	Progressive stiffening of hands and shoulders in first few years of life Mild facial coarsening Dysostosis multiplex with carpal tunnel syndrome Clinical findings stabilize after teens	Mild corneal haze Hyperopia Surface-wrinkling maculopathy Papilledema
MLIV	252650	Mucolipidin, an integral membrane protein, likely involved in endocytosis Two founder mutations account for 95% of the 70 or so known cases 19p13.3–p13.2	Most common in Ashkenazi Jews Athetosis Progressive motor and mental disability starting in first year of life in most cases Vacuolated cells in bone marrow No dysostosis multiplex Characteristic intracellular inclusions in all cells	Clouding of corneal epithelium Progressive retinal degeneration

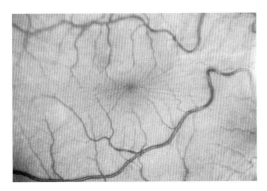

Mucolipopolysaccharidase III (MLIII) Epimacular membrane and striations in a patient with MLIII. (Reproduced with permission from *Am J Ophthalmol*)

OCULAR FINDINGS

See Table 18.

THERAPEUTIC ASPECTS

There is no specific treatment.

REFERENCES

Mucolipidosis I

Spranger J, Cantz M: Mucolipidosis I, the cherry red spot–myoclonus syndrome and neuroaminidase deficiency. *Birth Defects* Orig. Art. Series 1978; 14:105–112.

Spranger JW, Wiedemann HR: The genetic mucolipidoses: diagnosis and differential diagnosis. *Humangenetik* 1970;9:113–139.

Mucolipidosis II

Libert J, Van Hoof F, Farriaux JP, et al: Ocular findings in I-cell disease (mucolipidosis type II). *Am J Ophthalmol* 1977;83:617–627.

Mueller DT, Honey NK, Little LE, et al: Mucolipidosis II and III: the genetic relationships between two disorders of lysosomal enzyme biosynthesis. *J Clin Invest* 1983;72:1016–1023.

Mucolipidosis III

Mueller OT, Honey NK, Little LE, et al: Mucolipidosis II and III: the genetic relationships between two disorders of lysosomal enzyme biosynthesis. *J Clin Invest* 1983;72:1016–1023.

Traboulsi EI, Maumenee IH: Ocular findings in mucolipidosis III. *Am J Ophthalmol* 1986;102:592–597.

Mucolipidosis IV

Bargal R, Avidan N, Ben-Asher E, et al: Identification of the gene causing mucolipidosis type IV. *Nat Genet* 2000;26:118–123.

Bassi MT, Manzoni M, Monti E, et al: Cloning of the gene encoding a novel integral membrane protein, mucolipidin, and identification of the two major founder mutations causing mucolipidosis type IV. *Am J Hum Genet* 2000;67:1110–1120.

Berman ER, Livni N, Shapiro E, et al: Congenital corneal clouding with abnormal systemic storage bodies: a new variant of mucolipidosis. *J Pediatr* 1974;84:519–526.

Merin S, Livni N, Berman E, et al: Mucolipidosis IV: ocular, systemic, and ultrastructural findings. *Invest Ophthalmol* 1975;14:437–448.

Pradham SM, Atchaneeyasakul LO, Appukuttan B, et al: Electroretinogram in mucolipidosis IV. *Arch Ophthalmol* 2002;120:45–50.

Riedel KG, Zwaan J, Kenyon KR, et al: Ocular abnormalities in mucolipidosis IV. *Am J Ophthalmol* 1985;99:125–136.

RESOURCE

Mucolipidosis IV Foundation
www.ml4.org

Mucopolysaccharidoses

OMIM NUMBERS

See Table 19.

INHERITANCE

See Table 19.

GENE/GENE MAP

See Table 19.

EPIDEMIOLOGY

See Table 19.

CLINICAL FINDINGS

See Table 19.

OCULAR FINDINGS

See Table 19.

THERAPEUTIC ASPECTS

Bone marrow transplantation and gene therapy have been tried in a number of patients with

TABLE 19. Mucopolysaccharidoses

Type	OMIM Number	Epidemiology	Inheritance	Enzyme Defect	Gene Map	Ocular Findings
MPS I (Hurler, Scheie, and Hurler-Scheie syndromes)	252800	1 in 100,000 for Hurler syndrome 1 in 600,000 for Scheie syndrome	Autosomal recessive	α-L-iduronidase	4p16.3	Corneal clouding Pigmentary retinopathy Glaucoma Chronic papilledema Optic atrophy Nonrecordable electroretinogram
MPS II (Hunter syndrome)	309900	1 in 70,000 in Israel; rarer in British and British Columbian surveys	X-linked recessive	Iduronate sulfatase	Xq27–q28	Pigmentary retinopathy Abnormal electroretinogram Chronic papilledema Optic atrophy
MPS III (Sanfilippo syndrome) Types A, B, C, D	IIIA: 252900	1 in 24,000 (all types combined) in the Netherlands IIIA and IIIB most common A > B in northern Europe B > A in southern Europe	Autosomal recessive All four types nonallelic	IIIA: heparan N-sulfatase IIIB: α-N-acetyl-glucosaminidase IIIC: acetyl-coenzyme A α-glucosaminide acetyltransferase IIID: N-acetylglucosamine-6-sulfatase	17q25.3 17q21 Chr 14 12q14	Pigmentary retinopathy Optic atrophy
MPS IV (Morquio syndrome) Types A, B	IVA: 253000 IVB: 253010	1 in 300,000 worldwide	Autosomal recessive Both types nonallelic	IVA: galactose 6-sulfatase IVB: β-galactosidase	16q24.3 3p21–pter	Corneal clouding
MPS VI (Maroteaux-Lamy syndrome)	253200	1 in 200,000	Autosomal recessive	N-acetylgalactosamine 4-sulfatase (arylsulfatase B)	5q13–q14	Corneal clouding Papilledema Optic atrophy Abnormal electroretinogram
MPS VII (Sly syndrome)	253220	Very rare	Autosomal recessive	β-glucuronidase	7q21.1–q22	Mild corneal clouding Mild pigmentary retinopathy

limited success. (Discussion of this modality is beyond the scope of this monograph.)

REFERENCES

Collins ML, Traboulsi EI, Maumenee IH: Optic nerve head swelling and optic atrophy in the mucopolysaccharidoses. *Ophthalmology* 1990;97:1445–1449.

Gullingsrud EO, Krivit W, Summers CG: Ocular abnormalities in the mucopolysaccharidoses after bone marrow transplantation: longer follow-up. *Ophthalmology* 1998;105:1099–1105.

RESOURCE

The National MPS Society
www.mpssociety.org

Multiple Endocrine Neoplasia (MEN) Type IIB

OMIM NUMBER
162300

INHERITANCE
Autosomal dominant
Fifty percent of cases are sporadic

GENE/GENE MAP
Ninety-five percent of patients have a single point mutation that changes a methionine to a threonine at codon 918 of the *RET* tyrosine kinase receptor proto-oncogene.

All patients with medullary thyroid carcinoma have this mutation.

10q11.2

EPIDEMIOLOGY
Fewer than 1 in 20,000 individuals carry a mutation in the *RET* gene.

CLINICAL FINDINGS
Hyperplasia and/or neoplasia of multiple neural crest–derived tissues occurs. Type IIB (previously type III) shares some features with type IIA. Both diseases present with medullary carcinoma of the thyroid (90%) and pheochromocytoma (45%). Hyperparathyroidism is rare in type IIB.

Patients with type IIB characteristically have multiple superficial nodular hamartomatous neuromas of the face, lids, lips, tongue, and other mucosal and serosal body surfaces and cavities. This leads to thickened lips and everted upper lids.

There is a marfanoid body habitus but no cardiac or ocular features of the Marfan syndrome.

C-cell hyperplasia usually precedes medullary thyroid carcinoma by several years. If C-cell hyperplasia is present, the calcitonin level may be elevated. Measurement of the serum calcitonin level after induction with pentagastrin has been used traditionally as a screening method for type II.

Vanillylmandelic acid, metanephrine, and unconjugated catecholamine measurements in urine are used for the diagnosis of pheochromocytoma.

Genetic testing has replaced calcitonin testing as the preferred screening method for the Met 918 Thr mutation.

OCULAR FINDINGS
Prominent thickened corneal nerves in a clear stroma are characteristic and are detectable early in life.

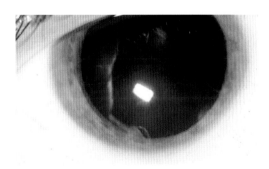

Multiple endocrine neoplasia (MEN) type IIB Prominent corneal nerves in a patient with MEN type IIB.

Neuromas that involve the lid margins lead to their thickening and occasional eversion. The nodules may involve the conjunctiva.

THERAPEUTIC ASPECTS

Surgery may be necessary for lid and conjunctival neuromas.

Monitoring for thyroid tumors and pheochromocytomas is mandatory.

Patients die in the second or third decade of life from metastatic carcinoma. The prognosis improves with early detection or prevention of thyroid cancer using prophylactic thyroidectomy.

REFERENCES

Jacobs JM, Hawes MJ: From eyelid bumps to thyroid lumps: report of a MEN type IIb family and review of the literature. *Ophthalmic Plast Reconstr Surg* 2001;17:195–201.

Jones BA, Sisson JC: Early diagnosis and thyroidectomy in multiple endocrine neoplasia, Type 2B. *J Pediatr* 1983;102:219–223.

Riley FC Jr, Robertson DM: Ocular histopathology in multiple endocrine neoplasia type 2b. *Am J Ophthalmol* 1981;91:57–64.

Schimke RN, Hartmann WH, Prout TE, et al: Syndrome of bilateral pheochromocytomas, medullary thyroid carcinoma and multiple neuromas. *N Engl J Med* 1968;279:1–7.

RESOURCE

Multiple Endocrine Neoplasia Type 2 resource site www.endocrineweb.com/men/men2.html

Myoclonus with Epilepsy and Ragged Red Fibers (MERRF)

OMIM NUMBER
545000

INHERITANCE
Mitochondrial

GENE/GENE MAP

MTTK (OMIM 590060) and *MTTL1* (OMIM 590050)

There is a point mutation in the gene coding for tRNA, resulting in a generalized defect in translation of all mtDNA-encoded genes and producing multiple deficiencies in the enzyme complexes of the respiratory chain, most prominently involving reduced nicotinamide adenine dinucleotide–coenzyme Q (NADH-CoQ) reductase (complex I) in cytochrome-c-oxidase (COX) (complex IV).

EPIDEMIOLOGY
Very rare

CLINICAL FINDINGS

Clinical variability, probably as the result of heteroplasty

Myoclonus
Generalized seizures
Ataxia
Dementia
Sensorineural hearing loss
Optic atrophy
Proximal weakness
Sensorimotor peripheral neuropathy
Cardiomyopathy
Cutaneous lipomas

OCULAR FINDINGS

Some patients develop chronic progressive external ophthalmoplegia.

THERAPEUTIC ASPECTS

Seizure disorders are treated.

Vitamin supplementation and antioxidants have been tried.

REFERENCES

Chang TS, Johns DR, Walker D, et al: Ocular clinicopathologic study of the mitochondrial encephalomyopathy overlap syndromes. *Arch Ophthalmol* 1993;111:1254–1262.

Isashiki Y, Nakagawa M, Ohba N, et al: Retinal manifestations in mitochondrial diseases associated with mitochondrial DNA mutation. *Acta Ophthalmol Scand* 1998;76:6–13.

RESOURCES

United Mitochondrial Disease Foundation
www.umdf.org
Washington University Department of Neurology: Mitochondrial Disorders resource site
www.neuro.wustl.edu/neuromuscular/mitosyn.html

Myotonic Dystrophy

OMIM NUMBERS

Dystrophia myotonica I (DMI): 160900
Dystrophia myotonica II (DMII): 602668

INHERITANCE

Autosomal dominant

Shows anticipation, that is, increasing severity of the phenotype in successive generations of the same family

GENE/GENE MAP

Dystrophia myotonica I: The dystrophia myotonica protein kinase gene (*DMPK*, OMIM 605377) on 19q13.2–q13.3. This protein has been called *myotonin*. The classic form of the disease, dystrophia myotonica I, is caused by an amplified trinucleotide (CTG) repeat in the 3′ untranslated region of the gene. Affected patients have more than 50 trinucleotide repeats. The severity of the disease is correlated to the number of trinucleotide repeats. Extensive amplification of repeats may occur in babies of women with the disease, resulting in a child with a severe congenital myotonic dystrophy.

Dystrophia myotonica II maps to 3q. No expansion of trinucleotide repeats was found in patients with dystrophia myotonica II.

EPIDEMIOLOGY

Most common muscular dystrophy
Incidence: 13.5 in 100,000 live births
Prevalence: 3 to 5 in 100,000 worldwide

CLINICAL FINDINGS

Dysfunction in muscle relaxation, cataracts, hypogonadism, and intellectual impairment

Muscle disease (skeletal, cardiac, and smooth muscles)

1. Unrelated patients often resemble each other more than they resemble their own relatives. They have a characteristic hollow, expressionless face, frontal balding, sagging chin, poor teeth, monotonous nasal speech, stooped appearance, and wasted limbs. A handshake with the patient makes the myotonic reaction (delayed muscle relaxation) apparent.
2. Cardiac conduction defects may be a cause of sudden death.
3. Involvement of respiratory muscle can produce respiratory difficulties.
4. Smooth muscle in the gastrointestinal tract can also be affected, resulting in dysphagia, reduced gut motility, and chronic pseudo-obstruction.
5. Incontinence sometimes occurs.

Endocrine anomalies

1. Testicular or ovarian atrophy, impotence, and a high rate of spontaneous abortions have been reported.
2. Multiple endocrine abnormalities have been described, including a marked reduction in the affinity of insulin receptors.

The clinical diagnosis is not difficult in severe or familial cases.

Subclinical cases are detected by observation of fine, multicolored crystals in the lens.

DNA testing is available, and the number of trinucleotide repeats can be measured to confirm the clinical diagnosis.

OCULAR FINDINGS

Typical cataracts are present in at least 90% of patients and may be present in family members without muscle involvement. Early in the disease, visual acuity is unaffected by small, closely packed white cortical opacities that are mixed with red, green, or blue crystals of varied shape, size, and optical properties. This results in the characteristic *Christmas-tree cataract*. With time, opacities increase in density along the lens sutures, and eventually water clefts appear in the anterior and posterior subcapsular areas, together with sclerosis of the nucleus. Progression to mature cataracts in midadulthood is not uncommon.

Ocular hypotension is characteristic and may be due to either increased outflow facility or decreased aqueous humor secretion, as in other glands. Intraocular pressure decreases with increasing age.

Children appear to be consistently hypermetropic and have a predisposition to accommodative esotropia.

Retinal pigmented streaks in the macula are fairly common and, in early cases, may be preceded by white lesions deep in the retina or in Bruch's membrane. Some patients have clumpy

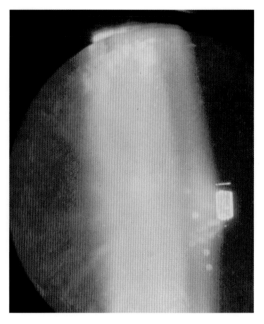

Myotonic dystrophy Fine diffuse lens opacities in a patient with myotonic dystrophy. These are best detected on retroillumination. Some of the opacities are multicolored and others are grayish-white.

(not bone-spicule) pigmentation in the retinal periphery. Narrowed arterioles have been described.

Electroretinographic abnormalities are present in most patients, and consist of subnormal scotopic responses in 82% of patients and photopic abnormalities in 35%. Dark-adaptation studies are frequently abnormal. Color vision is normal.

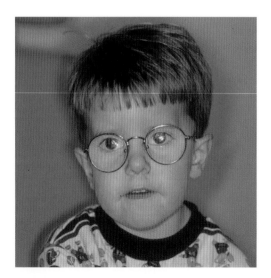

Myotonic dystrophy Facial appearance of a child with myotonic dystrophy; note the droopy mouth margins. The patient is highly hypermetropic.

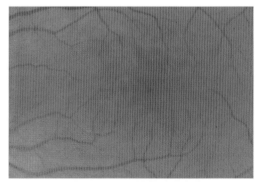

Myotonic dystrophy C-macular pigmentary changes in an adult with myotonic dystrophy. (Courtesy of Irene Maumenee, M.D.)

Unilateral or bilateral ptosis may be present, especially in patients with marked muscle disease. Weakness of the orbicularis muscle is present in almost all patients.

Abnormalities of the lacrimal system often account for the ocular symptoms that bring these patients to the ophthalmologist. Epiphora and dry eye have been documented.

Abnormalities in smooth ocular pursuit movements occur. Versions can be normal or limited.

Pupils show a sluggish reaction to both light and accommodation. There is no hypersensitivity to pharmacologic agents.

THERAPEUTIC ASPECTS

Annual electrocardiograms are recommended to detect cardiac conduction defects. A pacemaker may be necessary.

The visual outcome after cataract extraction is generally good. Ptosis repair may occasionally be needed. Other complications of atrophy of the levator palpebrae and orbicularis oculi (e.g., lagophthalmos, ectropion, and punctal eversion) may also require surgical attention.

REFERENCES

Brook JD, McCurrach ME, Harley HG, et al: Molecular basis of myotonic dystrophy: expansion of a trinucleotide (CTG) repeat at the 3-prime end of a transcript encoding a protein kinase family member. *Cell* 1992;68:799–808.

Burian HM, Burns CA: Ocular changes in myotonic dystrophy. *Am J Ophthalmol* 1967;63:22–24.

Tamai A, Holland HG: Ophthalmologic studies on myotonic dystrophy II electrophysiologic evaluation. *Folia Ophthalmol Jpn* 1975;26:194.

Thompson HS, Van Allen MW, von Noorden GK: The pupil in myotonic dystrophy. *Invest Ophthalmol* 1964;3:325–338.

von Noorden GK, Thompson HS, Van Allen MW: Eye movements in myotonic dystrophy. *Invest Ophthalmol* 1964;3:314–324.

RESOURCE

International Myotonic Dystrophy Organization www.myotonicdystrophy.org

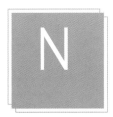

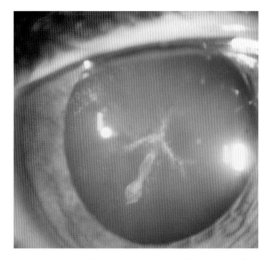

Nance-Horan syndrome Y-sutural opacities in lens of a female carrier of Nance-Horan syndrome.

Nance-Horan Syndrome

Also called cataract-dental syndrome

OMIM NUMBERS
302200
302300
302350

INHERITANCE
X-linked with mild ocular signs in female carriers

GENE/GENE MAP
Xp22.2–p22.13

Burdon et al. isolated the *NHS* gene and found mutations in Australian families with this syndrome. The gene encompasses approximately 650 kb of genomic DNA, coding for a 1630 amino acid putative nuclear protein. Although orthologs were found in other vertebrates, no sequence similarity to known genes was identified.

EPIDEMIOLOGY
Rare; fewer than 20 families in the literature

CLINICAL FINDINGS
Crown-shaped dental abnormalities (screwdriver-shaped, conical, or notched), supernumerary teeth, a central incisor, position and implantation anomalies, as well as other, less common abnormalities occur. Female carriers may also have mild dental abnormalities similar to those in males.

Facial dysmorphism, with a long narrow face, long protruding chin, long narrow nose, and protruding ears with simple helices is characteristic.

Mental retardation is found in 20% to 30% of patients.

Francis et al. mapped a gene for cataracts and complex cardiac defects to the same chromosomal region, suggesting allelic heterogeneity.

OCULAR FINDINGS
Microcornea is found in patients and female carriers.

Males have total cataracts. Carrier females have sutural opacities and presenile cataracts.

Glaucoma is common in males after cataract

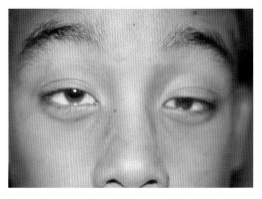

Nance-Horan syndrome Microcornea in a child with Nance-Horan syndrome.

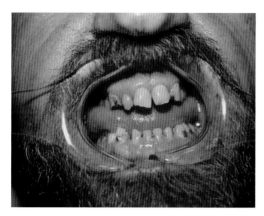

Nance-Horan syndrome Dental abnormalities in an adult with Nance-Horan syndrome. (Courtesy of Richard Lewis, M.D.)

extraction and may reflect the anterior segment maldevelopment in this condition.

THERAPEUTIC ASPECTS

Cataract extraction should be performed as needed, and lifelong monitoring for aphakic or pseudophakic glaucoma is necessary.

REFERENCES

Burdon KP, McKay JD, Sale MM, et al. Mutations in a novel gene, *NHS*, cause the pleiotropic effects of Nance-Horan syndrome, including severe congenital cataract, dental anomalies, and mental retardation. *Am J Hum Genet* 2003;73:1120–1130.

Francis PJ, Berry V, Hardcastle AJ, et al: A locus for isolated cataract on human Xp. *J Med Genet* 2002; 39:105–109.

Horan MB, Billson FA: X-linked cataract and Hutchinsonian teeth. *Aust Paediatr J* 1974;10: 98–102.

Lewis RA: Mapping the gene for X-linked cataracts and microcornea with facial, dental, and skeletal features to Xp22: an appraisal of the Nance-Horan syndrome. *Trans Am Ophthalmol Soc* 1989;87: 658–728.

Nance WE, Warburg M, Bixler D, et al: Congenital X-linked cataract, dental anomalies and brachymetacarpalia. *Birth Defects* Orig Art Ser 1974; 10:285–291.

Toutain A: Nance-Horan syndrome: linkage analysis in 4 families refines localization in Xp22.31–p22.13 region. *Hum Genet* 1997;99:256–261.

Walpole SM: Exclusion of *RAI2* as the causative gene for Nance-Horan syndrome. *Hum Genet* 1999; 104:410–411.

RESOURCE

Toutain A: Nance-Horan syndrome. *Orphanet Encyclopedia* January 2002: orphanet.infobiogen.fr/ data/patho/GB/uk-NHS.html

Neurofibromatosis Type 1 (NF1)

Also called **von Recklinghausen disease**

OMIM NUMBER
162200

INHERITANCE

Both central (NF2) and peripheral (NF1) types are inherited as autosomal dominant disorders with virtually 100% penetrance but wide variability in expression.

Nearly one-half of the patients have fresh mutations in the *NF1* gene, the highest value known for humans; one-half of these have fathers of advanced age.

GENE/GENE MAP

The *NF1* or neurofibromin gene is very large and extends over a 350 kb region. It contains three other genes within intron 27b (*EVI2A*, *EVI2B*, and *OMPG*) and one pseudogene (*AK3*) in intron 37. None of these genes appears to play a role in the pathogenesis of NF1. A very large number of private mutations have been reported (www.nf.org/nflgene) and include deletions, insertions, and point mutations. There does not appear to be a correlation between the type of mutation and the severity or character of the phenotype.

17q11.2

EPIDEMIOLOGY

1 in 3000 to 1 in 4000 live births without sexual or racial predilection

CLINICAL FINDINGS

This disorder is the most common of the neurocutaneous hamartoses. The physical manifestations may be minimal in childhood but become more apparent with age.

Café-au-lait patches are evident at birth or during the first year of life and are usually the presenting sign. They are present in almost all patients.

Freckling (small café-au-lait spots) is present in 70% to 80% of affected adults, especially in intertriginous flexures, inframammary creases, etc.

There is a high incidence of scoliosis and cyst-like destruction of bone.

There is a wide range of neurologic abnormalities, including tumors of the cranial or peripheral nerves. Hydrocephalus is present in 2% to 5% of patients.

Moderate to severe mental retardation is present in 30% to 45% of patients.

Endocrine problems, such as precocious puberty, can be a sign of perichiasmal gliomas. Patients can also develop pheochromocytomas and medullary carcinomas of the thyroid.

Although most tumors are benign, 3% of patients develop neurofibrosarcomas, malignant schwannomas, or malignant melanomas.

The clinical diagnosis is based on the presence of two or more of the minimal criteria as listed in Table 20.

TABLE 20. Neurofibromatosis Type 1: Diagnostic Criteria

1. Presence of six or more café-au-lait spots measuring 1.5 cm or more in diameter in adults, 0.5 cm or more in children
2. Axillary or inguinal freckling
3. More than one neurofibroma of any type or one plexiform neurofibroma
4. Characteristic osseous lesions such as sphenoid-wing dysplasia or thinning of long-bone cortices with or without pseudoarthrosis
5. One optic nerve glioma
6. More than one iris Lisch nodule
7. A first-degree relative with neurofibromatosis

Sixty-seven percent of optic gliomas in neurofibromatosis are not suspected clinically or detected by ophthalmologic examination; they can be detected only by neuroimaging, hence the need for routine neuroimaging between ages 2 and 3 years if the patient is otherwise normal.

Prenatal testing is available.

OCULAR FINDINGS

Lisch nodules are melanocytic hamartomas in the iris. They are smooth, round, dome-shaped, gelatinous-looking, elevated lesions on the surface of the iris. They are pale or medium brown in blue and green eyes and light tan in dark brown eyes.

Lisch nodules increase in number with age and are bilateral. They are present in 33% of patients at 2.5 years of age and in 90% of 25-year-olds. In children, they are highly specific for NF1.

Iris mammillations have also been described and should be differentiated from Lisch nodules.

Prominent corneal nerves are visualized in 22% of patients.

Conjunctival hamartomas have been reported.

Optic nerve gliomas are present in 15% of patients; 25% of patients with optic gliomas have NF. Bilateral optic nerve gliomas are pathognomonic of NF1. Patients with chiasmal tumors are on average 15 years younger than patients with tumors of the optic nerve only. Two-thirds of tumors produce no signs or symptoms. Magnetic resonance imaging is the neuroimaging study of choice to detect these lesions and shows a typical pattern of double-density tubular thickening along the optic nerve.

Fifty percent of patients of European ancestry have between 1 and 20 choroidal hamartomas. These are ill-defined yellow-white or light brown lesions scattered throughout the posterior pole. They are composed of a variety of melanocytic, neuronal, and fibrocytic components. *Ovoid bodies* consist of lamellae of Schwann cell processes arranged around axons.

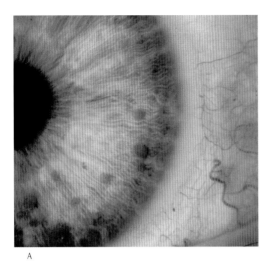

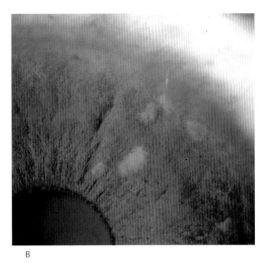

A   B

Neurofibromatosis Type 1 (NF1) Lisch nodules in a blue iris (A) and Lisch nodules in a dark iris (B).

Melanocytic and neuronal hamartomas are present in the trabecular meshwork, uvea, retina, and optic nerve.

Neurofibromas of the choroid are rare.

Sectoral retinal pigmentation, cone–rod dystrophy, and congenital hypertrophy of the retinal pigment epithelium may occur but are of doubtful significance.

A number of mechanisms have been implicated in the causation of glaucoma in NF1, including infiltration of the angle by neurofibromas, closure of the angle by neurofibromatous thickening of the ciliary body, secondary fibrovascular and synechial closure of the angle, and possibly a congenital malformation of the chamber angle. Most patients with congenital glaucoma in NF have a plexiform neuroma of the ipsilateral upper lid.

Eyelids are involved in 25% of patients. The most common lid lesion is a punctate neurofibroma. Plexiform neuromas are seen less frequently. Café-au-lait spots of the lid have also

Neurofibromatosis Type 1 (NF1) Plexiform neurofibroma of the eyelid with an S-shaped deformity.

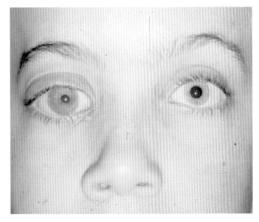

Neurofibromatosis Type 1 (NF1) Congenital glaucoma ipsilateral to a lid neurofibroma.

been described. When neuromas of the lid are present, they are accompanied by ipsilateral congenital glaucoma in 50% of patients.

Neurofibromas involving the orbit, lids, and temporal area may extend intracranially.

Absence of the greater wing of the sphenoid leads to prolapse of the temporal lobe into the orbit and pulsating exophthalmos. Enophthalmos may result from the increased size of the bony orbit and from enlarged superior and inferior orbital fissures.

Intracranial tumors may produce visual field defects, oculomotor and sensory nerve deficits, papilledema, and optic atrophy.

The differential diagnosis includes the McCune-Albright syndrome, in which jagged-edge skin lesions may be confused with café-au-lait lesions, and multiple endocrine neoplasia type IIB with prominent corneal nerves, pheochromocytoma, medullary thyroid adenocarcinoma, multiple mucous neuromas, and a marfanoid habitus.

THERAPEUTIC ASPECTS

The management of ocular complications includes surgery for large neurofibromas of the lids and orbits, medical or surgical therapy of glaucoma, and screening for the presence of optic nerve gliomas.

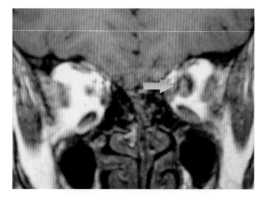

Neurofibromatosis Type 1 (NF1) Coronal magnetic resonance imaging view of the orbits showing glioma of the left optic nerve (*arrow*) in a patient with NF1.

REFERENCES

Gutmann DH: The neurofibromatoses: when less is more. *Hum Mol Genet* 2001;10:747–755.

Gutmann DH, Aylsworth A, Carey JC, et al: The diagnostic evaluation and multidisciplinary management of neurofibromatosis 1 and neurofibromatosis 2. *JAMA* 1997;278:51–57.

Klein RM, Glassman L: Neurofibromatosis of the choroid. *Am J Ophthalmol* 1985;99:367–368.

Lewis RA, Gerson LP, Axelson KA, et al: von Recklinghausen neurofibromatosis, II: incidence of optic gliomata. *Ophthalmology* 1984;91:929–935.

Lewis RA, Riccardi VM: Neurofibromatosis: incidence of iris hamartomata. *Ophthalmology* 1981; 88:348–354.

Ragge NK, Traboulsi EI: The phakomatoses. In: Traboulsi EI, ed: *Genetic Diseases of the Eye*. New York: Oxford University Press; 1998:733–775.

Riccardi VM: Von Recklinghausen neurofibromatosis. *N Engl J Med* 1981;305:1617–1626.

Stern J, Jakobiec FA, Housepian EM: The architecture of optic nerve gliomas with and without neurofibromatosis. *Arch Ophthalmol* 1980;98:505–511.

RESOURCE

Neurofibromatosis Clinics Association
　www.nfpittsburgh.org

Neurofibromatosis Type 2 (NF2)

OMIM NUMBER
101000

INHERITANCE
Autosomal dominant with almost complete penetrance and variable expressivity

GENE/GENE MAP
NF2 (merlin or schwannomin)
22q12.2

EPIDEMIOLOGY
1 in 33,000 to 40,000 live births

CLINICAL FINDINGS

Patients with NF2 tend to develop tumors in neural covers, whereas NF1 patients usually develop neural tumors. This disease is characterized by bilateral eighth nerve masses and multiple central nervous system tumors. Vestibular schwannomas develop after the first or second decade of life and have been reported as late as the seventh decade.

Patients usually present with unilateral or bilateral hearing loss. Diagnosis is frequently delayed for several years.

Café-au-lait spots may be present, but are much less common than in NF1, and their presence is not required for diagnosis.

The workup of a patient with documented or suspected NF2 includes a thorough skin examination, an ophthalmologic examination, neuroimaging studies with attention to the vestibular nucleus region, and an audiologic study.

Acoustic neuromas are best detected by magnetic resonance imaging.

First-degree relatives should be examined for stigmata of the disease.

Patients are diagnosed with NF2 if they have bilateral vestibular schwannomas (acoustic neuromas), are younger than 30 years of age, and have one first-degree relative with NF2 and a unilateral vestibular schwannoma or if they have any two of the following: neurofibroma, meningioma, glioma, schwannoma, juvenile posterior subcapsular cataract or juvenile cortical cataract, and a combined retinal hamartoma.

Individuals with the following clinical features should be evaluated for NF2 (presumptive or probable NF2): unilateral vestibular schwannoma, less than 30 years of age, and at least one of the following: meningioma, glioma, schwannoma, juvenile posterior subcapsular lenticular opacities or juvenile cortical cataract; or multiple meningiomas (two or more) plus unilateral vestibular schwannoma, less than 30 years of age, or one of the following: glioma, schwannoma, juvenile posterior subcapsular lenticular opacities, or juvenile cortical cataract.

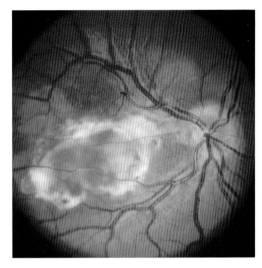

Neurofibromatosis Type 2 (NF2) Hamartoma of retina and retinal pigment epithelium in a young girl with NF2.

OCULAR FINDINGS

Ocular findings are present in 86% of patients.

Presenile or juvenile cataracts that have been described as posterior cortical occur in 69% of patients.

Combined hamartomas of the retina and retinal pigment epithelium have been reported and/or observed in over 25% of patients and are usually present around the optic disc or in the

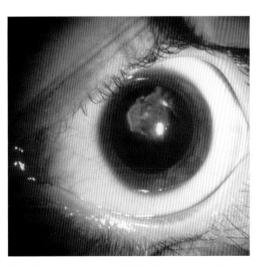

Neurofibromatosis Type 2 (NF2) Cortical cataract in a patient with NF2.

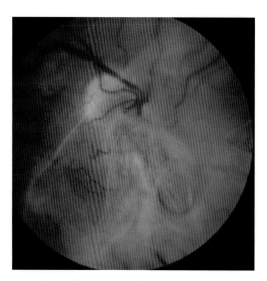

Neurofibromatosis Type 2 (NF2) Epiretinal membrane and "hamartomatous" changes in a patient with NF2.

posterior pole. They may take the form of epiretinal membranes or appear as a retinal fold from the disk or macula to a mass in a more peripheral location.

Intracranial and optic nerve sheath meningiomas are common causes of severe visual loss.

Oculomotor paresis occurs in 12% of patients.

Lisch nodules have been reported in only one patient.

THERAPEUTIC ASPECTS

The detection of characteristic ocular abnormalities assists in diagnosing the disease earlier, allowing surgical excision of smaller vestibular schwannomas and the preservation of hearing.

Cataract surgery may be necessary.

Gene testing is available at the Massachussets General Hospital laboratory.

REFERENCES

Good WV, Brodsky MC, Edwards MS, et al: Bilateral retinal hamartomas in neurofibromatosis type 2. *Br J Ophthalmol* 1991;75:190.

Gutmann DH: The neurofibromatoses: when less is more. *Hum Mol Genet* 2001;10:747–755.

Gutmann DH, Aylsworth A, Carey JC, et al: The diagnostic evaluation and multidisciplinary management of neurofibromatosis 1 and neurofibromatosis 2. *JAMA* 1997;278:51–57.

Kaiser-Kupfer MI, Freidlin V, Datiles MB, et al: The association of posterior capsular opacities with bilateral acoustic neuromas in patients with neurofibromatosis type 2. *Arch Ophthalmol* 1989;107: 541–544.

Landau K, MuciMendoza R, Dossetor FM, et al: Retinal hamartoma in neurofibromatosis 2. *Arch Ophthalmol* 1990;108:328–329.

Martuza RL, Eldridge R: Neurofibromatosis 2 (bilateral acoustic neurofibromatosis). *N Engl J Med* 1988;318:684–688.

National Institute of Health Consensus Development Conference Statement of Neurofibromatosis. *Arch Neurol* 1988;45:575–578.

RESOURCE

The NF2 Crew
  www.nf2crew.org

Neuronal Ceroid Lipofuscinoses (NCLs)

Includes **Batten disease, Vogt-Spielmeyer disease, Batten-Mayou disease, Kufs disease, Hagberg-Santavuori disease, Haltia-Santavuori disease, infantile NCL, Jansky-Bielschowsky disease, late-infantile NCL, juvenile NCL, adult NCL, cerebromacular degeneration, juvenile amaurotic idiocy**

OMIM NUMBERS

CLN I: 256730
CLN II: 204500
CLN III: 204200
CLN IV: 204300

INHERITANCE

Autosomal recessive

GENE/GENE MAP

CLN I gene encodes palmitoyl-protein thioesterase (PPT; OMIM 600722); 1p32

CLN II gene encodes a protease; 11p15.5

CLN III gene codes for a protein whose function is unknown; 16p12.1; 73% are due to a 1 kb deletion in the so-called 56 chromosome haplotype

EPIDEMIOLOGY

Three hundred affected children are born each year in the United States, most with the juvenile form.

The incidence in Finland is 1 in 13,000 newborns.

CLINICAL FINDINGS

The NCLs are characterized by progressive neurodegeneration and storage of lipopigments in the central nervous system and other organs. Dementia, seizures, and pigmentary retinopathy with progressive visual loss occur in all patients except those with Kufs disease.

Four major types and several less common forms have been described, depending on the age of onset and the temporal relation of visual loss to neurologic symptoms and the electron microscopic appearance of the storage material. As the genes for the different types have been mapped and discovered, a more precise classification, based on the gene defect, has emerged.

In the largest clinicopathologic study on the NCLs, Wisneiwski et al. reviewed the clinical and pathologic data on 319 patients from the Batten registry and from Staten Island to determine the degree of variability within the different forms and among and within families. Thirty-six patients (11.3%) had the infantile form; 116 (36.3%), the late infantile form; 163 (51.1%), the juvenile form; and 4 (1.3%), the adult form (Kufs disease). Clinical variability was found in all forms studied but was most striking in the juvenile and late-infantile forms. Seizures, dementia, blindness, or motor impairment were evident in 255 patients (80%). Rarer, less typical initial neurologic symptoms such as behavior abnormalities, psychoses, neuropathy, involuntary movements, and ataxia were seen mainly in the 64 patients (20%) with the juvenile form. Six juvenile and two adult pa-

tients had no detectable impairment of vision. All 319 patients had skin or conjunctival biopsies or buffy coats that showed the characteristic ultrastructural abnormalities of NCL. Variability was evident in 16.7% in that a combination of fingerprint, curvilinear, and membranous profile inclusion bodies was observed in storage lysosomes, although one type of inclusion was distinctly predominant for each form. Postmortem examination of the brains of 19 patients (3 with the infantile form, 6 with the late-infantile form, 9 with the juvenile form, and 1 with the adult form) revealed characteristic changes. Sixteen of the 19 brains (84%) showed pathologic variability in that they contained more than one kind of characteristic inclusion body in the neuronal lysosomal storage compartment. In all 19, small amounts of aging lipofuscin were also found.

The clinical characteristics of the four main clinical forms are:

1. Infantile (Haltia-Santavuori)

- Onset occurs at 8 to 18 months of age. Neurologic symptoms precede retinopathy and visual loss. Microcephaly, seizures, ataxia, visual impairment with a pigmentary retinopathy, and progressive profound developmental delay appear in the first 2 years of life; patients die in infancy or early childhood.
- Ocular findings include optic atrophy and a pigmentary retinopathy. The electroretinogram is reduced in amplitude or nonrecordable. Visual evoked potentials are abnormal. Cataracts have also been reported.

2. Late-infantile (Jansky-Bielschowsky)

- Onset occurs at 2 to 4 years of age. Progressive neurologic symptoms precede retinopathy and visual loss. Patients die in the first decade of life or in the early teenage years.
- Ocular findings include pigment mottling and granularity in the macular area, optic atrophy, and attenuation of retinal blood vessels.

3. Juvenile (Vogt-Spielmeyer and Batten)

• Onset occurs at 4 to 8 years. Neurologic deterioration follows visual loss. Patients have seizures and a variety of extrapyramidal and cerebellar disturbances. They become wheelchair-bound in their 20s, and most die in the third decade of life if not earlier.

• Patients have amaurotic pupils. A pigmentary retinopathy is present, often with a bull's-eye macular lesion, and may be the only finding for several months or a few years. Retinal vessel attenuation and optic atrophy may ensue.

4. Adult form (Kufs)

• Onset occurs in adulthood. The clinical picture is extremely variable, and the diagnosis is difficult to make. Neurologic symptoms start in the second and third decades of life and may take the form of psychological or motor disturbance. Extrapyramidal signs appear later, and some patients develop myoclonic seizures. The clinical course is slowly progressive.

• No ocular manifestations are found.

• The diagnosis is established by typical clinical symptomatology; computed tomography or magnetic resonance imaging of the head; neurophysiologic studies; electron microscopy of various body tissues, including lymphocytes, skin, muscle, rectal mucosa, and conjunctiva; and more recently, genetic testing.

The differential diagnosis includes metabolic diseases with progressive neurodegenerative disease and blindness such as Tay-Sachs disease, Refsum disease, cerebellar ataxia with retinal degeneration, and infantile adrenoleukodystrophy.

OCULAR FINDINGS
See Clinical Findings

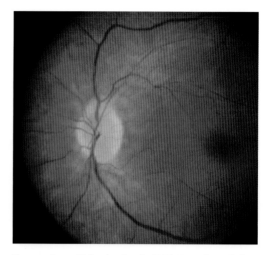

Neuronal ceroid lipofuscinosis (NCL) Posterior pole in a patient with juvenile NCL. Note the optic pallor, attenuated blood vessels, and fine pigmentary changes in the macula. Other patients present with typical bull's-eye maculopathy.

THERAPEUTIC ASPECTS

No specific therapies have been developed.

General supportive care and antiseizure medications are given.

Antioxidants such as vitamins E and C and selenium have also been tried.

Gene testing is available at the Massachussets General Hospital laboratory.

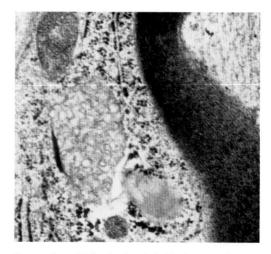

Neuronal ceroid lipofuscinosis (NCL) Electron microscopic view of Schwann cells in NCL demonstrating curvilinear inclusions.

REFERENCES

Boustany R-MN, Kolodny EH: The neuronal ceroid lipofuscinoses: a review. *Rev Neurol* 1987;145: 105–110.

Gillis WS, Bennet MJ, Galloway JH, et al: Lipid abnormalities in Batten's disease. *J Inherit Metab Dis* 1987;suppl 2:1–4.

International Batten Disease Consortium: Isolation of a novel gene underlying Batten disease, CLN3. *Cell* 1995;82:949–957.

McLeod PM, Dolman CL, Nickel RE, et al: Prenatal diagnosis of neuronal ceroid lipofuscinosis. *Am J Med Genet* 1985;22:781–789.

Traboulsi EI, Green WR, Luckenbach MW, et al: Neuronal ceroid lipofuscinosis: ocular histopathologic studies in the late infantile, juvenile and adult forms. *Graefes Arch Clin Exp Ophthalmol* 1987;225:391–402.

Weleber RG: The dystrophic retina in multisystem disease: the electroretinogram in neuronal ceroid lipofuscinosis. *Eye* 1998;12:580–590.

Wisneiwski KE, Kida E, Patxot OF, et al: Variability in the clinical and pathological findings in the neuronal ceroid lipofuscinoses: review of data and observations. *Am J Med Genet* 1992;42:525–532.

Zeman W: Studies in the neuronal ceroid lipofuscinoses. *J Neuropathol Exp Neurol* 1974;33:1–12.

RESOURCE

Batten Disease Support & Research Association www.bdsra.org

Niemann-Pick Disease

OMIM NUMBERS

Types A and B: 257200
Types C1 and C2: 257220 and 601015
Type D: 257250

INHERITANCE

Autosomal recessive

GENE/GENE MAP

Types A and B result from mutations in the gene for sphingomyelinase (*ASM*); at 11p15.4–

p15.1. Takahashi et al. showed that small deletions or nonsense mutations that truncated the *ASM* polypeptide or missense mutations that rendered the enzyme noncatalytic resulted in type A disease, whereas a missense mutation that produced a defective enzyme with residual catalytic activity caused the milder nonneuronopathic type B phenotype.

There is genetic heterogeneity in type C disease. The gene for the main form resides at 18q11–q12. The *NPC1* gene accounts for 95% of type C cases. *NPC1* functions as a pump to move lipids out of the lysosomes for storage in the endoplasmic reticulum. A gene called *HE1* on chromosome 14 is resopnsible for 5% of patients with type C disease. Mutations in *HE1* and *NPC1* have similar effects on cholesterol metabolism.

EPIDEMIOLOGY

Niemann-Pick disease affects all segments of the population, with cases reported from North America, South America, Europe, Africa, Asia, and Australia. However, a higher incidence has been found in certain populations: Ashkenazi Jews (types A and B), French Canadians of Nova Scotia (type D), residents of the Maghreb region (Tunisia, Morocco, and Algeria) of North Africa (type B), and Spanish Americans of southern New Mexico and Colorado (type C).

CLINICAL FINDINGS

This is a group of disorders of variable severity that share a defect in the enzyme sphingomyelinase. Sphingomyelin and cholesterol are stored in the central nervous system and the reticuloendothelial system.

Several clinical phenotypes of the disease are recognized, presumably from the effects of different mutations in the sphingomyelinase gene. The phenotypes are differentiated on the basis of age of onset, rate of disease progression, and sites of sphingomyelin storage:

1. Type A, the acute neuropathic form, is the most common and most severe pheno-

type. Moderate hepatosplenomegaly may be present at birth. Massive enlargement of the liver and spleen is universal before age 6 months. There is failure to thrive. Loss of motor and intellectual capacity occurs before the first birthday. Mental and physical deterioration is rapid, and patients die before the age of 4 years. There is massive foam-cell storage in the liver and spleen, as well as in bone marrow, lymph nodes, lungs, and other organs.

2. Type B, the chronic form, is characterized by splenomegaly but no central nervous system involvement. Survival has been noted for up to 20 years after the onset of symptoms. There is evidence of some sphingomyelinase activity.

3. Type C is similar to type A, except for delayed onset to 2 to 6 years of age, a more prolonged course, and survival to an older age.

4. Other variants have been reported and may be the result of other mutations at the sphingomyelinase locus.

The diagnosis is based on clinical features and the presence of leukocyte vacuolization in peripheral blood smears. The bone marrow contains foam cells. Sphingomyelinase activity in cultured fibroblasts is deficient in types A and B but is normal in type C. Prenatal diagnosis is possible.

Differential diagnosis includes storage diseases with hepatosplenomegaly such as GM_1 gangliosidosis, Wolman disease, and Gaucher disease. The exaggerated startle response to sound, common in infants with Tay-Sachs disease, is not seen in Niemann-Pick disease, nor do these children develop the coarse facial features that are present in some other storage diseases.

OCULAR FINDINGS

A cherry-red spot is present in one-half to two-thirds of patients. In type A, the spot has been observed as early as 10 weeks of age. The

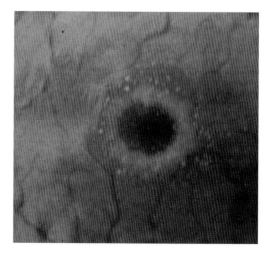

Niemann-Pick disease Cherry-red spot in the macula of a patient with Niemann-Pick disease type B.

white ring surrounding the spot is less sharply demarcated than in Tay-Sachs disease. The entire retina shows a mild milky appearance. Storage material accumulates primarily in retinal ganglion cells.

THERAPEUTIC ASPECTS

Research on therapies for types A and B progressed in the 1990s. Research on bone marrow transplantation, enzyme replacement therapy, and gene therapy is underway. Although some of these therapies have had some success in type B disease in the laboratory, none has been effective against type A. Bone marrow transplantation was effective in mouse models of type B when the transplant was performed early in life.

No specific treatment is available for type C disease. A healthy low-cholesterol diet is recommended. Symptoms, such as seizures and cataplexy, can be controlled or tempered by drugs.

Splenectomy may be required if symptoms of hypersplenism are present. No medications are particularly helpful.

REFERENCES

Naureckiene S, Sleat DE, Lackland H, et al: Identification of *HE1* as the second gene of Niemann-Pick C disease. *Science* 2000;290:2298–2301.

Takahashi T, Suchi M, Desnick RJ, et al: Identification and expression of five mutations in the human acid sphingomyelinase gene causing types A and B Niemann-Pick disease: molecular evidence for genetic heterogeneity in the neuronopathic and non-neuronopathic forms. *J Biol Chem* 1992; 267:12552–12558.

Walton DS, Robb RM, Crocker AC: Ocular manifestations of group A Niemann-Pick disease. *Am J Ophthalmol* 1978;85:174–180.

RESOURCE

National Niemann-Pick Disese Foundation, Inc. www.nnpdf.org

Norrie Disease

Includes X-linked familial exudative vitreoretinopathy

OMIM NUMBER
310600

INHERITANCE
X-linked

GENE/GENE MAP
Norrin, a protein believed to function in neuronal cell–cell interactions, is present. Most patients have private mutations. Deletions and other chromosomal rearrangements have been shown to cause the disease.

Xp11

EPIDEMIOLOGY
Worldwide distribution

CLINICAL FINDINGS
The principal sign is the presence of bilateral retrolental masses in a male child at birth.

Loss of mental function becomes apparent at an early age in some patients and is frequently significant. Psychosis occurs in over 25% of patients. In other patients, the dementia appears late and is not profound.

Auditory hallucinations are common, and hearing impairment may be severe.

The diagnosis is clinical and based on X-linked inheritance of bilateral blindness from neonatal retinal detachment and associated hearing problems and dementia or psychosis in some patients.

The differential diagnosis includes bilateral retinoblastoma, retinopathy of prematurity, juvenile retinoschisis, and familial exudative vitreoretinopathy or Criswick-Schepens syndrome; in older patients with phthisis, the differential diagnosis includes X-linked microphthalmos and X-linked cataract.

OCULAR FINDINGS
The bilateral retrolental masses are usually present at birth but may not be appreciated for days, weeks, or months. Microphthalmos is usually present. The anterior chamber is shallow, and the pupils are frequently dilated. The iris is hypoplastic, with posterior synechiae and ectropion uvae. The mass inside the eye appears as a gray membrane or a gray-yellow pink mass. The ciliary processes are elongated and often visible through the pupil.

If the fundus can be visualized, retinal folds or retinal detachments are frequently observed.

Carrier females may have peripheral retinal scars, folds, or pigmentary changes. Occasion-

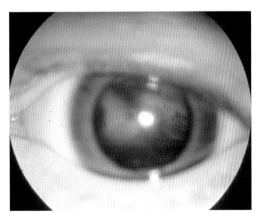

Norrie disease Hemorrhagic retinal detachment causing leukocoria in a patient with Norrie disease.

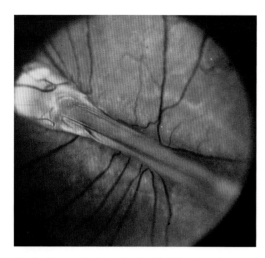

Norrie disease Peripheral retinal fold in a female carrier of Norrie disease. (Courtesy of Irene Maumenee, M.D.)

ally, they may be blind in one or both eyes because of unfavorable Lyonization.

THERAPEUTIC ASPECTS

Vitrectomy and retinal reattachment surgery are not helpful, and virtually all patients become blind.

Gene testing is available at the Massachusetts General Hospital.

REFERENCES

Berger W, Meindl A, van de Pol TJ, et al: Isolation of a candidate gene for Norrie disease by positional cloning. *Nat Genet* 1992;1:199–203.

Black G, Redmond RM: The molecular biology of Norrie's disease. *Eye* 1994;8:491–496.

Schuback DE, Chen ZY, Craig IW, et al: Mutations in the Norrie disease gene. *Hum Mutat* 1995; 5:285–292.

Shastry BS, Hejtmancik JF, Plager DA, et al: Linkage and candidate gene analysis of X-linked familial exudative vitreoretinopathy. *Genomics* 1995;27: 341–344.

Sims KB, Irvine AR, Good WV: Norrie disease in a family with a manifesting female carrier. *Arch Ophthalmol* 1997;115:517–519.

Warburg M: Norrie's disease: a new hereditary bilateral pseudotumor of the retina. *Acta Ophthalmol* (Copenhagen) 1961;39:757.

Zhu DP, Antonarakis SE, Schmeckpeper BJ, et al: Microdeletion in the X-chromosome and prenatal diagnosis in a family with Norrie disease. *Am J Med Genet* 1989;33:485–488.

RESOURCES

For a compendium of mutations reported until 1999: www.retina-international.org/sci-news/ndgmut. htm

For a forum of parents of patients with Norrie disease:
neuro-www.mgh.harvard.edu/forum_2/Norrie-DiseaseF/12.30.996.17PMParentsofch.html

North Carolina Macular Dystrophy

See **Retinal Dystrophies and Degenerations**

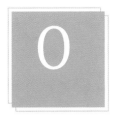

Oculocerebrocutaneous Syndrome

Also called Delleman-Oorthuys syndrome

OMIM NUMBER
164180

INHERITANCE
No familial occurrences
Mode of inheritance is unclear

GENE/GENE MAP
Not identified

EPIDEMIOLOGY
Very rare

CLINICAL FINDINGS
Areas of skin hypoplasia or aplasia are found in all patients and have no particular pattern of distribution.

Skin appendages were present in all reported cases and tend to appear in the periorbital or postauricular regions.

Intracranial findings include multiple intracranial cysts, hydrocephalus, and agenesis of the corpus callosum.

Delleman syndrome shares features with the Goltz (focal dermal hypoplasia) and Goldenhar syndromes. Encephalocraniocutaneous lipomatosis can be differentiated by the presence of cerebral calcifications and the absence of orbital cysts and agenesis of the corpus callosum.

OCULAR FINDINGS
Unilateral or bilateral orbital cysts are present in most patients.

Other findings include anophthalmos, microphthalmos, lid coloboma, dermoid cysts, and coloboma of the lateral canthal region.

THERAPEUTIC ASPECTS
Surgical interventions may be necessary to correct lid defects or excise skin appendages. Lubrication of the ocular surface is needed if the cornea is exposed.

REFERENCES

Al-Gazali LI, Donnai D, Berry SA, et al: The oculocerebrocutaneous (Delleman) syndrome. *J Med Genet* 1988;25:773–778.

McCandless SE, Robin NH: Severe oculocerebrocutaneous (Delleman) syndrome: overlap with Goldenhar anomaly. *Am J Med Genet* 1998;78: 282–285.

RESOURCES

None listed

Oculodento-Osseous Dysplasia

Also called oculodentodigital dysplasia

OMIM NUMBERS
ODDD, dominant 164200
ODOD, recessive 257850

INHERITANCE
Autosomal dominant
Probable autosomal recessive form

GENE/GENE MAP
The autosomal dominant form maps to 6q22–q24 and results from mutations in the connexin 43 gene (*GJA1*).

EPIDEMIOLOGY
The rare dominant form is much more "common" than the recessive form.

CLINICAL FINDINGS

The principal abnormalities are microcornea with iris anomalies, dental enamel hypoplasia, and syndactyly of two or more of the third, fourth, and fifth fingers or toes.

The characteristic face has a narrow nose, hypoplastic alae, and thin nostrils. Abnormal external ears, cleft lip, and cleft palate are occasional features.

The mandible is often thickened, and increased sclerosis of the long bones may be present.

The recessive form is more severe than the dominant form.

The diagnosis is based on clinical findings and can be supported by radiologic studies of the femur, hands, feet, and teeth.

Patients are often confused with those who have Hallermann-Streiff syndrome or mandibulofacial dysostosis (Treacher Collins syndrome).

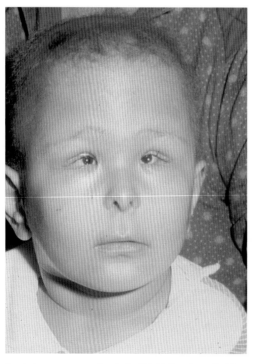

Oculodento-osseous dysplasia (ODOD form) Typical facial features of a patient with ODOD. (Reprinted with permission from *Am J Med Genet* 1986;24:95–100)

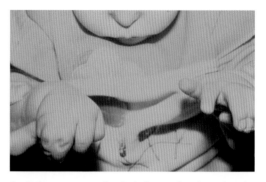

Oculodento-osseous dysplasia (ODOD form) Syndactyly in a patient with ODOD.

OCULAR FINDINGS

Microcornea (corneal diameter 6 to 10 mm) is a consistent finding. In the dominant form, the globe is generally of normal size; in the recessive form, microphthalmos and/or persistent hyperplasia of the primary vitreous can occur.

The distance between the outer canthi is decreased, whereas the distance between the inner canthi is normal. This may be related to the presence of small, shallow orbits. In addition, the palpebral fissures are shortened horizontally and vertically.

Infantile and juvenile glaucoma has been described in several patients and in more than one affected family member. This may be related to abnormal development of the anterior segment. The pupil may be eccentric and the iris hypoplastic.

THERAPEUTIC ASPECTS

Patients should be closely monitored for the development of glaucoma at any age.

REFERENCES

Gorlin RJ, Meskin LH, St Geme JW: Oculodentodigital dysplasia. *J Pediatr* 1963;63:69–75.

Holmes LB, Walton DS: Hereditary microcornea, glaucoma and absent frontal sinuses. *J Pediatr* 1969;74:968–972.

Meyer-Schwickerath G, Gruterich E, Weyers H: Mikrophthalmussyndrome. *Klin Mbl Augenheilk* 1957;131:18–30.

Paznekas WA, Boyadjiev SA, Shapiro RE, et al: Connexin 43 (*GJA1*) mutations cause the pleiotropic phenotype of oculodentodigital dysplasia. *Am J Hum Genet* 2003;72:408–418.

Traboulsi EI, Faris BM, Der Kaloustian VM: Persistent hyperplastic primary vitreous and recessive oculo-dento-osseous dysplasia. *Am J Med Genet* 1986;24:95–100.

Traboulsi EI, Parks MM: Glaucoma in oculo-dento-osseous dysplasia. *Am J Ophthalmol* 1990;109: 310–313.

RESOURCES

None listed

Oguchi Disease

See **Retinal Dystrophies and Degenerations**

Olivopontocerebellar Atrophy with Retinal Dystrophy

Also called **spinocerebellar ataxia 7, SCA7,** *or* **OPCA type III**

OMIM NUMBER
164500

INHERITANCE
Autosomal dominant

GENE/GENE MAP
SCA7 gene
3p21.1–p12

EPIDEMIOLOGY
Not applicable

CLINICAL FINDINGS
This is the only hereditary cerebellar ataxia that is not recessively inherited.

Patients typically have cerebellar ataxia and retinal degeneration. Cerebellar, pyramidal, extrapyramidal, and brain stem dysfunction signs are present and are accompanied by progressive external ophthalmoplegia and ptosis, dementia, deafness, occasional motor deficits, and bladder and bowel dysfunction.

There is great variability in age of clinical onset. Early onset is correlated with a more severe neurologic and ocular disease. Affected infants have developmental delay, ataxia, and poor vision. Seizures are uncommon. There is diffuse pigmentary mottling of the retina, with a diminished electroretinogram. Strabismus may be present. Death occurs in the first few years of life. In children or adolescents, the disease proceeds at a slower rate, with progressive cerebellar ataxia, dysarthria, and blindness. Adults have even slower progression, with gradually increasing ataxia and decreased vision.

This condition should be suspected in infants presenting with a neurodegenerative disease and retinal dystrophy. Molecular diagnosis is possible by assessing the number of trinucleotide CAG repeats in the *SCA7* genes. Normal individuals have up to 35 repeats, while patients have anywhere from 37 to 200. Neuroimaging reveals pontine and cerebellar atrophy.

This entity should be differentiated from metabolic diseases such as infantile phytanic acid storage disease, abetalipoproteinemia, recessive neonatal adrenoleukodystrophy, and the infantile form of neuronal ceroid lipofuscinosis. One parent is usually mildly affected in infants or children with *SCA7*, and the dominant mode of inheritance, along with the clinical presence of ataxia, is the best differential diagnostic clue. Epilepsy and microcephaly are frequently present in infantile neuronal ceroid lipofuscinosis and absent in olivopontocerebellar atrophy type III.

OCULAR FINDINGS
The appearance of the fundus and the extent of retinal involvement depend on the age of

clinical onset. In early onset, pigmentary changes involve the macula and retinal periphery. In adult onset, only the macula is affected and the macular lesion may appear as a circumscribed area of retinal pigment epithelial atrophy or a bull's-eye. In older children and adolescents, atrophic retinal pigment epithelial lesions appear in the posterior pole and retinal periphery and coalesce over time, along with the progressive appearance of bony spicules.

Electrophysiologic studies reveal diffuse cone and rod dysfunction.

Color vision may be affected.

Visual field testing may show central scotomas.

Ocular histopathologic studies show loss of outer and inner segments of the retinal photoreceptors. There is moderate to severe loss of photoreceptors, most marked in the macular area, and a striking variability in the melanin content of the retinal pigment epithelial cells.

Progressive ophthalmoplegia affects upward gaze initially, but progresses to involve convergence and eventually leads to a frozen globe.

Ptosis, abnormal optokinetic nystagmus, and abnormal pupillary responses have been described.

THERAPEUTIC ASPECTS
There is no specific therapy.

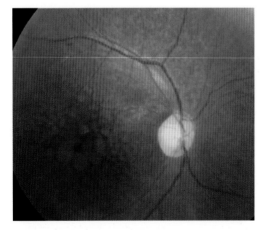

Olivopontocerebellar atrophy with retinal dystrophy
Fundus of a young adult with olivopontocerebellar atrophy with typical geographic atrophic macular lesions and generalized pigmentary retinopathy.

REFERENCES

Abe T, Abe K, Aoki M, et al: Ocular changes in patients with spinocerebellar degeneration and repeated trinucleotide expansion of spinocerebellar ataxia type 1 gene. *Arch Ophthalmol* 1997;115: 231–236.

Giunti P, Stevanin G, Worth PF, et al: Molecular and clinical study of 18 families with ADCA type II: evidence for genetic heterogeneity and de novo mutation. *Am J Hum Genet* 1999;64:1594–1603.

Harding AE: Classification of the hereditary ataxias and paraplegias. *Lancet* 1983;1:1151–1154.

Harding AE: The clinical features and classification of the late onset autosomal dominant cerebellar ataxias: a study of 11 families including descendants of "the Drew family of Walworth." *Brain* 1982;105:1–28.

Jampel RS, Okazaki H, Bernstein H: Ophthalmoplegia and retinal degeneration associated with spinocerebellar ataxia. *Arch Ophthalmol* 1961;66:123–135.

Konigsmark BW, Weiner LP: The olivopontocerebellar atrophies: a review. *Medicine* 1970;49:227–241.

Traboulsi EI, Maumenee IH, Green WR, et al: Olivopontocerebellar atrophy with retinal degeneration: a clinical and ocular histopathologic study. *Arch Ophthalmol* 1988;106:801–806.

RESOURCES
None listed

Organoid Nevus Syndrome

Also called linear nevus sebaceus of Jadassohn

OMIM NUMBER
163200

INHERITANCE
Most cases are isolated.

GENE/GENE MAP
Not mapped

EPIDEMIOLOGY
Incidence unknown; appears to be relatively rare

CLINICAL FINDINGS

This phakomatosis involves the skin, central nervous system, and eyes.

At birth, raised, hairless yellow-orange or tan plaques with irregular margins are present on the face, scalp, neck, body, or, occasionally, the oral mucosa. The lesions initially are composed of small papulae but become frankly verrucous and nodular at puberty. Scalp lesions are congenital and are accompanied by alopecia. Frequently, one nevus extends from the forehead to the tip of the nose. The nevi may be large but generally respect the midline. Malignant transformation of the nevi occurs in up to 15% to 20% of patients.

Mental retardation and seizures, which often begin in the first few weeks or months of life, are common. Milestones are normal in the first few months of life, but failure to thrive, poor growth, and delayed development become evident later. Some children may be severely affected, with multiple system involvement, while others have only linear sebaceous nevi, mental retardation, and seizures.

Electroencephalograms are often abnormal due to seizure activity or diffuse encephalopathy. The electrocardiogram may be abnormal due to cardiac involvement.

The nevi in the organoid nevus syndrome should not be confused with the flat red blanching nevus flammeus seen in Sturge-Weber syndrome, or with the flat, smooth-bordered café-au-lait spots of neurofibromatosis or McCune-Albright syndrome. Goldenhar syndrome has several features in common with this disorder, including asymmetry of the orbits, epibulbar dermoids, lipodermoids, and colobomas of the lids and irides. Other conditions to exclude in childhood are nevoxanthoendothelioma, juvenile melanoma, and scarring alopecia. In older patients, nevus verrucosus, verrucus vulgaris, scarring alopecia, and xanthoma should be considered.

OCULAR FINDINGS

The nevi may extensively involve the eyelids, and a large, vascularized choristomatous

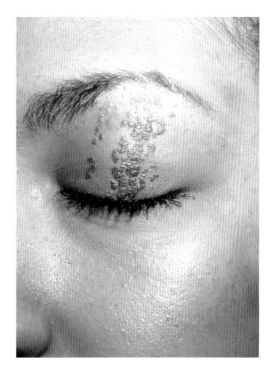

Organoid nevus syndrome Sebaceous nevus of the forehead and lid.

mass may involve the lids, conjunctiva, and cornea.

Nystagmus, strabismus, ptosis, third nerve palsy, and scarring and vascularization of the cornea may be present.

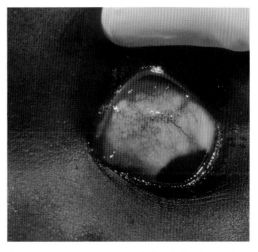

Organoid nevus syndrome Epibulbar lesion in a patient with organoid nevus syndrome.

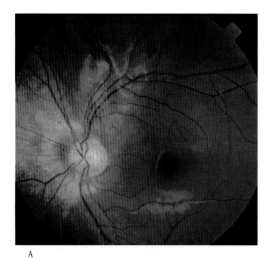

A

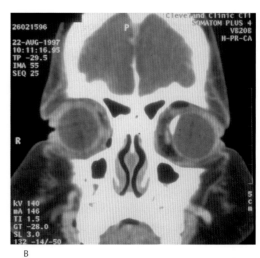

B

Organoid nevus syndrome Peripapillary choristomatous lesion in a patient with organoid nevus syndrome (A); computed tomography scan of the same patient showing bone density in the area of the choristoma (B).

Iris coloboma, choroidal coloboma, corectopia with an updrawn pupil, limbal dermoids, lipodermoids, and slanting palpebral fissures have all been described.

Biopsy of the conjunctival lesions demonstrates multiple choristomas with hyperplastic sebaceous glands, apocrine glands, and immature hair follicles.

Intrascleral cartilage and bone have been documented and appear as yellowish peripapillary or sectoral lesions deep to the retina and retinal pigment epithelium. They are highly reflective on ultrasonography and can be visualized on computed tomography.

THERAPEUTIC ASPECTS

Profoundly retarded patients may need institutionalization. The seizure disorder may be severe. Anticonvulsant medications and supportive care are necessary.

Surgical repair of the choristomatous scarring of the cornea and conjunctiva is rarely beneficial.

Malignant transformation of the nevus is possible, and excisional biopsies of any areas of growth are indicated.

REFERENCES

Alfonso I, Howard C, Lopez PF, et al: Linear nevus sebaceous syndrome: a review. *J Clin Neuroophthalmol* 1987;7:170–177.

Feuerstein RC, Mims LC: Linear nevus sebaceous with convulsions and mental retardation. *Am J Dis Child* 1962;104:675–679.

Jadassohn J: Mermerkungen zur histologie der systematisierten Naeri und uber Talgdrusen-Naevi. *Arch Dermatol Syphilis* 1885;33:355–394.

Shields JA, Shields CL, Eagle RC Jr, et al: Ocular manifestations of the organoid nevus syndrome. *Ophthalmology* 1997;104:549–557.

Stavrianeas NG, Katoulis AC, Stratigeas NP, et al: Development of multiple tumors in a sebaceous nevus of Jadassohn. *Dermatology* 1997;195:155–158.

Traboulsi EI, Zin A, Massicotte SJ, et al: Posterior scleral choristoma in the organoid nevus syndrome (linear nevus sebaceous of Jadassohn). *Ophthalmology* 1999;106:2126–2130.

RESOURCES

None listed

Osteogenesis Imperfecta

OMIM NUMBERS
Type I: 166200
Type II: 166210
Type III: 259420
Type IV: 166220

INHERITANCE
Types I and IV: autosomal dominant

Type III: generally sporadic, although some forms may be recessive

Type II: autosomal dominant, usually due to new mutation in gametes (likely germ line mosaicism)

GENE/GENE MAP
Mutation in genes for type I collagen, *COL1A1* (OMIM 120150) or *COL1A2* (OMIM 120160)

17q21.31–q22, 7q22.1

EPIDEMIOLOGY
The incidence is unknown. There are currently between 20,000 and 50,000 patients in the United States.

CLINICAL FINDINGS
Osteogenesis imperfecta is the name given to a heterogeneous group of generalized connective tissue disorders sharing clinical evidence of multiple fractures of the bones and, in some cases, blue sclerae, hearing loss, opalescent teeth, hypermobile joints, abnormal platelet function, and hypermetabolism. There are four main types:

1. Type I, previously called *osteogenesis imperfecta tarda*, is dominantly inherited. It may be suspected during the childhood years because of frequent fractures. The sclerae are blue. The bone disease is generally mild to moderate, although severe disability is known. Fifty percent of patients have hearing loss. At least two forms exist, depending on whether the teeth are opalescent or not.

2. Type II, previously called *osteogenesis imperfecta congenita*, presents at birth with a soft membranous skull, micromelia, ribs continuously beaded by fracture callus, and broad femurs. The sclerae are slate gray. Death usually occurs within a few hours or days after birth.

3. Type III, a heterogeneous group sharing early, frequent long bone fractures, is progressively deforming. Normal sclerae are the rule, although slate-gray sclerae may be noted in the first few months of life. Nearly all cases are sporadic, although a few recessive pedigrees are known. The severity of the bone disease separates these patients from type I.

4. Type IV patients have dominantly inherited disease and normal sclerae. The disorder is mild. Two different type IV syndromes exist, depending on the presence or absence of dental abnormalities.

The diagnosis of types II and III is based on clinical and radiologic criteria at the time of birth. The other types may be apparent only when the clinical history and course are well known. The color of the sclerae is the main differentiating point between types I and IV. The presence or absence of dental abnormalities serves to differentiate at least four osteogenesis imperfecta syndromes.

Prenatal diagnosis is possible for some forms of the disease.

Differential diagnosis includes Ehlers-Danlos syndrome type VI, in which patients may have gray sclerae. Rupture of the cornea and sclera is common in Ehlers-Danlos type VI but has rarely been reported in osteogenesis imperfecta. Joint hyperextensibility is present in both.

OCULAR FINDINGS
"Blue" sclerae, which in fact are slate gray, not blue, are the ocular finding in types I and II. At

times, blue sclerae may be the only feature of the disease in certain family members. The perilimbal region is often whiter than the remaining sclera, resulting in the so-called Saturn's ring.

Frequently associated abnormalities are a prominent Schwalbe's line or posterior embryotoxon.

The cornea is thinner than normal: on average 0.443 mm compared to 0.522.

Hyperopic refractive errors are frequent.

Rupture of the globe has been described in very few patients.

THERAPEUTIC ASPECTS

Vigorous orthopedic management of the fractures may prevent deforming abnormalities of the extremities.

Patients with the severe form (a membranous skull and multiple fractures at birth) rarely survive beyond the first few years of life. A normal life span can be anticipated for patients with the milder form, especially types I and IV. Many patients, especially those with type III, have multiple fractures with gross deformity of the extremities and are confined to a wheelchair.

REFERENCES

Baitner AC, Maurer SG, Gruen MB, Di Cesare PE: The genetic basis of the osteochondrodysplasias. *J Pediatr Orthop* 2000;20:594–605.
Byers PH: Osteogenesis imperfecta: perspectives and opportunities. *Curr Opin Pediatr* 2000;12:603–609.
Myllyharju J, Kivirikko KI: Collagens and collagen-related diseases. *Ann Med* 2001;33:7–21.

RESOURCES

Children's Brittle Bone Foundation
www.cbbf.org
Osteogenesis Imperfecta Foundation
www.oif.org

Osteopetrosis

Also called Albers-Schönberg disease

OMIM NUMBERS

Malignant recessive: 259700
Dominant: 166600
Benign recessive: 259710 and 259370

INHERITANCE

The malignant infantile form and the more benign form associated with renal tubular acidosis and mental retardation are recessively inherited. The other mild form is dominantly inherited.

GENE/GENE MAP

The autosomal recessive infantile malignant form is caused by a mutation in the *TCIRG1* subunit (OMIM 604592) of the vacuolar proton pump, a protein involved in bone resorption by osteoclasts, and has been mapped to 11q13.4–q13.5. It can also result from mutations in the *CLCN7* gene, a chloride channel protein that provides the chloride conductance required for proton pumping by the $H(+)$ adenosine triphosphatase of the osteoclast membrane (OMIM 602727).

The autosomal dominant form has been mapped to 1p21.

The autosomal recessive form with renal tubular acidosis is caused by a mutation in carbonic anhydrase II (CAII). This enzyme also has a role in bone resorption by osteoclasts and has been mapped to locus 8q22.

EPIDEMIOLOGY

The entity has been reported in most ethnic groups, although, as the disease is very rare, it is more frequently seen in ethnic groups where consanguinity is frequent.

The frequency of the dominant form in Brazil has been estimated to be 1 in 100,000.

CLINICAL FINDINGS

Osteopetrosis is a group of disorders of bone resorption. It is caused by the failure of osteoclasts to resorb immature bone. This leads to abnormal bone marrow cavity formation and to signs and symptoms of bone marrow failure and, in the severe recessive form, to bony narrowing of the cranial nerve foramina, which results in cranial nerve (especially optic nerve) compression. Pathologically, there is a persistence of the primary spongiosa, characterized by cores of calcified cartilage within bone. Abnormal remodeling of primary woven bone to lamellar bone results in *brittle* bone, which is prone to fracture. Thus, fractures, visual impairment, and bone marrow failure are the classical features of the disease.

Infantile-onset osteopetrosis should also be distinguished from the much milder autosomal dominant adult disease and the carbonic anhydrase II deficiency syndrome, which is associated with renal tubular acidosis and less severe osteopetrosis.

Three types of osteopetrosis have been clearly defined:

1. The severe recessive form has its onset at birth or in early infancy.

    • Neonatal hypocalcemia and secondary hyperparathyroidism may be present.
    • Severe anemia, infections, and bleeding result from hypersplenism and bone marrow dysfunction.
    • Small cranial foramina may cause optic, oculomotor, or facial nerve palsy.
    • Characteristic X-ray findings consist of a generalized sclerotic skeleton with failure of normal bone modeling. On radiography, bone density is generally found to be increased. Partial aplasia of distal phalanges, straight femora, and blocky *bone within bone* metacarpals are characteristic features. Macrocephaly with frontal bossing is usually present.

2. In the benign dominant form, in which abnormal radiologic appearance of the bones is consistently present, clinical disease severity is variable.

3. A third recessively inherited form, with onset in infancy and a more benign course, has been delineated. Renal tubular acidosis, calcification of the basal ganglia, and

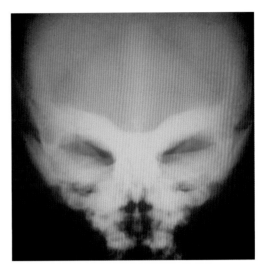

Osteopetrosis Mask-like radiologic appearance of the thickened base of the skull and orbit in a patient with osteopetrosis.

mental retardation are prominent features in the teenage or early adult years. Periodic hypokalemic paralysis is a major clinical manifestation.

OCULAR FINDINGS

Compression of the optic nerve as it emerges from the skull is common in the severe infantile form and leads to optic atrophy.

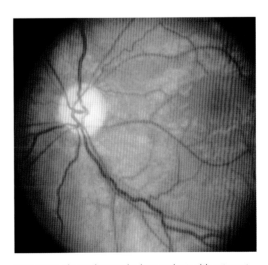

Osteopetrosis Optic atrophy in a patient with osteopetrosis.

Retinal dystrophy with reduced electro-retino-graphic responses and atrophic macular changes may be present in the mild recessive form.

THERAPEUTIC ASPECTS

Successful orbital decompression to relieve optic nerve pressure has been reported.

Corticosteroids, high-dose calcitriol, and interferon have been used with varying success.

Bone marrow transplantation is the only treatment that has been proven to significantly alter the course of the disease. Successful recipients continue to have minor orthopedic and dental problems, and their vision rarely improves. However, hemopoietic potential is restored and the long-term prognosis is favorable. There is a 79% 5-year disease-free survival in patients with human leukocyte antigen–identical sibling donors. Recipients of nongenotypically identical grafts have significantly worse results, with only a 13% 5-year disease-free survival.

REFERENCES

Felix R, Hofstetter W, Cecchini MG: Recent developments in the understanding of osteopetrosis. *Eur J Endocrinol* 1996;134:143–156.

Hoyt CS, Billson FA: Visual loss in osteopetrosis. *Am J Dis Child* 1979;133:955–958.

Thompson DA, Kriss A, Taylor D, et al: Early VEP and ERG evidence of visual dysfunction in autosomal recessive osteopetrosis. *Neuropediatrics* 1998;29:137–144.

Vanhoenacker FM, De Beuckeleer LH, Van Hul W, et al: Sclerosing bone dysplasias: genetic and radioclinical features. *Eur Radiol* 2000;10:1423–1433.

Wilson CJ, Vellodi A: Autosomal recessive osteopetrosis: diagnosis, management, and outcome. *Arch Dis Child* 2000;83:449–452.

RESOURCE

For families: www.osteopetrosis.org (resource site)

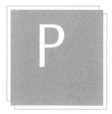

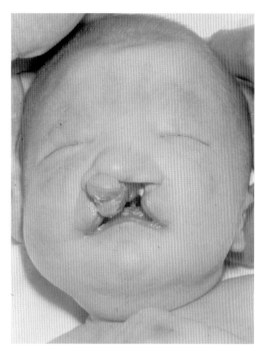

Patau syndrome Facial appearance and cleft lip/palate in a newborn with trisomy 13.

Patau Syndrome

Also called **trisomy 13**

OMIM NUMBERS
Not applicable

INHERITANCE
Non-Mendelian
A maternal age effect has been described. This does not apply to 20% of cases, which are due to unbalanced translocations. In these families, the risk of recurrence is much higher.

GENE/GENE MAP
Trisomy 13
The critical region seems to be located in the portion 13q14 to terminus.

EPIDEMIOLOGY
1 in 10,000 to 1 in 25,000 newborns

CLINICAL FINDINGS
Microcephaly and cerebral malformations, which may be very severe, such as holoprosencephaly
    Low-set ears
    Cleft lip and palate, often bilateral (80%)
    Polydactyly and clenched fist
    Rocker-bottom feet
    Rib abnormalities
    Severe cardiac malformations (80%)
    Renal and genital anomalies

OCULAR FINDINGS
    Hypotelorism
    Epicanthal folds

    Microphthalmos of varying degrees of severity, from isolated iris or choroidal coloboma to anophthalmos or cyclopia
    Anterior segment dysgenesis, including corneal opacities, Peters anomaly, congenital glaucoma, and cataracts

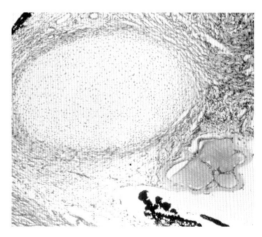

Patau syndrome Intraocular cartilage in the eye of a patient with Patau syndrome. (Courtesy of W. Richard Green, M.D.)

Persistent hyperplastic primary vitreous, retinal dysplasia, and optic nerve hypoplasia

THERAPEUTIC ASPECTS

About one-half of the patients die within the first month of life, and only 25% survive after the sixth month of life.

REFERENCE

Koole FD, Velzeboer CM, van der Harten JJ: Ocular abnormalities in Patau syndrome (chromosome 13 trisomy syndrome). *Ophthalmic Paediatr Genet* 1990;11:15–21.

RESOURCE

Support Organization for Trisomy 18, 13, and Related Disorders
www.trisomy.org

Pattern Dystrophy

See **Retinal Dystrophies and Degenerations**

Peroxisomal Disorders

OMIM NUMBERS

Disorders of peroxisomal biogenesis
1. Zellweger syndrome (ZS): 214100
2. Neonatal adrenoleukodystrophy (NALD): 202370
3. Infantile Refsum disease (IRD) (infantile phytanic acid storage disease): 266510
4. Rhizomelic chondrodysplasia punctata (RCDP): 215100
5. Hyperpipecolic acidemia (variant of ZS or NALD): 239400

Disorders of single peroxisomal proteins:
1. Adult-type Refsum disease: 266500

2. Adrenoleukodystrophy (ALD), adrenomyeloneuropathy: 300100
3. Pseudo-Zellweger syndrome, acetyl-CoA acyltransferase deficiency, 3-oxoacyl-CoA thiolase deficiency: 261510
4. Pseudoneonatal adrenoleukodystrophy, acyl-CoA oxidase deficiency: 264470; peroxisomal bifunctional protein deficiency: 261515
5. Pseudorhizomelic chondrodysplasia punctata, deficiency of dihydroxyacetonephosphate acetyltransferase: 222765
6. Oxalosis, primary hyperoxaluria type I, peroxisomal alanine glyoxalate aminotransferase deficiency: 259900
7. Acatalasemia: 115500

INHERITANCE

Autosomal recessive: ZS, NALD, IRD, RCDP, adult-type Refsum disease, oxalosis, acatalasemia
X-linked: adrenoleukodystrophy, adrenomyeloneuropathy

GENE/GENE MAP

Disorders of peroxisomal biogenesis:
1. Zellweger syndrome is caused by mutations in one of several genes: peroxin-1 (*PEX1*; OMIM 602136), 7q21; peroxin-2 (*PEX2*; OMIM 170993), 8q; peroxin-3 (*PEX3*; OMIM 603164), 6q; peroxin-5 (*PEX5*; OMIM 600414), chr 12; peroxin-6 (*PEX6*; OMIM 601498), 6p; peroxin-12 (*PEX12*; OMIM 601758). Other mapped loci for this disease: 2p15, chr 1.
2. Neonatal ALD: 2p15, chr 1, 12p13.3, 7q21–q22
3. Infantile Refsum disease: 8q21.1, 7q21–q22
4. Rhizomelic chondrodysplasia punctata: 6q22–q24
5. Hyperpipecolic acidemia

Disorders of single peroxisomal proteins:
1. Adult-type Refsum disease: 10pter–p11.2
2. Adrenoleukodystrophy, adrenomyeloneuropathy: Xq28

3. Pseudo-Zellweger syndrome-acetyl-CoA acyltransferase deficiency, 3-oxoacyl-CoA thiolase deficiency: 3p23–p22
4. Pseudoneonatal adrenoleukodystrophy: acyl-CoA oxidase deficiency: 17q25; peroxisomal bifunctional protein deficiency: 3q27
5. Pseudorhizomelic chondrodysplasia punctata, deficiency of dihydroxyacetonephosphate acetyltransferase: chr 1; deficiency of alkyl dihydroxyacetonphosphate synthase
6. Oxalosis, primary hyperoxaluria type I, peroxisomal alanine glyoxalate aminotransferase deficiency: 2q36–q37
7. Acatalasemia: 11p13

EPIDEMIOLOGY

Individually, all the peroxisomal disorders are extremely rare, although exact prevalences and incidences are unknown. They may be more common in populations in which consanguineous marriages are frequent.

CLINICAL FINDINGS

The peroxisomal disorders are due to dysfunction or absence of peroxisomes or of multiple or single peroxisomal enzymes. Disorders of isolated enzymatic deficiencies may present like disorders of peroxisomal biogenesis.

The biochemical hallmark of most peroxisomopathies is an elevated serum level of very long chain fatty acids (VLCFA) and pipecolic acid and decreased levels of plasmalogens. However, VLCFA are not elevated in RCDP, and phytanic acid and plasmalogen levels may not be abnormal in older patients with ZS, NALD, and IRD.

Zellweger syndrome is the prototype of peroxisomal diseases. Infantile hypotonia, psychomotor retardation, seizures, characteristic facies, impaired hearing, renal cortical cysts, hepatic interstitial fibrosis, and chondrodysplasia punctata are typical signs. Most patients die before 1 year of age.

Neonatal adrenoleukodystrophy presents with hypotonia, seizures, and psychomotor retardation in infancy. These patients have demyelination of the brain but no renal cysts or chondrodysplasia punctata. They generally die by 7 to 10 years of age.

Infantile Refsum disease is characterized by dysmorphic facies, mental retardation, hepatomegaly, severe progressive neurosensory deafness, and retinal dystrophy but no renal cysts, central nervous system demyelination, or chondrodysplasia punctata.

Rhizomelic chondrodysplasia punctata presents with craniofacial dysmorphism, dwarfism, mental retardation, and stippling of epiphyses.

Adult-type Refsum disease is characterized by cerebellar ataxia, polyneuropathy, retinitis pigmentosa, anosmia, deafness, ichthyosis, and cardiac myopathy with arrhythmias. There is an increased cerebrospinal protein concentration without pleocytosis. The diagnosis is often not made until adulthood, when elevated plasma levels of phytanic acid are demonstrated.

OCULAR FINDINGS

Zellweger syndrome: nystagmus, cloudy cornea, congenital glaucoma, cataract (80%), retinal dystrophy (71%), and, occasionally, optic nerve hypoplasia.

Neonatal adrenoleukodystrophy: nystagmus, cataracts (45%), and pigmentary retinopathy (82%) with optic atrophy; leopard spots can be seen in the fundus during the first or second year of life.

Infantile Refsum disease: possible severe visual impairment in infancy, nystagmus with progressive peripheral pigmentary retinopathy (100%) in the form of clumping rather than bone-spicule formation, optic nerve pallor, macular atrophic changes, arteriolar narrowing, late-onset cataracts (7%).

Rhizomelic chondrodysplasia punctata: congenital cataract (72%) but no retinal degeneration.

Adult-type Refsum disease: night blindness may be an early symptom. Atrophic maculopathy and pigmentary retinal changes develop with advancing disease.

Primary hyperoxaluria: crystalline deposits in the retina and retinal pigment epithelium

(RPE). Early macular changes reveal rings of hyperfluorescence around crystalline deposits in the RPE, followed by tiny refractile crystals in the neuroepithelium. With advancing disease come proliferation of pigment and eventual dense black discoloration of the macular area.

THERAPEUTIC ASPECTS

Dietary restriction of phytanic acid can prevent progression or allow improvement of some features of adult-type Refsum disease, such as ichthyosis, peripheral neuropathy, and cardiac conduction defects, but not visual or auditory function. No conclusive beneficial effect has been shown for IRD.

Dietary treatment with oleic acid/erucic acid (*Lorenzo's oil*) can reduce VLCFA levels in ALD, but no improvement in clinical symptoms has been shown in symptomatic patients. It may have a role in preventing deterioration in asymptomatic patients. Adrenal insufficiency in ALD responds to corticosteroid replacement therapy.

Patients with hyperoxalosis type I eventually require kidney transplants or combined liver-kidney transplants, but the disease recurs in the graft.

REFERENCE

Weleber RG: Peroxisomal disorders. In: Traboulsi EI, ed: *Genetic Diseases of the Eye*. New York: Oxford University Press; 1998:663–696.

RESOURCE

Kennedy Krieger Institute resource site
www.genetics.kennedykrieger.org/testlist.htm#pero

Peutz-Jeghers Syndrome

OMIM NUMBER
175200

INHERITANCE
Autosomal dominant, but a high percentage seem to be new mutations

GENE/GENE MAP
Serine/threonine kinase *STK11* gene
19p13.3

EPIDEMIOLOGY
Incidence unknown

CLINICAL FINDINGS
The most characteristic findings are deeply pigmented freckles on the lips, oral mucosa, and fingers, as well as hamartomas of the stomach and small bowel.

Intestinal polyps may cause pseudo-obstruction or intussusception and may necessitate surgery. These hamartomas are different from those of juvenile polyposis, and the risk of malignancy is smaller.

About one-half of patients develop some form of cancer in adulthood that may or may not be related to intestinal polyps. Pancreatic, ovarian, testicular, breast, and other types of cancers have been reported.

OCULAR FINDINGS
These patients do not have the pigmented ocular fundus lesions characteristic of familial adenomatous polyposis.

Pigmented spots can be seen on the lids, including lid margins, and conjunctiva.

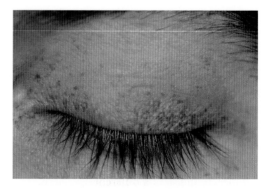

Peutz-Jeghers syndrome Pigmented lid lesions in a patient with Peutz-Jeghers syndrome. The patient also had a few pigmented lesions on the bulbar and palpebral conjunctiva. There were also pigmented lesions on his lips and buccal mucosa.

THERAPEUTIC ASPECTS

Monitoring for cancers and signs of gastrointestinal obstruction is necessary.

REFERENCES

Gruber SB, Entius MM, Petersen GM, et al: Pathogenesis of adenocarcinoma in Peutz-Jeghers syndrome. *Cancer Res* 1998;58:5267–5270.

Jenne DE, Reimann H, Nezu J, et al: Peutz-Jeghers syndrome is caused by mutations in a novel serine threonine kinase. *Nat Genet* 1998;18:38–43.

Traboulsi EI, Maumenee IH: Periocular pigmentation in the Peutz-Jeghers syndrome. *Am J Ophthalmol* 1986;102:126–127.

RESOURCE

The Network for Peutz Jeghers and Juvenile Polyposis Syndrome
www.epigenetic.org/~pjs/homepage.html

Prader-Willi Syndrome

OMIM NUMBER

176270

INHERITANCE

Autosomal dominant with imprinting, but the vast majority of cases are sporadic

This syndrome is a classical example of abnormalities in imprinting, resulting in different phenotypes, depending on whether the chromosomal material that is lacking belongs to the maternal or paternal line. The syndrome can originate from the inheritance of a deletion of 15q11–q13 from the father or from uniparental disomy, in which both chromosomes 15 are inherited from the mother. In Angelman syndrome, the same deletion is inherited from the mother, resulting in a different phenotype.

From 70% to 80% of cases result from an interstitial deletion. A minority of cases are due to an unbalanced translocation. The rest are caused by maternal disomy.

GENE/GENE MAP

Deletion of the transcription unit of the paternal copies of the imprinted *SNRPN* gene (small nuclear ribonucleoprotein polypeptide N), the *Necdin* gene, and possibly other genes
15q11–q13

EPIDEMIOLOGY

Between 1 in 16,000 and 1 in 25,000
Considered the most frequent cause of syndromic obesity

CLINICAL FINDINGS

Diagnostic criteria include infantile hypotonia, hypogonadism, truncal obesity, intellectual impairment, dysmorphic facies, and short stature.

Additional features include small hands and feet, poor fetal activity, early-onset childhood hyperphagia, carbohydrate intolerance, skin picking with persistent sores, abnormal dentition, scoliosis, and behavioral problems.

OCULAR FINDINGS

Strabismus (more commonly, esotropia) occurs in one-half of patients. It may be secondary to central nervous system anomalies, characteristic general hypotonia, or orbital anatomic factors.

Refractive errors are common, including moderate myopia, astigmatism, or anisometropia, and may be a cause of amblyopia.

Iris transillumination without other signs of albinism, like macular hypoplasia or nystagmus, has been described in one-third of patients. Abnormal visual evoked potentials have been explained by misrouting of optic nerve fibers.

Optic nerve hypoplasia occurs.

Rarely, it has been associated with cataracts, congenital ocular fibrosis syndrome, and congenital ectropion uvea.

Patients should be differentiated from those with the Bardet-Biedl syndromes.

THERAPEUTIC ASPECTS

Short stature seems to be responsive to growth hormone.

Weight loss may allow menarche in affected females.

REFERENCES

Cassidy SB: Prader-Willi syndrome. *J Med Genet* 1997;34:917–923.

Khan NL, Wood NW: Prader-Willi and Angelman syndromes: update on genetic mechanisms and diagnostic complexities. *Curr Opin Neurol* 1999; 12:149–154.

Kuslich CD, Kobori JA, Mohapatra G, et al: Prader-Willi syndrome is caused by disruption of the SNRPN gene. *Am J Hum Genet* 1999;64:70–76.

RESOURCE

Prader-Willi Syndrome Association (USA)
www.pwsausa.org

Pseudoxanthoma Elasticum

Also called Grönblad-Strandberg syndrome

OMIM NUMBERS

177850
177860
264800
264810

INHERITANCE

Autosomal dominant and recessive modes have been described, but all appear to result from mutations in the same *ABCC6* gene.

GENE/GENE MAP

The disease seems to be caused by mutations in the *ABCC6* gene, which codes for a protein belonging to the superfamily of adenosine triphosphate–binding cassette proteins.

16p13.1

EPIDEMIOLOGY

1 in 100,000 to 1 in 25,000

The disease is frequently underdiagnosed, and data on prevalence may not be accurate.

CLINICAL FINDINGS

This is a connective tissue disorder that affects mainly the skin, eyes, and blood vessels.

Skin lesions: The disease is named after the typical skin lesions, yellow papules (pseudoxanthomas) that occur on flexion surfaces, such as the neck, axilla, or groin, or behind the elbows and knees. The skin in these regions is often thick, lax, and redundant, with surface grooves like coarse-grained leather. The appearance of these areas has been compared to plucked chicken skin.

Vascular degeneration: Calcification of the internal elastic laminae of the arterial wall results in accelerated atherosclerosis. Coronary insufficiency, hypertension, and hemorrhages are frequent. Massive gastrointestinal bleeding can be the presenting sign of the disease and occurs before age 10 years. Mucous membranes may show clusters of small yellow intramucosal nodules resting on a background of dilated and tortuous capillaries.

Ocular features include angioid streaks and mottled (*peau d'orange*) fundus.

The clinical picture of skin change, angioid streaks, and gastrointestinal hemorrhages is diagnostic. However, skin lesions are not necessary for the diagnosis. The microscopic changes in affected skin are characteristic.

OCULAR FINDINGS

A mottled fundus, angioid streaks, and later development of choroidal neovascularization and macular degeneration are typical. Mottled fundus always occurs first and may be seen in the first decade.

Angioid streaks eventually develop in 80% to 95% of patients. They consist of cracks in Bruch's membrane. Skip areas and calcium deposits can be demonstrated histopathologically in the membrane. Choroidal neovascularization may develop, and eventually a hemorrhagic disciform macular degeneration may result. Retinal pigment epithelium proliferation is usually evident in or near the macula. Atrophic macular degeneration is commonly seen as well.

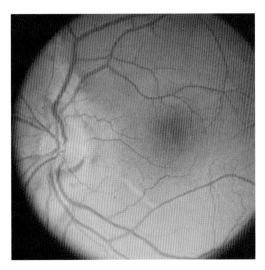

Pseudoxanthoma elasticum *Peau d'orange* appearance of the fundus and angioid streaks in a patient with pseudoxanthoma elasticum.

Areas of punched-out lesions in the peripheral fundus (*salmon spots*), with or without surrounding pigment, may also be seen.

Pseudoxanthoma elasticum is the most common cause of angioid streaks (66% of cases).

McDonald et al. reported 14 consecutive patients with pseudoxanthoma elasticum, of whom 9 (64%) had a spectrum of peculiar, sometimes reticular, pigmentary changes in the retina. Ten of 18 (56%) eyes had a random scattering of small, round pigment dots throughout the macula and around the optic nerve, sometimes extending to the equator. In 4 of the 18 (22%) eyes, the pigment clumps appeared in lines, resembling a string of pearls. These strings occasionally radiated from the macula in a spoke-like fashion. In 4 of the 18 (22%) eyes, the pigment clumping occurred in a fishnet, or truly reticular, pattern. Of the 18 eyes in these nine patients, 12 (67%) had subretinal neovascularization. Of the 10 eyes in the five patients

who did not show this pigmentary change, 2 (20%) had subretinal neovascularization.

The mottled fundus may simulate fundus albipunctatus or fundus flavimaculatus, especially when it occurs in the absence of angioid streaks.

Other diseases in which angioid streaks are occasionally seen include Paget disease, sickle cell disease, familial hyperphosphatasia, idiopathic thrombocytopenic purpura, and lead poisoning.

The skin changes may resemble those of senile elastosis.

THERAPEUTIC ASPECTS

Photocoagulation of neovascularization associated with the angioid streaks may be necessary.

Death may occur early in some patients from arterial occlusion or hemorrhage. Other patients have a normal life span.

REFERENCES

Connor PJ Jr, Juergens JL, Perry H, et al: Pseudoxanthoma elasticum and angioid streaks: a review of l06 cases. *Am J Med* 1961;30:537–543.

Deutman AF, Kovacs B: Argon laser treatment in complications of angioid streaks. *Am J Ophthalmol* 1979;88:12–17.

McDonald HR, Schatz H, Aaberg TM: Reticular-like pigmentary patterns in pseudoxanthoma elasticum. *Ophthalmology* 1988;95:306–311.

Secretan M, Zografos L, Guggisberg D, et al: Chorioretinal vascular abnormalities associated with angioid streaks and pseudoxanthoma elasticum. *Arch Ophthalmol* 1998;116:1333–1336.

Shimizu K: Mottled fundus in association with pseudoxanthoma elasticum. *Jpn J Ophthalmol* 1961; 5:l-l3.

RESOURCE

Pseudoxanthoma Elasticom (PXE) International www.pxe.org/index.html

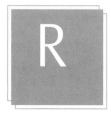

Refsum Disease

OMIM NUMBER
266500

INHERITANCE
Autosomal recessive

GENE/GENE MAP
10pter–p11.2
Phytanic acid-alpha-hydroxylase deficiency

EPIDEMIOLOGY
Prevalence unknown

CLINICAL FINDINGS
Phytanic acid, a 20-carbon branched-chain fatty acid, is excessively stored in all tissues, and its serum levels are elevated.

The three major clinical components of this disease are:
1. Progressive pigmentary retinopathy
2. Chronic polyneuropathy
3. Cerebellar signs

Night blindness appears in the teens, followed by peripheral neuropathy with gradual loss of sensations, muscle atrophy, and loss of deep tendon reflexes. Ataxia, nerve deafness, mental deterioration, and tetraplegia may occur. Patients may have ichthyosis.

Cerebrospinal fluid protein is elevated.

A number of radiologic abnormalities are present, including flattening of the femoral condyles, the tibias, and the dome of the talus.

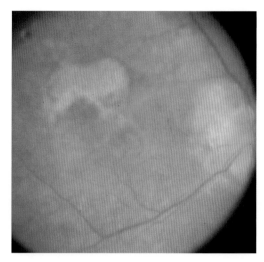

Refsum disease Posterior pole of the right eye of a patient with Refsum disease showing macular atrophic lesions and pigmentary retinopathy.

The metatarsals are shortened, and the distal phalanges are hypoplastic.

Heterozygotes may have elevated plasma phytanic acid levels.

OCULAR FINDINGS
The retinopathy is variable and may resemble that of typical retinitis pigmentosa or may consist of salt-and-pepper pigmentary changes.

Atrophic posterior pole and macular lesions with pigmented edges develop with advancing age.

THERAPEUTIC ASPECTS
Plasmapheresis has been used to reduce levels of serum phytanic acid.

A diet low in phytanic acid may result in reversal of some neurologic abnormalities.

Death ensues in middle age.

REFERENCES

Folz SJ, Trobe JD: The peroxisome and the eye. *Surv Ophthalmol* 1991;35:353–368.

Refsum S: Heredopathia atactica polyneuritiformis. *J Nerv Ment Dis* 1952;116:1046–1050.

Refsum S: Heredopathia atactica polyneuritiformis. *Arch Neurol* 1981;38:605–606.

Rinaldi E, Cotticelli L, Dimeo A, et al: Ocular findings in Refsum's disease. *Metab Pediatr Ophthalmol* 1981;5:149–154.

Robertson EF, Poulos A, Sharp P, et al: Treatment of infantile phytanic acid storage disease: clinical, biochemical and ultrastructural findings in two children treated for 2 years. *Eur J Pediatr* 1988;147: 133–142.

RESOURCE

University of Texas School of Public Health at Houston resource site
www.sph.uth.tmc.edu/Retnet.home.htm

Reticular, Macroreticular, and Butterfly-Shaped Pigment Dystrophies

See Pattern Dystrophy *under* Retinal Dystrophies and Degenerations

Retinal Dystrophies and Degenerations

Discussion of all clinical and molecular genetic aspects of retinal dystrophies is beyond the scope of this monograph. Although the clinical features of most of these disorders have been well described in the literature for several decades, new findings pertaining to the natural history, genotype–phenotype correlations, and management of some of these diseases continue to appear. The reader is referred to the Web site for Refsum disease under Resources for a continual update of new genetic loci and cloned genes for retinal dystrophies. The Web site also provides reference citations for the gene mapping and cloning information for each disease. Table 21 summarizes the clinical data on some of the retinal dystrophies. For additional information, the reader is referred to more specialized books.

Retinitis Pigmentosa

See Retinal Dystrophies and Degenerations

Retinoblastoma

OMIM NUMBER
1802000

INHERITANCE

Forty percent of cases are heritable and include patients with bilateral multifocal disease, a positive family history (including family member with retinoma, spontaneously regressed tumor, or pinealoma), second malignant neoplasms, chromosome 13q14 deletions in somatic cells, and about 15% of those with unilateral unifocal disease.

Most heritable cases are due to new germline mutations. Although recessive at the cellular level (abnormal tumor-suppressor gene), the disease behaves as a dominant trait because when a mutation inactivates one of the two *RB* alleles, the chance that the second allele will be inactivated by a variety of mechanisms is so high that effectively one germinal mutation is enough to ensure the occurrence of the disease. In nonheritable cases, the two genetic events have to take place in the same photoreceptor precursor cell, and the chance of such a combination of events occurring is so low that they can occur in only one retinal cell; hence, patients with nonheritable *RB* alleles develop only one tumor in one eye.

TABLE 21. Retinal Dystrophies and Degenerations

Inheritance Pattern OMIM Numbers Gene/Gene Map Protein	Clinical and Laboratory Findings
Achromatopsia, Congenital *Also called* **rod monochromacy**	Decreased central vision (20/200); no color perception; infantile nystagmus; photophobia
AR	Nonprogressive; nystagmus is a constant feature; histopathologic studies show many missing cones and many abnormally structured cones
	OF: macula usually normal, but may have hypoplastic appearance or show mild RPE thinning
ACHM2	FA: normal or may show RPE transmission defects
216900	ERG: photopic—abnormal to nonrecordable; scotopic—normal;
2q11	flicker fusion frequency—generally below 20 Hz
CNGA3	EOG: normal
ACHM3	DA: cone segment—abnormal and may be absent; rod segment—normal
262300	CV: no color perception; all colors appear as shades of gray
CNGB3	VF: ±central scotoma; normal peripheral fields
8q21–q22	
ACHM1 *Also called* **blue-cone monochromacy**	
603096	
Xq28	
Red and green pigment genes	
Ch. 14	
Central Areolar Choroidal Dystrophy	Symptoms appear in third to fifth decade
Also called **central areolar choroidal atrophy, central areolar choroidal sclerosis**	Decreased central vision (20/25–20/200)
	OF: mild nonspecific foveal granularity early; later, develops into circumscribed zone of neurosensory retina; RPE and choriocapillaris atrophy within central macula
	FA: early lesions may show faint RPE transmission defects within fovea; later lesions demonstrate a well-circumscribed zone of choriocapillaris atrophy within central macula
AD	ERG: photopic—normal to slightly subnormal; scotopic—normal
215500	EOG: normal to slightly subnormal
CACD	CV: moderate protan-deutan defect
17p13	VF: large central scotoma

Inheritance Pattern OMIM Numbers Gene/Gene Map Protein	Clinical and Laboratory Findings	
Central Areolar Choroidal Dystrophy continued	Histopathologic studies show well-demarcated area of RPE and choriocapillaris atrophy, with no evidence of choroidal "sclerosis"	**Choroideremia** Posterior pole view of left eye in patient with choroideremia. Note healthy-appearing optic nerve head and blood vessels. The choriocapillaris and choroids are well preserved in the macular area. Outside the macula, there is choroid and choriocapillaris atrophy, together with some coarse pigment clumps.
Choroideremia	Visual loss starts in second to third decade	
X-LINKED	Night blindness followed by loss of peripheral and later central vision	
303100		
CHM	OF: progressive atrophy of choroid, RPE and neurosensory retina in periphery with preservation of macular area until late in the course of the disease. Coarse pigment clumps. Heterozygous females are asymptomatic but have ocular fundus changes similar to those of affected males	
Xq21.2		
Rab escort protein-1		
	FA: peripheral areas of choroidal and choroicapillaris loss	
	ERG: reduced scotopic and photopic amplitudes	
	CV: normal until late in disease	
	VF: peripheral ring scotoma	
Dominant Cystoid Macular Dystrophy	Onset in first to second decade	
AD	Decreased central vision (20/25–20/80); progression to 20/200 or count fingers vision late in disease	
153880	Early cystoid macular edema; late macular RPE changes and atrophy; some cases may have RPE changes in bull's-eye configuration that progress to atrophy; whitish punctate deposits in vitreous; moderate to high hypermetropia	
7p21–p15		
	FA: cystoid macular edema; increased retinal capillary permeability within posterior pole	
	ERG: normal	
	EOG: normal to subnormal	
	DA: normal to subnormal	
	CV: mild to moderate deutan-tritan defect	
	VF: ± central scotoma	

continued

TABLE 21. Retinal Dystrophies and Degenerations (*Continued*)

Inheritance Pattern OMIM Numbers Gene/Gene Map Protein	Clinical and Laboratory Findings
Dominant Progressive Foveal Dystrophy *Also called* **autosomal dominant Stargardt disease** AD 600110 *ELOVL4* 6q14	Onset in first to third decade Decreased central vision; mild color and night vision changes; no photophobia Clinical findings similar to those of Stargardt disease, except for AD inheritance pattern, later onset, and generally less severe clinical course OF: fundus may be normal early; later macular dystrophic changes; ± flecks in posterior pole and midperipheral retina FA: irregular RPE transmission within fovea ERG: photopic—normal to subnormal; scotopic—normal EOG: normal to subnormal DA: normal to subnormal CV: mild to moderate deutan-tritan defect VF: central scotoma
Enhanced S-Cone Syndrome *Also called* **Goldmann-Favre syndrome** AR 268100 and 604485 *NR2E3* or *PNR* 15q23	Night blindness since early childhood; reduced visual acuity becomes evident with age; Goldmann-Favre syndrome refers to severe end of disease spectrum OF: fundus findings include pigmentary changes and subretinal dot-like flecks in peripheral retina and cystic lesions similar to those of juvenile retinoschisis in fovea of some patients; liquefied vitreous with veils One hypothesis concerning pathogenesis is that cone cells become blue (S cones) by default unless they receive a signal to become red or green; another hypothesis is that *NR2E3* mutations alter the photoreceptor's fate, causing cells that would normally develop as rods to become cones instead FA: depends on severity of retinal dystrophic changes ERG: scotopic—ERG does not reveal any rod-driven responses; large, slow waveforms are detected in response to bright flashes; photopic—more sensitive to blue than to red or white stimuli EOG: reduced light peak

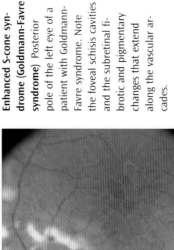
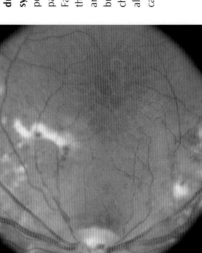

Enhanced S-cone syndrome (Goldmann-Favre syndrome) Posterior pole of the left eye of a patient with Goldmann-Favre syndrome. Note the foveal schisis cavities and the subretinal fibrotic and pigmentary changes that extend along the vascular arcades.

Inheritance Pattern OMIM Numbers Gene/Gene Map Protein	Clinical and Laboratory Findings	
Familial Radial Drusen *Also called* **Doyne honeycomb choroiditis, Holthouse-Batten superficial choroiditis, Hutchinson-Tays central guttate choroiditis, Malattia Leventinese** AD 126600 *EFEMP1* 2p16–p21	Onset in the second to fourth decade; rare congenital cases Asymptomatic unless degenerative change occurs in macula OF: round yellow-white deposits within posterior pole and midperiphery that tend to coalesce with time; later may show associated degenerative change within macula (RPE pigmentary disturbance, RPE detachment, and subretinal neovascularization) FA: early blockage of transmission and possible late staining; irregular dye transmission, leakage and pooling within macula, depending on degree of associated degenerative change ERG: normal EOG: subnormal DA: normal CV: normal VF: normal; central scotoma if macular degeneration is present	**Familial radial drusen** Two patients from the same family with familial radial drusen and mutation in *EFEMP1* gene. (A) Early disease. (B) Fine irregular drusen, some of which are associated with pigmentary changes, are present in a radial fashion in the macular area. Other drusen can be seen at the edge of the optic nerve head, a finding characteristic of this condition.

A

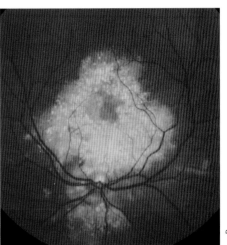

B

continued

TABLE 21. Retinal Dystrophies and Degenerations (*Continued*)

Inheritance Pattern OMIM Numbers Gene/Gene Map Protein	Clinical and Laboratory Findings
Fundus Albipunctatus AR 136880 *RDH5* 12q13–q14	Congenital night blindness OF: distinctive small, discrete round dots uniformly distributed in posterior pole and midperiphery, sparing macula ERG: delayed cone and rod adaptation; a- and b-wave amplitudes increase slowly with dark adaptation and reach normal levels after about 3 hours
Fundus Flavimaculatus *Subtype of* **Stargardt disease** (*see below*) AR 248200 *ABCA4* 1p21–p13	Onset in first to sixth decade Asymptomatic if no flecks in fovea; otherwise, slowly progressive reduction of vision Angulated (pisciform) yellow-white flecks within posterior pole and midperipheral retina; histopathologic studies show that yellow flecks are groups of enlarged RPE cells packed with granular substance with ultrastructural, autofluorescent, and histochemical properties consistent with lipofuscin FA: generalized decreased choroidal fluorescence (dark choroid sign) in most but not all patients; flecks demonstrate early blockage and late hyperfluorescent staining ERG: photopic—normal to subnormal; scotopic—normal

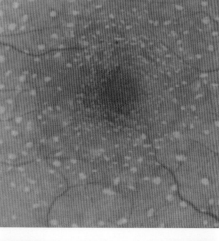

A   B

Fundus albipunctatus
Myriad small, round white lesions are present in the periphery (A) and macula (B) of this patient with fundus albipunctatus.

Inheritance Pattern
OMIM Numbers
Gene/Gene Map Protein

Clinical and Laboratory Findings

Fundus Flavimaculatus
continued

EOG: subnormal

DA: usually normal

CV: may be abnormal as
disease progresses

VF: normal

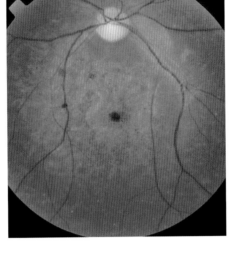

Stargardt disease/fundus flavimaculatus Advanced
Stargardt disease with an atrophic lesion occupying the
area between arcades. Note presence of a few pigment
clumps.

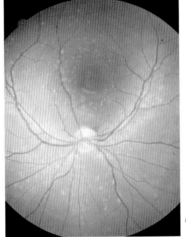

B

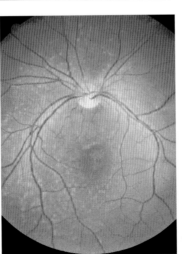

A

Stargardt disease/fundus flavimaculatus (A) Numerous fish-tail-like flecks are present in the
midperiphery of the fundus in this patient with Stargardt disease. Macular flecks are also present.
(B) Silent choroid sign with macular transmission defects in patient with Stargardt disease.

continued

TABLE 21. Retinal Dystrophies and Degenerations (*Continued*)

Inheritance Pattern OMIM Numbers Gene/Gene Map Protein	Clinical and Laboratory Findings
Leber Congenital Amaurosis (LCA)	Onset at birth
AR	Very poor vision; light sensitivity in 50%; high hypermetropia in some; ocu- lodigital sign; keratoconus in some at the end of the first decade
204000	OF: fundus may be normal early in life; progressive pigmentary changes that take a variety of appearances; macular "colobomas" in some
1q31	FA: variable findings, depending on ophthalmoscopic changes
LCA1	ERG: nonrecordable
17p13.1	EOG: abnormal
LCA2	DA: abnormal
RPE65	CV: abnormal
14q23	VF: severely restricted
LCA3	
14q11	
6q11–q16	
LCA1	
Guanylate cyclase	
204100	
1p31	
LCA2	
RPE65	
604232	
14q24	
LCA3	
604393	
17p13.1	
LCA4	
AIPL1	
604537	
6q11–q16	
LCA5	
605446	
14q11	
LCA6	
RPGRIP1	

continued

Inheritance Pattern
OMIM Numbers
Gene/Gene Map Protein

Clinical and Laboratory Findings

Leber Congenital Amaurosis (LCA) continued

604210
CRB1
1q31–q32.1

60225
CRX
19q13.3

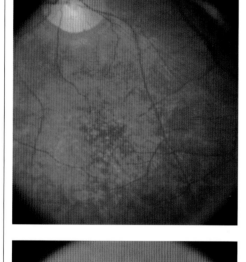

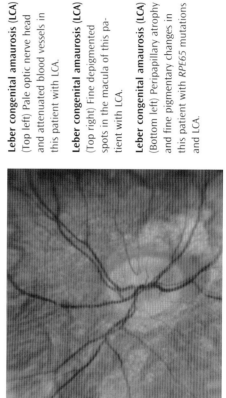

Leber congenital amaurosis (LCA) (Top left) Pale optic nerve head and attenuated blood vessels in this patient with LCA.

Leber congenital amaurosis (LCA) (Top right) Fine depigmented spots in the macula of this patient with LCA.

Leber congenital amaurosis (LCA) (Bottom left) Peripapillary atrophy and fine pigmentary changes in this patient with *RPE65* mutations and LCA.

TABLE 21.　Retinal Dystrophies and Degenerations (*Continued*)

Inheritance Pattern OMIM Numbers Gene/Gene Map Protein	Clinical and Laboratory Findings	
North Carolina Macular Dystrophy (NCMD) *Also called* **Lefler-Wadsworth-Sidbury dystrophy** AD 136550 and 600790 *MCDR1* 6q14–q16.2	Onset in first decade Normal central vision early, unless atrophic macular "colobomas"; possible late progression to 20/200 or worse in some patients with choroidal neovascular membranes; typically nonprogressive; visual acuity normal in patients with grade I lesions; grade III lesions may resemble coloboma; initial reports of associated aminoaciduria later refuted Grade I—drusen-like lesions and pigment dispersion in fovea; grade II—confluent drusen-like lesions in fovea; grade III—atrophy of RPE and choriocapillaris within central macula FA: grades I and II—RPE transmission defects and late staining of drusen-like lesions; grade III—nonperfusion of choriocapillaris ERG: normal EOG: normal DA: normal CV: normal in patients tested VF: ± central scotoma; normal peripheral fields	 **North Carolina macular dystrophy (NCMD)** Characteristic macular colobomatous lesion of NCMD.
Oguchi Disease *One form of* **congenital stationary night blindness** AR 181031 and 258100 Oguchi 1 Arrestin/*SAG* 2q37.1 Oguchi 2 Rhodopsin kinase (*RHOK*) 13q34	Onset at birth Congenital stationary night blindness OF: diffuse golden-brown, yellow, or gray discoloration of fundus that reverts to normal coloration after 2–3 hours in darkness (Mizuo phenomenon) FA: normal ERG: electronegative; no b-wave; a-wave increases with dark-adaptation time	

Inheritance Pattern OMIM Numbers Gene/Gene Map Protein	Clinical and Laboratory Findings	
Pattern Dystrophy *Also called* **reticular,** *macroreticular, and* **butterfly-shaped pigment dystrophies** AD 169150 Peripherin/*RDS* 6p21.1–cen	Onset in second to fifth decade Asymptomatic or slight decrease in central vision (20/25–20/40) until late in disease OF: subtle RPE mottling in younger patients; butterfly or net-like pigment pattern in macular area in older patients FA: ovoid area of hyperfluorescence and late staining surrounding central hypofluorescent spot; ± hyperfluorescence of posterior pole flecks ERG: photopic—normal to subnormal; scotopic—normal to subnormal EOG: usually normal CV: normal VF: ± relative central scotoma; normal peripheral fields	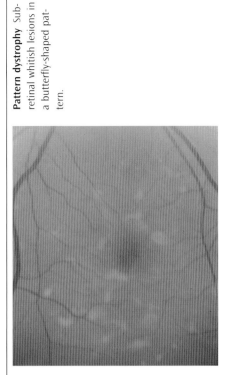 **Pattern dystrophy** Subretinal whitish lesions in a butterfly-shaped pattern.
Progressive Cone-Rod Dystrophies AR 1q12–q24 CORD8 8p11 CORD9	First or second decades; may not be detected early in course of disease Decreased central vision (20/40–20/100); defective color vision; photophobia; ± fine pendular nystagmus OF: macula may be normal or show nonspecific foveal granularity early; bull's-eye maculopathy frequent in AD type; salt-and-pepper maculopathy in AR type; ± macular and midperipheral pigmentation, arteriolar attenuation; temporal optic disc pallor	**Progressive cone-rod dystrophy** Slight optic nerve head pallor and attenuated retinal arterioles in association with circumscribed area of chorioretinal atrophy in the macula of this patient with cone-rod dystrophy.

continued

TABLE 21. Retinal Dystrophies and Degenerations (*Continued*)

Inheritance Pattern OMIM Numbers Gene/Gene Map Protein	Clinical and Laboratory Findings
Progressive Cone-Rod Dystrophies continued	FA: bull's-eye transmission pattern within macula; diffuse, irregular RPE transmission defects throughout posterior pole; ± diffuse, irregular RPE transmission defects throughout midperiphery
AD	
603649 6q CORD7	ERG: photopic—abnormal to nonrecordable; scotopic—often subnormal to abnormal; flicker fusion frequency reduced
	EOG: normal to subnormal
600977 17p13–p12 CORD5	DA: cone segment—abnormal; rod segment—normal (may be subnormal to abnormal later in disease)
601777 17p13.1 CORD6 GUCY2D	CV: severe deutan-tritan defect out of proportion to visual acuity; no color perception
	VF: central scotoma; normal peripheral fields (there may be midperipheral relative scotomas late)
120970 19q13.3 CORD2 CRX	
Retinitis Pigmentosa	Variable from first to fifth decade
AD	
601414 HPRP3	Night blindness; progressive loss of peripheral vision; late loss of central vision; cataracts; pigmented cells in vitreous; cystoid macular edema
1q21.1 180380 RHO 3q21–q24	OF: progressive narrowing of retinal vasculature, optic atrophy and pigmentary changes in fundus periphery, some in bony-spicule fashion

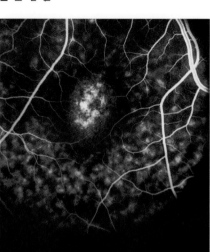

Retinitis pigmentosa Fundus of 70-year-old man with X-linked retinitis pigmentosa.

Inheritance Pattern
OMIM Numbers
Gene/Gene Map Protein

Gene/Gene Map Protein	Clinical and Laboratory Findings
Retinitis Pigmentosa continued	
179605 *RDS* 6q21.2–cen	Extreme variability in clinical manifestations; genotype–phenotype correlation not consistent, except for very few mutations
180104 *RP9* 7p15.1–p13	15,000 units of vitamin A supplementation indicated in patients with AD disease; Diamox may be useful in treatment of cystoid macular edema
146690 and 180105 *IMPDH1* 7q31.1	FA: depends on extent of retinal and RPE degenerative changes; patients may have cystoid macular edema
180100 and 603937 *RP1* 8q11–q13	ERG: subnormal scotopic amplitudes precede reduction of photopic amplitudes
180721 *ROM1* 11q13	EOG: subnormal
162080 *NRL* 14q11.2	DA: elevated rod and cone thresholds
600059 *PRPC8* 17p13.3	CV: normal except very late in disease
600852 *RP17* 17q22	VF: midperipheral ring scotoma; progresses to total loss except for central islands, which disappear at very end of disease process
No OMIM number *FSCN2* 17q25	
600138 and 606419 *PRPF31* 19q13.4	

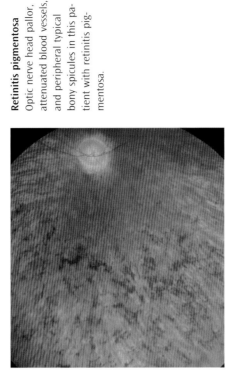

Retinitis pigmentosa
Optic nerve head pallor, attenuated blood vessels, and peripheral typical bony spicules in this patient with retinitis pigmentosa.

continued

TABLE 21. Retinal Dystrophies and Degenerations (Continued)

Inheritance Pattern OMIM Numbers Gene/Gene Map Protein		Inheritance Pattern OMIM Numbers Gene/Gene Map Protein		Inheritance Pattern OMIM Numbers Gene/Gene Map Protein	
Retinitis Pigmentosa continued		*Retinitis Pigmentosa continued*		*Retinitis Pigmentosa continued*	
AR		180071	*PDE6A*	XLR	
600105 and 604210 and 268030		5q31.2–q34		No OMIM number	*RP23*
CRB1		600132 and 602280	*TULP1*	Xp22	
1q31–q32.1		6p21.3		312612	*RP6*
No OMIM number		602772	*RP25*	Xp21.3–p21.2	
RP28		6cen–q15		21610	*RPGR*
2p11–p16		600342	*RGR*	Xp21.1	
604705	*MERTK*	10q23		304020	
2q14.1		180090	*RLBP1*	*COD1* same as *RPGR*	
604365	*PROML1*	15q26		Xp21.1	
4p		602594	*RP22*	300029	
163500 and 180072	*PDE6B*	16p12.1–p12.3		*RP15* same as *RPGR*	
4p16.3		123825		Xp21.1	
		600724	*CNGB1*	312600	*RP2*
CNGA1		16q13–q21		Xp11.3	
4p12–cen				300155	*RP24*
604863	*LRAT*			Xq26–q27	
4q31.2					
No OMIM number					
RP29					
4q32–q34					

continued

Inheritance Pattern OMIM Numbers Gene/Gene Map Protein	Clinical and Laboratory Findings
Stargardt Disease *Also called* **juvenile macular degeneration** 248200 and 601691 and 601718 AR *ABCA4* 1p21–p22	Onset usually in first or second decade; many cases dismissed as functional visual loss because of decreased central vision (± 20/200) out of proportion to macular changes; moderately defective color vision; no photophobia OF: vitreous is clear; fundus may be normal early; later, beaten-bronze macula followed by oval zone of RPE and choriocapillaris atrophy or bull's-eye maculopathy; ± flecks in posterior pole and midperiphery of fundus FA: irregular RPE transmission within fovea; occasional bull's-eye pattern of transmission; nonperfusion of choriocapillaris in advanced cases; when flecks present, pattern is similar to that of fundus flavimaculatus ERG: Ganzfeld photopic—normal to subnormal; Ganzfeld scotopic—normal; multifocal ERG subnormal in macular region EOG: normal to subnormal DA: normal to subnormal CV: mild to moderate deutan-tritan defect VF: central scotoma
Stationary Night Blindness, Nougaret Type AD 139330 *GNAT1* 3p21 Transducin	Onset at birth Night blindness but no reduction in central vision OF: retina totally normal ophthalmoscopically FA: normal ERG: photopic—normal; scotopic—subnormal EOG: normal CV: normal VF: none May affect taste perception

TABLE 21. Retinal Dystrophies and Degenerations (*Continued*)

Inheritance Pattern OMIM Numbers Gene/Gene Map Protein	Clinical and Laboratory Findings
Vitelliform Dystrophy *Also called* **Best disease, polymorphic macular degeneration of Braley, vitelliruptive macular dystrophy** AD 153700 *VMD2* 11q13 bestrophin	Onset in first decade; decreased central vision (20/30–20/50) at variable age; vision may remain relatively stable for many years OF: fundus appearance is variable; egg-yolk lesion in fovea in classic cases, but infrequently present; some patients have multifocal whitish lesions in posterior pole; lesions eventually degenerate, with associated RPE disturbance and pigment clumping; subretinal neovascularization and scarring may develop FA: blockage by vitelliform lesion; transmissionwhen cyst ruptures; irregular RPE transmission and staining, depending on presence of pigmentary disturbance, subretinal neovascularization, and scarring ERG: normal EOG: abnormal (even in otherwise normal-appearing carriers); necessary for diagnosis DA: normal CV: color defects proportional to degree of visual loss VF: relative central scotoma early; more dense scotomas may be noted following degeneration and organization of lesion

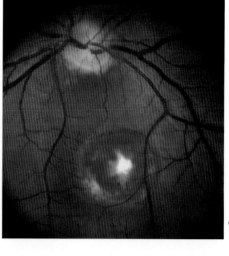

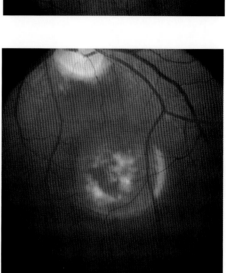

Vitelliform dystrophy: Best disease Three stages of Best disease: vitelliform (A), scrambled egg (B), and subretinal scar (C).

continued

Inheritance Pattern OMIM Numbers Gene/Gene Map Protein	Clinical and Laboratory Findings
X-Linked Congenital Stationary Night Blindness, Complete or Type 1 XLR 300278 and 310500 *NYX* Xp11.4	Congenital night blindness; nonprogressive; distinguished from dominant Nougaret type by presence of myopia and by mode of inheritance; some patients have nystagmus OF: fundus shows myopic changes, some pigment washout, and some fine pigmentary changes in periphery; may be normal FA: normal or minor transmission defects ERG: scotopic—no rod function; photopic—normal; electronegative scotopic bright flash ERG (Schubert-Bornsheim tracing or electronegative ERG) DA: abnormal
X-Linked Congenital Stationary Night Blindness, Incomplete or Type 2 XLR 300071 and 300110 *CACNA1F* Xp11.23	Congenital night blindness; nonprogressive; may have hyperopia or myopia OF: fundus generally normal ERG: scotopic—some residual rod function; photopic—subnormal b wave; electronegative scotopic bright flash ERG (Schubert-Bornsheim tracing or electronegative ERG) DA: abnormal
X-Linked Juvenile Retinoschisis XLR 312700 Xp22.2 *RS1* Retinoschisin	Onset in first decade; may even be present at birth Decreased central vision (20/25–20/50 or worse); slowly progressive OF: foveal retinoschisis 100%; peripheral retinoschisis ("vitreous veils") 50% FA: no abnormality within posterior pole until late in disease, then transmission defects within central macula ERG: photopic—selective decrease in b-wave amplitude; scotopic—selective decrease in b-wave amplitude (Schubert-Bornsheim tracing or electronegative ERG) EOG: normal in mild cases; may become subnormal in advanced cases DA: cone segment—normal to subnormal; rod segment—normal to subnormal

TABLE 21.　Retinal Dystrophies and Degenerations (*Continued*)

Inheritance Pattern
OMIM Numbers
Gene/Gene Map Protein　　　**Clinical and Laboratory Findings**

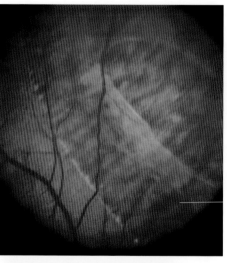

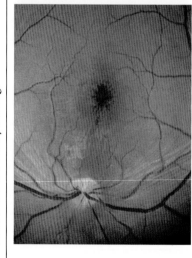

X-linked retinoschisis (XLRS) Posterior pole of a patient with XLRS showing the characteristic cartwheel-like foveal schisis.

X-linked retinoschisis (XLRS) Peripheral schisis cavity in a patient with XLRS. Note the large inner layer retinal break and posterior demarcation line.

CV: initial tritan defect followed by deutan-tritan defect (less severe than for cone-rod dystrophy)

VF: absolute scotomas corresponding to areas of schisis

Histopathologic studies show splitting of retina in nerve fiber layer

AD = autosomal dominant; AR = autosomal recessive; CV = color vision; DA = dark adaptation; EOG = electro-oculogram; ERG = electroretinogram; FA = fluorescein angiography; OF = ophthalmoscopic findings; RPE = retinal pigment epithelium; VF = visual fields; XLR = X-linked recessive.

Patients with 13q− syndrome have a number of congenital malformations, including peculiar facies (with a broad, prominent nasal bridge, hypertelorism, epicanthus, and ptosis), protruding upper incisors, micrognathia, prominent and low-set ears, imperforate anus, and hypoplastic thumbs. From 10% to 15% develop retinoblastoma. Some of these patients may also have microphthalmos. In general, retinoblastoma occurs in normal-sized eyes. When it is present in a microphthalmic eye, a 13q− syndrome should be suspected.

GENE/GENE MAP

RB is a tumor-suppressor gene, or recessive oncogene

13q14.1–q14.2

EPIDEMIOLOGY

1 in 15,000 live newborns worldwide

CLINICAL AND OCULAR FINDINGS

The great majority of cases are diagnosed before age 4 years. Males and females are equally affected. Mortality rates are very low if treatment is instituted before metastases occur, with 5-year survival rates of >90% in unilateral cases and >80% in bilateral cases.

The average age at diagnosis is about 1 year for bilateral disease and 18 months for unilateral disease. When there is a positive family history, affected infants are discovered earlier because of examinations shortly after birth and in the first few years of life. Patients most commonly present with leukocoria or strabismus. A white or tan reflex from the pupil is most often noted by parents when the child is looking in a direction that puts the white tumor in the path of the incident light. Other presenting signs and symptoms include pseudohypopyon, hyphema, periorbital swelling, and red eye.

The diagnosis should be suspected if a relative or sibling has had an eye enucleated in infancy or childhood. Because strabismus is the second most common sign of retinoblastoma, a search for retinal disease or tumor should be routinely made in infants and children with ocular misalignment.

Age at presentation, sex, laterality of ocular involvement, and family history are good clues to the differential diagnosis because the various simulating conditions appear in characteristic age groups and may be predominantly male (as in the case of Coats disease) or may have predominantly uniocular involvement (such as persistent hyperplastic primary vitreous or toxocariasis) or binocular involvement (Norrie disease, retinopathy of prematurity). More than 90% of retinoblastomas can be diagnosed easily using indirect ophthalmoscopy, ultrasonography, or computed tomography. In the past, about 50% of patients referred to tertiary specialized ophthalmic oncology centers with a suspicion of retinoblastoma turned out to have the tumor.

Flexner-Wintersteiner rosettes are characteristic of the tumor. Almost all tumors have areas of poorly differentiated cells and others of less well differentiated cells. Areas of necrosis and calcification are seen in the majority of tumors. Calcification is characteristic when demonstrated on ultrasonography or radiographic studies. The prognosis does not depend on the degree of tumor differentiation except in one situation, in which the entire tumor consists of benign cells that show areas of fleurette (bunch of flowers) formation. Such tumors have been termed *retinomas* or *retinocytomas*. These tumors, which look more like scars with areas of retinal pigment epithelial hyperplasia around the tumor, have been observed in parents of children with typical retinoblastoma. Retinomas carry the same genetic implication as retinoblastomas. Occasionally, retinoblastomas regress spontaneously and are accompanied by a severe inflammatory reaction; the eye harboring the tumor becomes phthisic. Vascular and immunologic mechanisms have been implicated in this process.

Secondary nonocular tumors in survivors of heritable retinoblastoma include osteosarcoma of the skull and long bones, soft-tissue sarcoma, cutaneous melanoma, adenocarcinoma, oat-cell carcinoma, sebaceous carcinoma, Wilms' tumor, neuroblastoma, and leukemia. Estimates for the incidence of secondary malignant neoplasms (SMNs) have varied from 2% at 12 years, using actuarial data, to 90% at 30 years, using extrapolated lifetime analysis. DerKinderen et al. report an incidence of 19% at 35 years, using material from the national registry in the Netherlands. In a study of 215 patients with bilateral retinoblastoma at the Armed Forces Institute of Pathology (AFIP), in which criteria for inclusion in the study were that (1) the first enucleated eye had to be submitted primarily to the AFIP for histopathologic examination and (2) that adequate clinical follow-up was available, Roarty et al. found SMNs in 24 instances (11.2%). Osteogenic sarcoma and chondrosarcoma represent the largest category of SMNs in most large series. The next most common malignancy appears to be cutaneous malignant melanoma, which accounts for about 7% of SMNs. Osteosarcoma and chondrosarcoma tend to occur in the second decade of life, while malignant melanoma manifests in the third or fourth decade of life. It is presumed that the secondary tumors develop because of loss of the tumor-suppressor activity of the retinoblastoma gene. Occasional patients develop two or three secondary neoplasms, sometimes within the field of irradiation. Radiation therapy definitely increases the risk of SMNs, even in sites remote from the orbit. All patients who develop SMNs have the heritable form of retinoblastoma. Mortality from osteogenic sarcoma in survivors of heritable retinoblastoma was formerly 100%. New advances in combination chemotherapy have resulted in occasional long-term survivors.

Two categories of intracranial neoplasms are seen in patients who have, or have been treated for, retinoblastoma:

1. The first category comprises midline tumors in the pineal or parasellar regions. Because these tumors have histologic features of retinoblastoma and almost always occur in association with bilateral retinoblastoma, they have been called *trilateral retinoblastoma*. More rarely, they may be seen in association with unilateral disease or in siblings of patients with retinoblastoma.

2. The second category includes all other intracranial neoplasms. Brain tumors reported in survivors of heritable retinoblastoma include glioblastomas, astrocytomas, a spongioblastoma, and meningiomas.

THERAPEUTIC ASPECTS

Examination under anesthesia is performed with scleral depression to detect anteriorly located small tumors. The treatment strategy depends on the size and location of the tumors. Computed tomography of the orbit and head, magnetic resonance imaging, and ocular ultrasonography are performed to detect intraocular calcifications and possible optic nerve and intracranial involvement by the tumor. Imaging studies are most helpful when the ocular media are not clear. Lumbar puncture and bone marrow aspiration are not routinely performed because of their extremely low yield if the optic nerve is not involved. A karyotype is obtained. If an eye is enucleated, a frozen section should preferably be submitted for DNA analysis, along with a blood sample to study the DNA from lymphocytes for mutations in the retinoblastoma gene (*RB*). In infants with a positive family history in a parent or sibling, frequent examinations are performed (under anesthesia, if needed) in the first 3 to 5 years and less frequently thereafter. Examinations under anesthesia may alternate with examinations in the office if such examinations are satisfactory, especially in young infants.

Enucleation is performed for advanced retinoblastoma if there is no chance of salvaging vision. Enucleation is also performed if there is

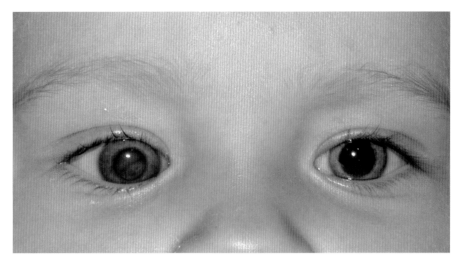

Retinoblastoma Leukocoria of the right eye in a child with retinoblastoma.

iris involvement, tumor-induced glaucoma, a flat anterior chamber, a pseudohypopyon, total retinal detachment, or optic nerve head involvement without obvious extension beyond the lamina cribrosa. If extension beyond the lamina cribrosa is suspected by imaging, then radiotherapy with or without chemotherapy is given prior to enucleation. Enucleation should be performed if tumor fills more than 50% of the vitreous cavity. Macular involvement, vitreous seeding, and localized retinal detachment are not indications for enucleation. Mortality is not affected in patients with stage 2 or stage 3 disease if enucleation is performed after external-beam radiotherapy fails to control tumor growth. This is probably also the case with stage 4 and stage 5 tumors. Tumor tissue should always be submitted for DNA analysis, which allows determination of the mechanisms of tumorigenesis, classification as sporadic versus heritable retinoblastoma, and accurate genetic counseling.

If external-beam radiation therapy is necessary, it is best given using an anterior and a lateral port approach, although the lens is exposed and cataract may develop. A total of 3500 to 4000 cGy is given in daily divided doses over 3 weeks. Side effects of external-beam therapy include local skin and ocular surface abnormalities, enophthalmos, failure of the bone to grow, cataracts (which typically develop 2 to 4 years following therapy), and, most importantly, an increased risk of developing SMNs in patients with heritable retinoblastoma. This has led all experts to favor chemotherapy over external-beam irradiation whenever possible.

Episcleral radioactive plaques are used to treat localized tumors that are not accessible to

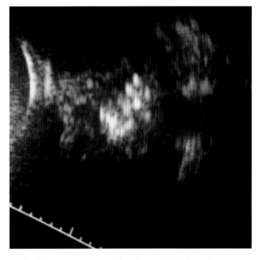

Retinoblastoma B-scan showing calcifications in retinoblastoma.

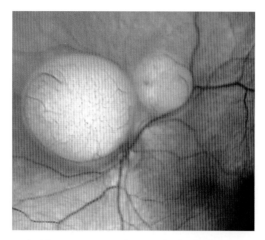

Retinoblastoma Retcam photograph of retinoblastoma. Two tumors are present nasal to the optic nerve head.

cryotherapy or laser treatment. Plaques can also be used in combination with external-beam ir-radiation. Materials used include cobalt 60, irid-ium 192, iodine 125, and ruthenium 106. Plaques are sutured to the globe over the area of the tumor and are left in place for calculated pe-riods of time to deliver a certain amount of ra-diation at the apex of the tumor. The advantage of plaque therapy is the avoidance of unneces-sary radiation exposure to remote ocular and ex-traocular sites that do not need to be irradiated.

Photocoagulation is used for small tumors. Laser spots are applied around the tumor to close its blood supply. Direct treatment to the

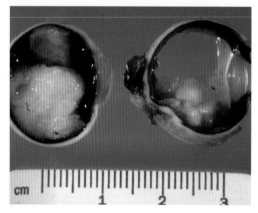

Retinoblastoma Sectioned eye with retinoblastoma.

tumor can be given with the diode laser at low power and long duration, using a microscope delivery system through a contact lens.

Cryotherapy is used to destroy small tumors measuring less than 10 mm in diameter and less than 3 to 5 mm in height. A triple freeze-thaw technique is used, leaving the ice ball over the tumor long enough to ensure destruction of all tumor cells. Small residual tumor foci after ex-ternal-beam radiation therapy may be treated by cryotherapy.

Chemotherapeutic agents are very effective, even as primary modalities of treatment. Initial chemotherapy to shrink the tumor, followed by photocoagulation or cryotherapy, is currently used by retinoblastoma experts. Others are in-vestigating the role of combining chemother-apy and phototherapy.

Vector-mediated gene therapy is in clinical trial.

REFERENCES

Abramson DH, Greenfield DS, Ellsworth RM: Bilat-eral retinoblastoma: correlations between age at diagnosis and time course for new intraocular tu-mors. *Ophthalmic Paediatr Genet* 1992;13:1–7.

Baud O, Cormier-Daire V, Lyonnet S, et al: Dys-morphic phenotype and neurological impairment in 22 retinoblastoma patients with constitutional cytogenetic 13q deletion. *Clin Genet* 1999;55:478–482.

Bremner R, Du DC, Connolly-Wilson MJ, et al: Dele-tion of RB exons 24 and 25 causes low-penetrance retinoblastoma. *Am J Hum Genet* 1997;61:556–570.

DerKinderen DJ, Koten JW, Wolterbeek R, et al.: Non-ocular cancer in hereditary retinoblastoma survivors and relatives. *Ophthalmic Paediatr Genet* 1987;8:23–25.

Draper GJ, Sanders BM, Brownbill PA, et al: Patterns of risk of hereditary retinoblastoma and applica-tions to genetic counselling. *Br J Cancer* 1992;66:211–219.

Dryja TP, Rapaport J, McGee TL, et al: Molecular etiology of low-penetrance retinoblastoma in two pedigrees. *Am J Hum Genet* 1993;52:1122–1128.

Eng C, Li FP, Abramson DH, et al: Mortality from second tumors among long-term survivors of

retinoblastoma *J Natl Cancer Inst* 1993;85:1121–1128.

Gallie BL, Budning A, DeBoer G, et al: Chemotherapy with focal therapy can cure intraocular retinoblastoma without radiotherapy [published erratum appears in *Arch Ophthalmol* 1997;115: 525]. *Arch Ophthalmol* 1996;114:1321–1328.

Moll AC, Kuik DJ, Bouter LM, et al: Incidence and survival of retinoblastoma in the Netherlands: a register based study 1862–1995. *Br J Ophthalmol* 1997;81:559–562.

Murphree AL: Retinoblastoma. In Traboulsi EI, ed: *Genetic Diseases of the Eye.* New York: Oxford University Press, 1998:813–849.

Roarty JD, McLean IW, Zimmerman LE: Incidence of second neoplasms in patients with bilateral retinoblastoma. *Ophthalmology* 1988;95:1583–1587.

Shields JA, Shields CL, Parsons HM: Differential diagnosis of retinoblastoma. *Retina* 1991;11:232–243.

Wong FL, Boice JD Jr, Abramson DH, et al: Cancer incidence after retinoblastoma: radiation dose and sarcoma risk *JAMA* 1997;278:1262–1267.

RESOURCES

A Parent's Guide to Understanding Retinoblastoma www.retinoblastoma.com/frameset1.htm

For a complete list of centers providing molecular genetic testing for retinoblastoma, go to www. geneclinics.org, sign up as a new user, and search the Web site. This Web site can also be searched for testing for other diseases.

The American Society of Clinical Oncology has issued a statement about genetic testing for susceptibility to cancer. The document can be viewed at www.asco.org/pro/pp/html/m ppgenetic.htm.

Retinoschisis, Juvenile X-Linked

See X-Linked Juvenile Retinoschisis *under* Retinal Dystrophies and Degenerations

Rod Monochromacy

See Achromatopsia *under* Retinal Dystrophies and Degenerations

Rubinstein-Taybi Syndrome

OMIM NUMBER
180849

INHERITANCE
Autosomal dominant

GENE/GENE MAP
16p13.3

cAMP Response Element Binding protein (CREB)–binding protein, a transcription factor

EPIDEMIOLOGY
1 in 700 to 1 in 300 institutionalized individuals

CLINICAL FINDINGS
Patients have characteristic facial features, broad thumbs, great toes, growth retardation, and mental deficiency.

Other clinical findings include high arched palate, delayed closure of the anterior fontanelle,

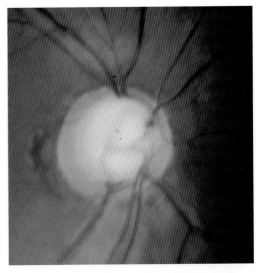

Rubinstein-Taybi syndrome Optic nerve head appearance in Rubinstein-Taybi simulates that of glaucomatous damage or of a colobomatous defect.

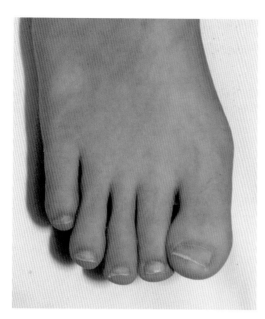

Rubinstein-Taybi syndrome Broad big toe in a patient with Rubinstein-Taybi syndrome.

hirsutism, short stature, and delayed skeletal maturation.

OCULAR FINDINGS

Almost all patients have antimongoloid (downslanting) lid slants. Strabismus is common, and refractive errors are present in 55% of patients.

Occasional patients have cataracts, colobomas of the iris and/or uvea, ptosis, enophthalmos, optic atrophy, and glaucoma.

The optic nerve head is frequently excavated, and its appearance simulates that of glaucomatous damage. Because of the established occurrence of glaucoma in this syndrome, large cups should not be assumed to be due to disc dysplasia; measurements of intraocular pressure are necessary in all patients. Infantile, juvenile, and adult-onset glaucoma have been reported.

In a study of 24 patients with the syndrome,

van Genderen et al. found visual acuity of less than 0.3 (5 patients), nasolacrimal duct problems (6 patients), cataract (6 patients, 4 congenital), and retinal abnormalities (18 patients). Visually evoked potentials showed an abnormal waveform in 15 patients. The electroretinogram was abnormal in 14 of 18 patients.

THERAPEUTIC ASPECTS

Correction of refractive errors and strabismus and screening for glaucoma

REFERENCES

Brei TJ, Burke MJ, Rubinstein JH: Glaucoma and findings simulating glaucoma in the Rubinstein-Taybi syndrome. *J Pediatr Ophthalmol Strabismus* 1995;32:248–252.

Ge N, Crandall BF, Shuler JD, et al: Coloboma associated with Rubinstein-Taybi syndrome. *J Pediatr Ophthalmol Strabismus* 1995;32:266–268.

Petrij F, Giles RH, Dauwerse HG, et al: Rubinstein-Taybi syndrome caused by mutations in the transcriptional co-activator CBP. *Nature* 1995;376:348–351.

Quaranta L, Quaranta CA: Congenital glaucoma associated with Rubinstein-Taybi syndrome. *Acta Ophthalmol Scand* 1998;76:112–113.

Roy FH, Summitt RL, Hiatt RL, et al: Ocular manifestations of the Rubinstein-Taybi syndrome: case report and review of the literature. *Arch Ophthalmol* 1969;79:272–278.

Rubinstein JH: Broad thumb-hallux (Rubinstein-Taybi) syndrome 1957–1988. *Am J Med Genet* 1990;6(suppl):3–16.

Rubinstein JH, Taybi H: Broad thumbs and toes and facial abnormalities. *Am J Dis Child* 1963;105:588–608.

van Genderen MM, Kinds GF, Riemslag FC, Hennekam RC: Ocular features in Rubinstein-Taybi syndrome: investigation of 24 patients and review of the literature. *Br J Ophthalmol* 2000;84:1177–1184.

RESOURCE

Rubinstein-Taybi Syndrome resource site
www.rubinstein-taybi.org

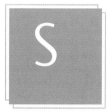

Smith-Lemli-Opitz Syndrome

OMIM NUMBER
270400

INHERITANCE
Autosomal recessive

GENE/GENE MAP
Caused by mutations in the sterol delta-7-reductase gene
11q12–q13

EPIDEMIOLOGY
This is one of the most common autosomal recessive disorders. Most studies in Europe, the United States, and Canada have found an incidence of 1 in 20,000 births. In some regions, the disorder may occur as often as 1 in 10,000 births. The incidence appears to be much lower in Asian and African populations.

CLINICAL FINDINGS
The syndrome affects development before and after birth. It was described in three boys with poor growth, developmental delay, and a pattern of congenital malformations, including cleft palate, genital malformation, and polydactyly. Other clinical abnormalities include microcephaly, low-set ears, small upturned nose, webbing between the second and third toes, abnormal palmar creases (usually single), ambiguous male genitalia with hypospadias and undescended testicles, cataracts, blepharoptosis, heart defects, micrognathia, pyloric stenosis, short thumbs, and Hirschsprung disease.

There is extreme variability of clinical expression, with some children having only one or two minor malformations and others having almost all of the defects listed.

Most patients have failure to thrive, and even children who are vigorous and feed well do not grow normally and tend to be small as children and adults.

At diagnosis, patients typically have cholesterol levels less than 50 mg/dL and abnormally high levels of a precursor of cholesterol, 7-dehydrocholesterol (7DHC). These abnormalities result from abnormally low levels of the enzyme 7DHC-reductase, which converts 7DHC into cholesterol. Carrier testing is now possible by measurement of 7DHC or enzyme levels in cultured cells.

OCULAR FINDINGS
The most common ocular findings include ptosis, epicanthal folds, absence of lacrimal puncta, cataracts, and posterior synechiae.

Occasional findings include photosensitivity, optic pits, choroidal hemangiomas, and pale optic discs.

Cataracts are present in 15% of patients.

Atachaneyasakul et al. evaluated the ophthalmologic findings in eight children and documented abnormal concentrations of cholesterol and cholesterol precursors in the ocular tissues in one patient. Mild to moderate blepharoptosis was found in six of eight patients. None demonstrated cataracts or amblyopia from blepharoptosis. Optic atrophy was found in one patient, and bilateral optic nerve hypoplasia was found in another. Sterol analysis from ocular tissues of an aborted fetus showed increased 7- and 8-DHC and a low cholesterol concentration in the retinal pigment epithelium, lens, cornea, and sclera.

THERAPEUTIC ASPECTS
Death usually occurs in early childhood due to severe psychomotor retardation and the multitude of medical problems associated with this syndrome. Few patients survive past puberty.

With the discovery that patients cannot make adequate amounts of cholesterol, many children and adults with Smith-Lemli-Opitz are being given supplementary cholesterol, either in a natural form, such as egg yolks and cream, or in the form of purified cholesterol given as part of several research protocols. Early results of cholesterol supplementation are encouraging.

REFERENCES

Atachaneyasakul LO, Linck LM, Connor WE, et al: Eye findings in 8 children and a spontaneously aborted fetus with RSH/Smith-Lemli-Opitz syndrome. *Am J Med Genet* 1998;80:501–505.

Kelley RI: RSH/Smith-Lemli-Opitz syndrome: mutations and metabolic morphogenesis [editorial]. *Am J Hum Genet* 1998;63:322–326.

Kretzer FL, Hittner H, Mehta RS: Ocular manifestations of the Smith-Lemli-Opitz syndrome. *Arch Ophthalmol* 1981;99:2000–2006.

Lowry RB: Variability in the Smith-Lemli-Optiz syndrome: overlap with the Meckel syndrome [editorial comment]. *Am J Med Gen* 1983;14:429–433.

Lowry RB, Yong SL: Borderline normal intelligence in the Smith-Lemli-Optiz (RSH) syndrome. *Am J Med Genet* 1980;5:137–143.

Nwokoro NA, Wassif CA, Porter FD: Genetic disorders of cholesterol biosynthesis in mice and humans. *Mol Genet Metab* 2001;74:105–119.

Smith DW, Lemli L, Opitz JM: A newly recognized syndrome of multiple congenital anomalies. *J Pediatr* 1964;64:210–217.

RESOURCES

members.aol.com/slo97/index.html
UNC School of Medicine resource site
www.med.unc.edu/%7Ehwaage/SLO.html

Sphingolipidoses

OVERVIEW

The sphingolipidoses are caused by a deficiency of the lysosomal enzymes necessary for the degeneration of sphingolipids: gangliosides, cerebrosides, and sphingomyelin.

The gangliosides are important constituents of cerebral gray matter. In the brain, they are localized primarily in nerve-ending membranes, with a high content in synaptic membranes. Cerebrosides are found both in the brain and in systemic tissues. Sphingomyelin is an important component of cell membranes.

The defect in sphingolipid catabolism results in the intralysosomal accumulation of sphingolipid breakdown products, which can be identified by electron microscopy as multimembranous inclusion bodies.

OMIM NUMBERS

See Table 22.

INHERITANCE

Autosomal recessive

GENE/GENE MAP

Tay-Sachs disease *HEXA* gene at 15q23–24
Niemann-Pick *SMPD1* gene at 11p15.4–p15.1
Gaucher disease *GBA* gene at 1q21

EPIDEMIOLOGY

Frequent in the Jewish population

CLINICAL FINDINGS

See Table 22.

OCULAR FINDINGS

See also Table 22.

The principal ocular abnormalities are caused by the accumulation of sphingolipids in the retinal ganglion cells, leading to a whitish appearance of the retina. Because there are a large number of ganglion cells in the parafoveal and perifoveal areas, the foveola, which has no ganglion cells, appears reddish, because it allows the normal orange-red color of the choroid and retinal pigment epithelium to be seen. This appearance of the macular area has been termed the *cherry-red spot*.

With atrophy of the ganglion cells, the cherry-red spot may disappear. Ganglion cell dysfunction causes subsequent optic atrophy.

TABLE 22. Sphingolipidoses: Clinical and Ocular Findings

Disease	OMIM Number	Genetic Defect	Clinical Findings	Ocular Findings
Tay-Sachs disease (GM2 gangliosidosis type I)	272800	Subunit A of hexosaminidase A	*See* **Tay-Sachs Disease**	Cherry-red spot
Sandhoff disease (GM2 gangliosidosis type II)	268800	Subunits A and B of hexosaminidase A *HEXB* gene at 5q11	Similar to Tay-Sachs disease	Cherry-red spot
Generalized gangliosidosis (GM1 gangliosidosis type I)	230500	Subunits A, B, and C of beta-galactosidase *GLB1* gene at 3p21.33	Severe cerebral degeneration leading to death within first 2 years of life Accumulation of ganglioside in neurons, in hepatic, splenic, and other histiocytes, and in renal glomerular epithelium Skeletal deformities resembling those of Hurler disease	Cherry-red spot
Gaucher disease	230800	Acid beta-glucosidase	Accumulation of glucosyl ceramide in liver, spleen, and skin Bone marrow is filled with Gaucher cells, resulting in anemia, thrombocytopenia, bleeding, and frequent bone fractures	Some patients have cherry-red spot, and others show whitish subretinal lesions in midperiphery of fundus Patients have peculiar wedge-shaped thickening of bulbar conjunctiva, which, with time, darkens to brownish hue
Niemann-Pick disease type B (chronic Niemann-Pick disease, sea-blue histiocyte syndrome)	257200	Sphingomyelinase	Usually diagnosed in teenage years or early adulthood Although there is no functional involvement of central nervous system, systemic findings include massive hepatosplenomegaly, bony changes, diffuse infiltration of lungs, and foam cell in bone marrow	Macular halo, which is said to be diagnostic
Niemann-Pick disease type A (acute neuronopathic)		Sphingomyelinase		Cherry-red spot in 50% of cases

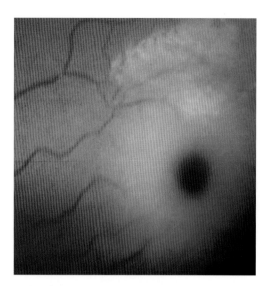

Sphingolipidoses: Tay-Sachs disease Cherry-red spot in a patient with hexosaminidase deficiency.

Interestingly, although there is a block in sphingolipid degradation in both Krabbe disease and Fabry disease, in neither is there a gross accumulation of lipid and neither features a cherry-red spot.

THERAPEUTIC ASPECTS
Not applicable

REFERENCES

None listed

RESOURCES

None listed

Spondyloepiphyseal Dysplasia Congenita

OMIM NUMBER
183900

INHERITANCE
Most cases are isolated

Genetic heterogeneity: autosomal dominant, autosomal recessive

GENE/GENE MAP
Defect in the *COL2A1* gene on 12q13.11–q13.2

EPIDEMIOLOGY
Very rare; fewer than 50 reported cases

CLINICAL FINDINGS
Truncal dwarfism with normal skull, hands, and feet is found.

Radiologic findings are characteristic.

Differential diagnosis includes Morquio syndrome mucopolysaccharidosis-IV (MPS-IV).

OCULAR FINDINGS
Hamidi-Toosi and Maumenee studied the ocular features of 18 patients: 7 had nonprogressive myopia of 5.00 or more diopters; 6 had vitreoretinal degeneration. A liquefied vitreous was present in all patients. Although the original report did not include any patients with retinal detachment, two later developed this complication (I. H. Maumenee, personal communication).

THERAPEUTIC ASPECTS
Routine eye examinations should be performed every 6 months. The retina should be scrutinized for breaks or detachments.

Appropriate management of orthopedic problems is necessary.

REFERENCES

Anderson IJ, Goldberg RB, Marion RW, et al: Spondyloepiphyseal dysplasia congenita: genetic linkage to type II collagen (*COL2A1*). *Am J Hum Genet* 1990;46:896–901.

Hamidi-Toosi S, Maumenee IH: Vitreoretinal degeneration in spondyloepiphyseal dysplasia congenita. *Arch Ophthalmol* 1982;100:1104–1107.

RESOURCES

None listed

Stargardt Disease

See Retinal Dystrophies and Degenerations

Stationary Night Blindness, Nougaret Type

See Retinal Dystrophies and Degenerations

Stickler Syndrome

Also called hereditary arthro-ophthalmopathy
Includes Marshall syndrome

OMIM NUMBERS
108300
604841
184840

INHERITANCE
Autosomal dominant

GENE/GENE MAP
Type I, STL1, is the most common, maps to 12q13.11–q13.2, and is due to mutations in the *COL2A1* gene.

Type II, STL2, maps to 1p21 and is due to mutations in the *COL11A1* gene. Mutations in this gene also cause Marshall syndrome, a condition that bears a close resemblance to Stickler syndrome, with prominent midfacial hypoplasia, a thin calvarium, intracranial calcifications, hearing loss, progressive myopia, cataracts, and a liquefied vitreous. Hence, Marshall syndrome is allelic to STL2.

Type III, STL3, maps to 6p21.3 and is due to mutations in the *COL11A2* gene. It has no ocular manifestations and is not discussed in this section.

There is evidence of at least one additional locus for Stickler syndrome.

EPIDEMIOLOGY
The most common disorders of connective tissue in the United States, they occur in 1 in 10,000 individuals.

Stickler syndrome is distinct from Wagner syndrome, with which it has been confused and associated for a number of decades.

CLINICAL FINDINGS
Patients with the full-fledged syndrome have characteristic ophthalmologic and orofacial features, as well as deafness and degenerative arthropathy.

Nonocular features show great variation in expression. Children typically have a flat midface, with depressed nasal bridge, short nose, anteverted nares, and micrognathia. These features become less pronounced with age. If midline clefting is present, it ranges in severity from a cleft of the soft palate to a Pierre-Robin sequence. There is joint hypermobility, which declines with age. Osteoarthritis develops typically in the third or fourth decade. Mild spondyloepiphyseal dysplasia is often apparent radiologically. Sensorineural deafness, with hightone loss, may be asymptomatic or mild. Occasional findings include slender extremities and long fingers, leading to confusion with Marfan syndrome in some patients. Stature and intellect are generally normal. Mitral valve prolapse was found to be a common finding in one series but not in the author's experience.

Stickler, Hughes, and Houchin sent questionnaires to 612 patients. Of those who returned 316 usable replies, 95% had eye problems (retinal detachment occurred in 60%, myopia in 90%, and blindness in 4%); 84% had problems with facial structures, such as a flat face, small mandible, or cleft palate; 70% had hearing loss; and 90% had joint problems, primarily early joint pain from degenerative joint disease. Treatment included cryotherapy and laser therapy for retinal detachment, repair of cleft palate, use of hearing and mobility aids, and joint replacements. The authors found wide variations in symptoms and signs among affected persons, even within the same family. There were delays in diagnosis, lack of understanding among family members, denial about the risk of serious eye problems, and joint disease.

The majority of families have mutations in the *COL2A1* gene and show the characteristic type 1 or synergetic vitreous phenotype. Patients with the type 2 or beaded vitreous phenotype have mutations in *COL11A1* or other loci yet to be identified. Mutations in *COL11A2* can give rise to a syndrome with the systemic features of Stickler syndrome but no ophthalmologic abnormalities.

The diagnosis of premature syneresis of the vitreous is obvious by slit-lamp examination by age 3 to 4 years in affected individuals. Questions about a family history of arthritis, retinal detachment, cleft palate, and hearing loss should be routine. Hand, hip, elbow, and shoulder X-rays are helpful if the diagnosis is suspected. Diagnostic X-ray findings in childhood consist of mild epiphyseal dysplasia, with widening of the proximal ends of the long bones. In older patients, irregular articular surfaces and other features of degenerative arthritis are present.

OCULAR FINDINGS

Abnormalities of vitreous gel architecture are pathognomonic and are associated with high myopia, which is congenital and nonprogressive in the majority of patients. An optically empty, liquefied vitreous is associated with vitreous veils inserting into the retina in the equatorial region. With time, the region of vitreoretinal adhesion develops a lattice-like degeneration with retinal holes. Radial perivascular lattice degeneration and punched-out areas of depigmentation are common.

There is a substantial risk of spontaneous or postcataract extraction retinal detachment.

Presenile cataracts are common.

Chronic open-angle glaucoma occurs in 5% to 10% of patients.

Rarely, congenital glaucoma can occur.

Subluxation of the lenses is rare.

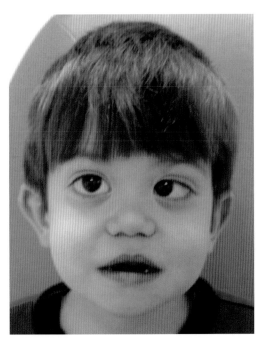

Stickler syndrome Characteristic facial appearance with malar hypoplasia and prominent globes.

THERAPEUTIC ASPECTS

A presumptive diagnosis should be made, and careful periodic retinal examinations should be instituted in persons with premature syneresis of the vitreous, dominant high myopia (with or without retinal detachment), and skeletal dysplasia.

If there has been retinal detachment in one eye, prophylactic cryoretinopexy should be considered for the other eye.

REFERENCES

Annunen S, Korkko J, Czarny M, et al: Splicing mutations of 54-bp exons in the *COL11A1* gene cause Marshall syndrome, but other mutations cause overlapping Marshall/Stickler phenotypes. *Am J Hum Genet* 1999;65:974–983.

Opitz J, France T, Herrmann J, et al: The Stickler syndrome. *N Engl J Med* 1972;286:546.

Shanske AL, Bogdanow A, Shprintzen RJ, et al: The Marshall syndrome: report of a new family and review of the literature. *Am J Med Genet* 1997;70:52–57.

Snead MP, Yates JR: Clinical and molecular genetics of Stickler syndrome. *J Med Genet* 1999;36:353–359.

Stickler GB, Belau PG, Farrell FJ, et al: Hereditary progressive arthro-ophthalmopathy. *Mayo Clin Proc* 1965;40:433–455.

Stickler GB, Hughes W, Houchin P: Clinical features of hereditary progressive arthroophthalmopathy (Stickler syndrome): a survey. *Genet Med* 2001; 3:192–196.

RESOURCES

Stickler Involved People
  www.sticklers.org
Stickler Syndrome Support Group
  www.stickler.org.uk

Sturge-Weber Syndrome

Also called encephalotrigeminal angiomatosis

OMIM NUMBER

185300

INHERITANCE

There is no evidence for an inherited form of the syndrome. It is considered to be one of the phakomatoses.

GENE/GENE MAP

There is one report of an association between a fragile site on chromosome 10 with Sturge-Weber syndrome. This is likely coincidental.

EPIDEMIOLOGY

The true prevalence is unknown. One in 200 individuals are born with a port-wine stain in the United States; it is said that 8% to 15% of them have the syndrome.

CLINICAL FINDINGS

The syndrome consists of facial venous angiomatosis (usually a port-wine stain), with ipsilateral angiomatosis of the leptomeninges.

Eighty percent of patients develop focal or generalized seizures because of central nervous system involvement, 54% are mentally retarded, and 31% have contralateral hemiplegia.

The majority of patients have intracranial calcifications.

The syndrome is presumably caused by the failure of regression of a vascular plexus between the cephalic portion of the neural tube and the ectoderm destined to become the facial skin. The facial nevus usually occurs in the area of distribution of the trigeminal nerve; however, cerebral involvement may be present without the facial port-wine stain. The lesion usually stops along the midline but may cross it. The flat angioma may become nodular or verrucous with age. The port-wine stain does not regress and does not respond to sclerosing agents or topical corticosteroids, but is currently treated cosmetically, with some success, with the carbon dioxide laser.

Macrocephaly has been described as an association.

Data on 52 adults aged 18 to 63 years, ascertained through the Sturge-Weber Foundation, were obtained via written questionnaires, telephone interviews, and reviews of medical records. The distributions of port-wine stains (cranial 98%, extracranial 52%) and the prevalence of glaucoma (60%), seizures (83%), neurologic deficits (65%), and other complications were established. The age of onset of glaucoma (0 to 41 years), the age of onset of seizures (0 to 23 years), and the correlation between the distribution of port-wine stains and the prevalence of seizures was identified. The relationship between the age of onset of seizures and seizure control was established. In patients with and without seizures, the prevalence of developmental delay (43% vs. 0%), emotional and behavioral problems (85% vs. 58%), special education requirements (71% vs. 0%), and employability (46% vs. 78%) were analyzed. Overall, 39% were financially self-sufficient, and 55% were or could be married. Ten participants produced 20 liveborn offspring; 17 were healthy; tuberous sclerosis, a café-au-lait spot, and a "birthmark" were found in 1 child each. The results of this study can be used for genetic counseling.

The Klippel-Trénaunay-Weber syndrome (unilateral or bilateral gigantism) may be seen in association with Sturge-Weber syndrome. It is possible that the two syndromes represent the same basic disorder. Other entities that should be considered are disseminated hemangiomatosis, neurofibromatosis, Beckwith-Wiedemann syndrome, and cutis marmorata telangiectatica congenita. Ocular disorders in the differential diagnosis include Wyburn-Mason syndrome and hereditary hemorrhagic telangiectasia.

The diagnosis should be reserved for patients who, in addition to the facial nevus flammeus, have evidence of intracranial involvement.

Skull X-rays and computed tomography scans may show ipsilateral gyriform calcifications of the cerebral cortex. If these are present, the double contour cortical calcifications are pathognomonic.

The electroencephalogram usually shows abnormalities over the involved hemisphere early in the disease.

OCULAR FINDINGS

Thirty percent of patients develop glaucoma (60% before age 2 years with buphthalmos and 40% in late childhood or young adulthood). Congenital glaucoma is often associated with involvement of the upper lid by the port-wine stain. The glaucoma is most often unilateral, but may rarely be bilateral in bilateral disease or if the angioma crosses the midline. The proposed mechanisms for the development of glaucoma include outflow obstruction because of abnormal angle development and vascularization of the iris; secondary angle closure in older patients with choroidal hemangioma, retinal detachment, and neovascular glaucoma; elevated episcleral pressure with reduced outflow; hypersecretion; hyperpermeability of blood vessel walls in choroidal hemangioma; and adult open-angle glaucoma mechanism.

Although gonioscopy reveals a pattern suggestive of goniodysgenesis, histopathologic studies reveal changes similar to those seen in open-angle glaucoma of elderly individuals.

Choroidal cavernous hemangiomas occur in 40% of patients and may be isolated or diffuse. They are most often located temporal to the optic disc and are most elevated in the macular area. Hemangiomas do not cause any visual disturbances early in life, but may later lead to overlying retinal cystoid changes or exudative retinal detachment.

Retinal venous anastomoses are occasionally present. The visual field frequently shows a homonymous hemianopsia contralateral to the cerebral and facial lesions.

Other ocular findings include heterochromia iridis, conjunctival angioma, dilation of episcleral vessels, and retinal aneurysms associated with an arteriovenous angioma of the thalamus and midbrain.

THERAPEUTIC ASPECTS

Older patients should have a fluorescein angiogram. Argon laser photocoagulation has been used to treat localized choroidal hemangiomas. Goniotomy, trabeculotomy, trabeculectomy, and drainage valved devices have been used in different sequences and combina-

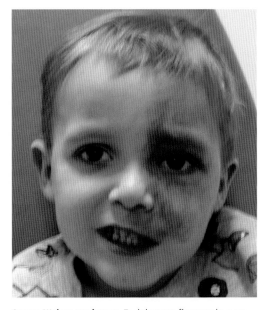

Sturge-Weber syndrome Facial nevus flameus in a patient with Sturge-Weber syndrome.

tions with a reasonable expectation for control of intraocular pressure. Topical medications should be tried before surgical interventions and may be the only therapy needed. Complications of glaucoma surgery in these patients include excessive bleeding, recurrent choroidal effusion, and massive choroid hemorrhage.

Early neurosurgical intervention is indicated if seizures and mental deterioration progress.

Significant neurologic problems may disrupt a normal life. Psychiatric problems are not uncommon.

REFERENCES

Awad AH, Mullaney PB, Al-Mesfer S, et al: Glaucoma in Sturge-Weber syndrome. *J AAPOS* 1999; 3:40–45.

Enjolras O, Riche MC, Merland JJ: Facial port-wine stains and Sturge-Weber syndrome. *Pediatrics* 1985;76:48.

Font RL, Ferry AP: The phakomatoses. *Int Ophthalmol Clin* 1972;12:1–50.

Hamush NG, Coleman AL, Wilson MR: Ahmed glaucoma valve implant for management of glaucoma in Sturge-Weber syndrome. *Am J Ophthalmol* 1999;128:758–760.

Olsen KE, Huang AS, Wright MM: The efficacy of goniotomy/trabeculotomy in early-onset glaucoma associated with the Sturge-Weber syndrome. *J AAPOS* 1998;2:365–368.

Phelps CD: The pathogenesis of glaucoma in Sturge-Weber syndrome. *Trans Am Acad Ophthalmol Otolaryngol* 1978;85:276–286.

Shihab ZM, Kristan RW: Recurrent intra-operative choroidal effusion in Sturge-Weber syndrome. *J Pediatr Ophthalmol Strabismus* 1983;20:250–252.

Sujansky E, Conradi S: Outcome of Sturge-Weber syndrome in 52 adults. *Am J Med Genet* 1995; 57:35–45.

Traboulsi EI, Dudin GE, To'nay KF, et al: The association of a fragile site on chromosome 10 with the Sturge-Weber syndrome and congenital glaucoma. *Ophthalmol Paediatr Genet* 1983;3:135–140.

RESOURCE

The Sturge-Weber Foundation
www.sturge-weber.com

Tay-Sachs Disease

OMIM NUMBER
272800

INHERITANCE
Autosomal recessive

GENE/GENE MAP
Deficient activity of the enzyme hexosaminidase A leads to the accumulation of GM_2 ganglioside in ganglion cells of the brain and retina, with subsequent cell destruction, demyelination, and reactive gliosis.

15q23–q24

EPIDEMIOLOGY
The gene is common in the Jewish population of eastern European origin. The carrier rate among the Jewish population of New York was estimated as 1 in 30 in 1964 versus 1 in 300 among non-Jews.

The disease occurs in all ethnic groups.

Consanguinity is significantly higher among non-Jewish parents of affected children.

CLINICAL FINDINGS
The affected child may be slow to achieve normal milestones in the first year of life. Sounds frequently cause an exaggerated startle response. There is a delayed ability to sit unassisted, and listless behavior and poor head control are seen.

Seizures are common in the first year of life.

Neurologic deterioration is rapid and leads to paralysis, deafness, and blindness by age 3 to 4 years.

During the end stage of the disease, cranial measurements may progressively increase and precocious puberty may develop because of hyperpituitarism.

The diagnosis is difficult to establish during the first 6 months of life by clinical criteria alone. The macular cherry-red spot, hypotonia, and failure to thrive in the absence of hepatosplenomegaly suggest the diagnosis. A definitive diagnosis must be based on demonstration of deficient hexosaminidase A activity in both serum and cultured fibroblasts.

Heterozygote detection and prenatal diagnosis are possible by examining hexosaminidase A levels in amniotic fluid and uncultured amniotic cells.

Other sphingolipidoses with cherry-red spots in the retina include Niemann-Pick disease, metachromatic leukodystrophy, generalized gangliosidosis, and mucolipidosis type I.

OCULAR FINDINGS
A macular cherry-red spot is present by age 3 to 4 months in virtually all children with an enzyme diagnosis of Tay-Sachs disease (see figure under "Sphingolipidoses"). It may be absent, however, during the first 2 months of life.

Blindness occurs by age 1.5 years, and pale discs are noted by age 2 years.

The pupillary reaction may remain normal.

The electroretinogram becomes abnormal late in the disease.

At about 6 months of age, voluntary or exploratory eye movement is lost. Subsequently, in order, there occur loss of following movements, loss of optically elicited movement, and, finally, loss of vestibular movements. In the last stages of the disease, the eyes are invariably deviated downward. Eye movement in this stage can be elicited by horizontal, but not vertical, doll's-head maneuvers.

THERAPEUTIC ASPECTS
Management is supportive only.

Rapid neurologic deterioration leads to paralysis, deafness, and blindness by age 3 to 4 years.

REFERENCES

Jampel RS, Quaglio ND: Eye movements in Tay-Sachs disease. *Neurology* 1964;14:1013–1019.

Kivlin JD, Sanborn GE, Myers GG: The cherry-red spot in Tay-Sachs and other storage diseases. *Ann Neurol* 1985;17:356–360.

Neufeld EF: Natural history and inherited disorders of a lysosomal enzyme, beta-hexosaminidase. *J Biol Chem* 1989;264:10927–10930.

RESOURCE

National Tay-Sachs & Allied Diseases Association www.ntsad.org

Treacher Collins Syndrome

Also called mandibulofacial dysostosis, Franceschetti syndrome

OMIM NUMBER

154500

INHERITANCE

Autosomal dominant. Sixty percent of cases represent new mutations, in which advanced paternal age plays a role. The gene is almost 100% penetrant. There is wide variability in expression of the disorder among family members.

GENE/GENE MAP

Treacle gene (*TCOF1*)
5q32–q33.1

EPIDEMIOLOGY

Prevalence is unknown

CLINICAL FINDINGS

This syndrome represents the most extensive abnormality of the first branchial arch.

Patients have antimongoloid (downslanting) palpebral fissures, mandibular and malar hypoplasia, malformed external ears, and lower-lid colobomas.

Additional findings include macrostomia, malocclusion, high palate, and a high nasal root.

Hair growth patterns are unusual, with tongue-like extensions of hair onto the cheeks. There may be grooves, clefts, or pits on the cheek between the mouth and the ear.

Deafness occurs in almost one-half of patients.

Most patients are of normal intelligence.

There is wide variance in expression of the disorder.

OCULAR FINDINGS

Ophthalmic features are consistent and diagnostic. They include antimongoloid lid slants and lateral lower-lid colobomas, with partial to total absence of the lower eyelashes.

Microphthalmia and defects of the orbital rim are occasionally seen.

THERAPEUTIC ASPECTS

Prognosis for life is not impaired, nor is vision threatened.

Hearing aids are helpful.

Craniofacial and plastic surgery may be of functional and cosmetic benefit.

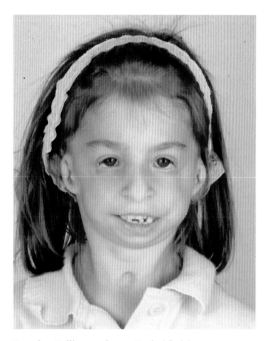

Treacher Collins syndrome Typical facial appearance. Note the lower lid colobomas and hearing aids.

REFERENCES

Cohen MM Jr: Mandibulofacial dysostosis. In: Bergsma D, ed: *Birth Defects Compendium.* 2nd ed. New York: Alan R. Liss, Inc.; 1979:678–679.

Dixon MJ: Treacher Collins syndrome. *Hum Mol Genet* 1996;5:1391–1396.

Edwards SJ, Gladwin AJ, Dixon MJ: The mutational spectrum in Treacher Collins syndrome reveals a predominance of mutations that create a premature-termination codon. *Am J Hum Genet* 1997; 60:515–524.

Franceschetti A, Klein D: *The Mandibulofacial Dysostosis, a New Hereditary Syndrome.* Copenhagen: E. Munksgaard; 1949.

Rovin S, Dachi SF, Borenstein DB, et al: Mandibulofacial dysostosis, a familial study of five generations. *J Pediatr* 1964;65:215–221.

Treacher Collins E: Case with symmetrical congenital notches in the outer part of each lower lid and defective development of the malar bones. *Trans Ophthalmol Soc UK* 1900;20:191–192.

Treacher Collins Syndrome Collaborative Group: Positional cloning of a gene involved in the pathogenesis of Treacher Collins syndrome. *Nat Genet* 1996;12:130–136.

RESOURCES

Reflections on Treacher Collins Syndrome resource site
www.treachercollins.org
Treacher Collins Foundation
www.treachercollinsfnd.org
Treacher Collins Syndrome—A Personal View resource site
www.treachercollins.co.uk

Tuberous Sclerosis

OMIM NUMBERS
191100
191090
191091
191092

INHERITANCE
Autosomal dominant, with a high rate of new mutations and variable expressivity, and with difficulty in detecting mildly affected cases.

GENE/GENE MAP
TSC1 on 9q34; gene product is hamartin.
TSC2 on 16p13; gene product is tuberin.
TSC3 is not localized.
TSC4 is not localized.

EPIDEMIOLOGY
Incidence is estimated at 1 in 7,000 to 1 in 10,000.

CLINICAL FINDINGS
The triad of hamartomatous skin nodules (adenoma sebaceum), seizures, and retinal glial hamartomas is characteristic. Hamartomas are present in multiple organ systems.

The terms *tuberous sclerosis* (potato-like sclerotic lesion) and *adenoma sebaceum* (describing the skin lesions) are inaccurate because the sebaceous glands are not directly involved.

Characteristic amelanotic spots or *ash-leaf* lesions may be present in the skin at birth or appear within the first 2 years of life. These can be accentuated with a Wood's light. The facial rash in the malar distribution is composed of two types of lesions: seed-like reddish angiofibromatous growths and yellow to brown primary fibromatous nodules. In most cases, skin lesions appear in the first 10 years of life. Ash-leaf spots were present in 11 of 18 patients (61%) in one series and in 11 of 71 (15%) in another series. Other skin lesions include shagreen plaques in 21% of patients in one series and 83% in another series. These are confluent areas of skin tumor with a waxy yellowish-brown or flesh-colored appearance. They are most often seen on the forehead, back, or legs. Other lesions include subungual fibromas and longitudinally grooved nails. Seventy-one percent of patients have pits of the tooth enamel, usually on the outer surfaces of the teeth and away from the gingiva.

Neurologic manifestations include epilepsy, learning difficulties, autism, and behavioral problems. Seizures tend to develop early in childhood. The seizures and mental deficiency seem to be related to the extent of the hamartomatous changes in the brain. On neuroimaging, the most typical abnormality is a high-signal lesion involving the cerebral cortex and corresponding to the cortical hamartomas (tubers). Giant-cell astrocytomas of the brain occur in 2% of patients.

Severely affected patients die early from brain or visceral tumors, infections, or status epilepticus. Patients who survive to the third decade tend to be of normal intelligence.

Many patients have renal lesions, usually angiomyolipomas, which can cause hemorrhage into or compression of healthy renal tissue, leading (rarely) to end-stage renal failure. Cysts, polycystic renal disease, and renal carcinoma can also occur.

Cardiac rhabdomyomas are most often asymptomatic. They occur in 43% of patients, mostly in the interventricular septum or ventricular wall.

OCULAR FINDINGS

The characteristic retinal lesion is a retinal hamartoma at the edge of the optic disc or elsewhere in the posterior pole. Hamartomas are present in one-half to two-thirds of patients. Retinal hamartomas are seen mostly in type 2 tuberous sclerosis. They are bilateral in one-third and unilateral in two-thirds. The typical late *mulberry* appearance of the tumor is due to the accumulation of calcium in the hamartoma. One-third of retinal hamartomas are flat or only slightly elevated, have a filmy grayish-white to yellow color, and have indistinct margins. Some lesions become calcified and progress to the mulberry appearance. Tumors are rarely complicated by vitreous hemorrhage or glaucoma, and they never undergo malignant degeneration. Histologically, they are composed of astrocytes with small oval nuclei and long processes; they contain large blood vessels and calcific deposits. The tumors arise from retinal ganglion cells but later involve all retinal layers. The ophthalmoscopic appearance of early astrocytic hamartomas may be similar to that of small retinoblastomas. More common are

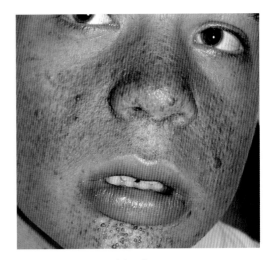

Tuberous sclerosis Facial rash.

achromic lesions of the retinal pigment epithelium. They are more common than hamartomas and are diagnostically significant.

Optic atrophy may occur, and ash-leaf spots of the pigment epithelium may be observed.

Other ocular findings include peripheral depigmented lesions of the retinal pigment epithelium, atypical colobomas, optic atrophy, eyelid angiofibromas, white patches of the iris or eyelashes, and strabismus. Papilledema and sixth nerve palsy may result from hydrocephalus secondary to brain tumors.

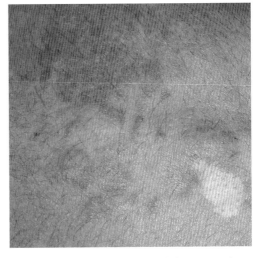

Tuberous sclerosis Ash-leaf spot and shagreen patch.

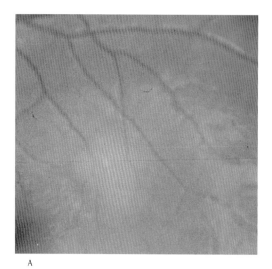

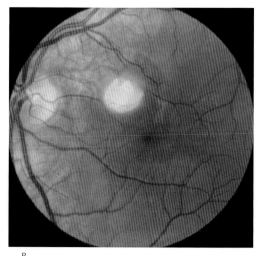

A   B

Tuberous sclerosis Retinal astrocytic hamartoma: (A) early lesions; (B) advanced lesion.

THERAPEUTIC ASPECTS

Seizures are controlled with appropriate medications.

Retinal lesions do not need any specific treatment unless they are complicated by vitreous hemorrhage.

REFERENCES

Dabora SL, Jozwiak S, Franz DN, et al: Mutational analysis in a cohort of 224 tuberous sclerosis patients indicates increased severity of TSC2, compared with TSC1, disease in multiple organs. *Am J Hum Genet* 2001;68:64–80.

Harris-Stith R, Elston DM: Tuberous sclerosis. *Cutis* 2002;69:103–109.

Lygidakis NA, Lindenbaum RH: Pitted enamel hypoplasia in tuberous sclerosis patients and first-degree relatives. *Clin Genet* 1987;32:216–221.

Roach ES, Williams DP, Laster DW: Magnetic resonance imaging in tuberous sclerosis. *Arch Neurol* 1987;44:301–303.

Robertson DM: Ophthalmic manifestations of tuberous sclerosis. *Ann NY Acad Sci* 1991;615:17–25.

Williams R, Taylor D: Tuberous sclerosis. *Surv Ophthalmol* 1985;30:143–154.

RESOURCES

The Tuberous Sclerosis Association
www.tuberous-sclerosis.org
www.ntsa.org

Turner Syndrome

OMIM NUMBERS

Not applicable

INHERITANCE

Part of one or all of one X chromosome is missing.

GENE/GENE MAP

Not applicable

EPIDEMIOLOGY

1 in 2000 to 2500 female newborns

CLINICAL FINDINGS

The common anomalies include short stature, epicanthal folds, low nuchal hairline, shield-like chest, webbed neck, high arched palate, coarctation of the aorta, ventricular septal defect, renal anomalies, pigmented nevi, lymphedema, hypoplastic nails, and inverted nipples.

Patients have a characteristic neurocognitive profile that includes impaired visuospatial/perceptual abilities.

OCULAR FINDINGS

Chrousos et al. examined 30 consecutive patients: 23 had 45XO and 7 had 45XO/46XX karyotypes (mosaicism). Nonfamilial strabismus, the most prominent ocular abnormality, was present in 33% of patients. Other eye findings included ptosis (16%), hypertelorism (10%), epicanthus (10%), and antimongoloid slants (10%). Red-green color deficiency was found in 10%, and one patient had congenital periodic alternating nystagmus.

Rarely reported ocular abnormalities include conjunctival lymphedema, retinal detachment, distichiasis, keratoconus, ocular melanoma, and anterior segment dysgenesis.

Prevalence of X-linked traits such as color vision deficiency is the same as that in males.

THERAPEUTIC ASPECTS

Hormone replacement therapy as needed because of ovarian hypoplasia.

Strabismus and ptosis management is necessary.

REFERENCE

Chrousos GA, Ross JL, Chrousos G, et al: Ocular findings in Turner syndrome: a prospective study. *Ophthalmology* 1984;91:926–928.

RESOURCE

Turner Syndrome Society of the United States
www.turner-syndrome-us.org

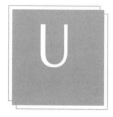

Usher Syndrome

OMIM NUMBERS
See Table 23.

INHERITANCE
Autosomal recessive in all types

GENE/GENE MAP
See Table 23.

EPIDEMIOLOGY
Hallgren estimated the frequency of Usher syndrome to be 3.0 in 100,000 in Scandinavia. According to Boughman et al., the prevalence in the United States is 4.4 in 100,000. The Usher syndromes constitute 2.5% of families with retinitis pigmentosa, and 24% to 54% of deaf-blind persons registered at the Helen Keller National Center for Deaf-Blind Youths and Adults have the syndrome. Thirty percent of deaf French Acadians in Louisiana have Usher syndrome, now identified as type 1C.

There is genetic heterogeneity for USH1 in France. The gene in the families originating from the Poitou-Charentes region in western France (*USH1A*) maps to 14q32. The Acadian variety in Louisiana (*USH1C*) maps to 11p15.1, and the non-Acadian, non-14q variety (*USH1B*) maps to 11q13.5.

CLINICAL FINDINGS
The name *Usher syndrome* encompasses a group of genetically and clinically distinct autosomal recessive conditions in which sensorineural hearing loss is accompanied by a retinal dystrophy indistinguishable from retinitis pigmentosa.

Hallgren reported on 177 patients from 102 families. Most developed cataracts by age 40, one-fourth had mental retardation or psychosis, and a majority had gait disturbances that were attributed to labyrinthine dysfunction.

From their studies of 133 Finnish patients, Forsius et al. concluded that there were two distinct forms of the disease (see Table 24). The criteria for the clinical diagnosis that were adopted by the Usher Syndrome Consortium are given by Smith et al., who stressed the importance of excluding intrauterine infections and perinatal problems that may cause profound hearing loss and retinal damage before making a diagnosis of Usher syndrome.

There is a structural abnormality of the axoneme (a component of ciliated cells, such as photoreceptors, auditory hair cells, and vestibular cells). Weil et al. demonstrated mutations in the gene coding for myosin VIIA, which maps to 11q13.5, in 75% of patients with type 1, suggesting that 75% of type 1 patients are type 1B.

TABLE 23. Usher Syndrome: Genetic Types

Type	OMIM Number	Gene/Gene Map
USH1A	276900	14q32
USH1B	276903	Myosin VIIA 11q13.5
USH1C	605242	Harmonin 11p15.1
USH1D	601067	Cadherin 23 10q21–q22
USH1E	602097	21q21
USH1F	602083	Procadherin 15 10q21–q22
USH1G	606943	SANS 17q24–q25
USH2A	276901	Usherin 1q41
USH2B	276905	3p24.2–p23
USH2C	605472	5q14–q21
USH3A	276902	Clarin 1 3q21–q25

TABLE 24. Usher Syndrome: Clinical Characteristics of Three Main Types

Characteristic	Type 1	Type 2	Type 3
Retinal dystrophy	Present	Present	Present
	Visual loss in first decade	Visual loss in teens	
	Electroretinogram is unrecordable	Electroretinogram is recordable	
Hearing loss	Profound and congenital	Mild and of later onset	Present
Vestibular dysfunction	Present	Absent	Present
Mental retardation	May develop	Absent	Absent
Psychosis	May develop	Absent	Absent
Percentage of all patients	75%	23%	2%

Delayed walking and vestibular dysfunction are characteristic findings in individuals suspected to have Usher syndrome.

OCULAR FINDINGS

Night blindness starts in childhood or the early teens in type 1 and later in types 2 and 3. Central visual acuity is often decreased late in the course of type 1, while it may remain at acceptable levels for a longer period in types 2 and 3.

Ophthalmoscopy reveals findings of typical retinitis pigmentosa, but in many patients and especially early in the course of the disease, the ophthalmoscopic changes may not be pronounced and the pigment migration may be very mild.

The electroretinogram is nonrecordable in type 1 disease, but a waveform may be present in type 2. Seeliger et al. demonstrated substantial timing differences of implicit time measurements between types 1 and 2 and suggested their usefulness as a diagnostic test.

THERAPEUTIC ASPECTS

There is no specific therapy for the visual loss, except for low-vision evaluation and assistance with mobility.

The hearing loss cannot be corrected by middle ear surgery. Patients with mild to moderate hearing loss may benefit from hearing aids, and those with severe hearing loss from cochlear implant surgery, especially those with type 1.

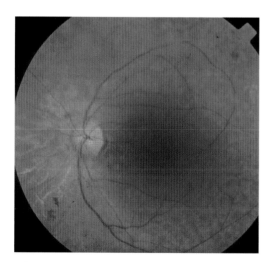

Usher syndrome type 2A (USH2A) Fundus photograph of an adult with Usher type 2. There is widespread peripheral retinal degeneration and bony spicule formation.

REFERENCES

Ahmed ZM, Riazuddin S, Riazuddin S, Wilcox ER: The molecular genetics of Usher syndrome. *Clin Genet* 2003;63:431–444.

Bitner-Glindzicz M, Lindley KJ, Rutland P, et al: A recessive contiguous gene deletion causing infantile hyperinsulinism, enteropathy and deafness identifies the Usher type *1C* gene. *Nat Genet* 2000; 26:56–60.

Boughman JA, Vernon, M, Shaver KA: Usher syndrome: definition and estimate of prevalence from two high-risk populations. *J Chronic Dis* 1983; 36:595–603.

Forsius H, Erikkson A, Nuutila A, et al: A genetic

study of three rare retinal disorders: dystrophia retinae dysacusis syndrome, X-chromosomal retinoschisis and grouped pigments of the retina. *Birth Defects Orig Art Ser* 1971;7:83–98.

Hallgren B: Retinitis pigmentosa combined with congenital deafness; with vestibulo-cerebellar ataxia and mental abnormality in a proportion of cases: a clinical and genetico-statistical study. *Acta Psychiatry Neurol Scand* 1959;138:5–101.

Hunter D, Fishman G, Mehta R, et al: Abnormal sperm and photoreceptor axonemes in Usher's syndrome. *Arch Ophthalmol* 1986;104:385–389.

Kimberling WJ, Orten D, Pieke-Dahl S: Genetic heterogeneity of Usher syndrome. *Adv Otorhinolaryngol* 2000;56:11–18.

Seeliger MW, Zrenner E, Apfelstedt-Sylla E, Jaissle GB: Identification of Usher syndrome subtypes by ERG implicit time. *Invest Ophthalmol Vis Sci* 2001;42:3066—3071.

Smith R, Berlin C, Hejmancik J, et al: Clinical diagnosis of the Usher syndromes. *Am J Med Genet* 1994;50:32–38.

Weil D, Blanchard S, Kaplan J, et al: Defective myosin *VIIA* gene responsible for Usher syndrome type 1B. *Nature* 1995;374:60–61.

Weston MD, Eudy JD, Fujita S, et al: Genomic structure and identification of novel mutations in usherin, the gene responsible for Usher syndrome type IIa. *Am J Hum Genet* 2000;66:1199–1210.

RESOURCES

National Center for the Study and Treatment of Usher Syndrome
www.boystownhospital.org/UsherSyndrome/index.asp

Usher Syndrome hub (resource site)
www.genomelink.org/usher

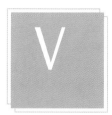

Vitelliform Dystrophy

See Retinal Dystrophies and Degenerations

Vitelliruptive Macular Dystrophy

See Vitelliform Dystrophy *under* Retinal Dystrophies and Degenerations

Vitreoretinopathy with Myelinated Nerve Fibers and Skeletal Findings

OMIM NUMBER
Not listed

INHERITANCE
Autosomal dominant or X-linked

GENE/GENE MAP
Unknown

EPIDEMIOLOGY
Only one family with a mother and daughter reported

CLINICAL FINDINGS
Malformations of the hands and feet in the daughter resembling ectrodactyly

OCULAR FINDINGS
High myopia

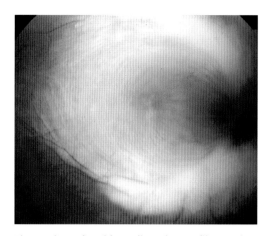

Vitreoretinopathy with myelinated nerve fibers and skeletal findings Fundus photograph of a young woman with this syndrome.

Vitreous and retinal degeneration with night blindness
Extensive bilateral myelinated nerve fibers
Vitreous cyst in the mother
Electroretinogram severely attenuated

THERAPEUTIC ASPECTS
Correct the error of refraction.
Rehabilitate the orthopedic deformity.

REFERENCE

Traboulsi EI, Lim JI, Pyeritz R, et al: A new syndrome of myelinated nerve fibers, vitreoretinopathy and skeletal malformations. *Arch Ophthalmol* 1993; 111:1543–1545.

RESOURCES
None listed

Von Hippel-Lindau Disease

OMIM NUMBER
193300

INHERITANCE
Autosomal dominant with incomplete penetrance

GENE/GENE MAP
Tumor-suppressor gene
3p26–p25

EPIDEMIOLOGY
1 in 40,000 births in Europe

CLINICAL FINDINGS
Retinal angiomas tend to appear before the third decade of life.

Cerebellar signs from cystic hemangioblastomas in the cortical area of the cerebellum occur in 35% to 75% of patients and are diagnosed in the second to fourth decade of life.

Hemangioblastomas can be found in the spinal cord or in the brain and may become calcified.

Other clinical symptoms include seizures and ataxia.

Cherry hemangiomas of the face, liver, lung, and adrenal gland are occasionally present.

Renal cell carcinoma is clinically evident in one-third of patients and most often presents as hematuria, obstructive nephropathy, or an abdominal mass. It tends to be the last of the major manifestations of the disease to appear.

Pheochromocytoma occurs in less than 10% of patients, is usually symptomatic, and is mutation-specific. Polycythemia occurs in 10% to 25% of patients; its cause is obscure.

Diagnostic workup includes a dilated fundus examination, careful history, and neurologic examination.

Neuroimaging is necessary to identify intracranial tumors.

If the diagnosis is established, a search for other tumors is initiated. Polycythemia or paroxysmal hypertension may result from either a cerebellar tumor or a pheochromocytoma.

The differential diagnosis includes Wyburn-Mason syndrome (arteriovenous aneurysms of the retina and midbrain).

OCULAR FINDINGS
Retinal hemangioblastomas are histologically identical to lesions found in the central nervous system.

Between 45% and 59% of patients have retinal tumors; about 50% are bilateral. These tumors have been diagnosed in 1- and 2-year-olds, but only about 5% are discovered before age 10. New lesions may develop at 2-year intervals, so frequent monitoring is important.

Histologically, hemangioblastomas are composed of vascular channels lined by cuboidal endothelial cells. Foamy stromal cells and pericytes comprise the remainder of the tumors. The lesions are usually peripheral in the retina but can involve the optic disc or ora serrata directly. A dilated feeding artery and vein are typically present, and microaneurysms can be seen. Very small peripheral angiomas can also be present but are not diagnostic. Early lesions take the form of small capillary clusters. Advanced lesions are globular, raised, pink, fed by a dilated tortuous arteriole, and drained by a dilated venule. Lipid exudation may develop around the lesion or distantly around the disc or in the macula. Exudative retinal detachment, neovascularization, rubeosis, or phthisis bulbi may ensue. The clinical course of untreated lesions is variable, with some causing no visual impairment and others leading to blindness and enucleation.

THERAPEUTIC ASPECTS
Photocoagulation, cryotherapy, and diathermy are more successful in small lesions. Treatment of larger tumors may be complicated by retinal detachment, retinal tears, vitreous hemorrhage, and neovascularization.

Argon laser burns are applied directly to the surface of lesions measuring less than 2.5 disc diameters in diameter.

Cryotherapy is useful in slightly larger tumors, in anteriorly located tumors, and in eyes with semiopaque media. Combined laser therapy and cryopexy may be necessary for larger tumors.

Diathermy with or without a scleral buckle may be used in larger tumors.

The prognosis for good vision is guarded even with appropriate diagnosis and treatment, except for tumors on the optic disc. Patients must be continually scrutinized for the presence of associated malignancies.

The disease is often lethal, with cerebellar hemangioblastoma and renal cell carcinoma being the most common causes of death.

When an individual is identified with this disease, a geneticist should be consulted to coordinate the various tests needed to completely evaluate the proband and to detect asymptomatic carriers among other family members. A database that includes the data on each family member, as well as reminders about testing dates and results, is useful.

Patients should know that some forms of genetic testing are now available. If the genetic test is successful in excluding the disease (with 99% certainty), only occasional screening is needed. If the genetic test is not definitive, the discovery of the disease may depend on imaging and ophthalmologic testing, which must be continued to at least age 60. Testing can be performed for specific genetic mutations.

For patients known to carry the gene or for patients at risk for the disease, a number of screening regimens employing clinical laboratory, imaging, and ophthalmoscopic tests have been proposed. All screening protocols require periodic testing throughout most, if not all, of

the patient's life. Any new symptoms should be studied immediately, without waiting for the next scheduled test.

Two support groups have been formed in the United States and are good sources of information for patients and for health care professionals involved with treatment of the disease (see Resources below). Affiliated chapters are forming in many other countries.

Two DNA testing laboratories are available (see Resources below).

REFERENCES

Annesley WH, Leonard BC: Fifteen year review of treated cases of retinal angiomatosis. *Trans Am Acad Ophthalmol Otolaryngol* 1977;83:446–453.

Choyke PL, Glenn GM, Walther MM, et al: Von Hippel-Lindau disease: genetic, clinical and imaging features. *Radiology* 1995;146:629–642. And for a complete text: http://www.cc.nih.gov/ccc/papers/vonhip/toc.html

Fearon ER: Human cancer syndromes: clues to the origin and nature of cancer. *Science* 1997;278: 1043–1050.

Gass JD: Treatment of retinal vascular anomalies. *Trans Am Acad Ophthalmol Otolaryngol* 1977;83: 432–442.

Goldberg MF, Duke JR: von Hippel-Lindau disease: histopathologic findings in a treated and untreated eye. *Am J Ophthalmol* 1968;66:693–705.

Hes F, Zewald R, Peeters T, et al: Genotype–phenotype correlations in families with deletions in the von Hippel-Lindau (VHL) gene. *Hum Genet* 2000; 106:425–431.

Latif F, Tory K, Gnarra J, et al: Identification of the von Hippel-Lindau disease tumor suppressor gene. *Science* 1993;260:317–1320.

Lindau A: Studien ueber Kleinhirnsystem: bon Pathogenese und Beziehungen zur ecngiomatosis retinae. *Acta Pathol Microbiol Scand* 1926(suppl);1:1.

Welch RB: Von Hippel-Lindau disease: the recognition and treatment of early angiomatosis retinae and the use of cryosurgery as an adjunct to therapy. *Trans Am Ophthalmol Soc* 1970;68:367–424.

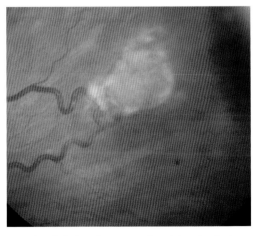

Von Hippel-Lindau disease Small peripheral retinal angioma with a feeder arteriole and draining venule.

RESOURCES

DNA Diagnostics Laboratory
    Center for Medical Genetics
    Johns Hopkins University
    Baltimore, MD 21205
    410-955-0483

Genetic Diagnostic Referral Center
  University of Pennsylvania School of Medicine
  Department of Genetics
  Philadelphia, PA 19104-6145
  215-573-9161
  Fax: 215-573-7760
VHL Family Alliance
  171 Clinton Rd.
  Brookline, MA 02146
  617-232-5946
  800-767-4VHL
  vhl@pipeline.com
  www.vhl.org

Von Hippel Lindau Syndrome Foundation
  35 Beaverson Blvd.
  Building 2, Suite B
  Brick, NJ 08723
  908-262-9708
  Voice mail: 908-244-7635

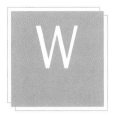

Waardenburg Syndrome

OMIM NUMBERS
193500 for type I
193510 for type IIA
600193 for type IIB

INHERITANCE
Autosomal dominant

GENE/GENE MAP
Mutations in *PAX3* on 2q35 cause type I
Mutations in *MITF* on 3p14–3p12.3 cause type IIA
Gene for type IIB maps to 1p21–p13.3
There is a paternal age effect for new mutations.
Germ-line mosaicism may occur.

EPIDEMIOLOGY
Type I occurs in 1 in 40,000 live births.

CLINICAL FINDINGS
The three features most commonly associated with type I are lateral displacement of the medial canthi, white forelock, and sensorineural deafness.

Freckles on the face and premature graying of the hair are frequent.

In a review of 1285 cases, Hageman and Delleman defined two types of Waardenburg syndrome: type I with dystopia canthorum (lateral displacement of inner canthi) and type II without this manifestation. There is a tendency in many patients for the nasal root to be broad and for the eyebrows to flare medially. Deafness is found in 20% of affected individuals. The characteristic pigmentary abnormalities are a white forelock, with or without hypoplastic pale-blue irides. Unilateral or sector heterochromia of the iris may be present. Other expressions of the pigmentary abnormalities include vitiligo.

Congenital deafness is the most serious feature of the disease and, when present, is usually bilateral and severe. Variants of the syndrome have been described. Bard reported affected patients in three generations of one family who had ocular albinism characterized by foveal hypoplasia and iris transillumination and who lacked lateral displacement of the medial canthi. Shah et al. reported 12 neonates in five families in which a white forelock and white eyebrows and eyelashes were associated with intestinal obstruction, later proved by biopsy to be long-segment Hirschsprung disease. Eight of the 12 patients had heterochromatic irides, but none of six in whom it was sought had dystopia canthorum or a broad nasal root.

DeStefano et al. assessed the relationship between phenotype and gene defect in 48 families containing 271 individuals with the syndrome collected by members of the Waardenburg Consortium. They grouped the 42 unique mutations previously identified in the *PAX3* gene in these families into five mutation categories:
1. Amino acid substitution in the paired domain
2. Amino acid substitution in the homeodomain
3. Deletion of the ser-thr-pro-rich region
4. Deletion of the homeodomain and the ser-thr-pro-rich region
5. Deletion of the entire gene

This classification of mutations was based on the structure of *PAX3* and was chosen to group mutations predicted to have similar defects in the gene product. DeStefano et al. found that the odds for the presence of eye pigment abnormality, white forelock, and skin hypopigmentation were two, eight, and five times greater, respectively, for individuals with deletions of the homeodomain and the ser-thr-pro-rich region compared to individuals with an amino acid substitution in the homeodomain. Odds ratios that differed significantly from 1.0 for these traits may indicate that the gene products resulting from different classes of mutations act differently in the expression of the syndrome. Although a suggestive association was detected for hearing loss with an odds ratio of 2.6 for amino acid substitution in the paired domain compared with the homeodomain, this odds ratio did not differ significantly from 1.0.

Mutations in *MITF*, another transcription factor, are responsible for type II. *MITF* transactivates the gene for tyrosinase and is critically involved in melanocyte differentiation. Absence of melanocytes affects hearing function in the cochlea and pigmentation in the skin, hair, and eyes. Therefore, hypopigmentation and hearing loss in type II are likely to be the result of an anomaly of melanocyte differentiation caused by *MITF* mutations. However, the molecular mechanism by which *PAX3* mutations cause the auditory-pigmentary symptoms in types I and III have not been explained. Watanabe et al. showed that *PAX3* transactivates the *MITF* promoter. They further showed that *PAX3* proteins associated with type I in either the paired domain or the homeodomain failed to recognize and transactivate the *MITF* promoter. These results provided evidence that *PAX3* directly regulates *MITF* and suggested that the failure of this regulation due to *PAX3* mutations causes the auditory-pigmentary symptoms in at least some individuals with type I.

In a personally studied series of 81 individuals from 21 families with type II in comparison with 60 personally studied patients from 8 families with type I, Liu et al. concluded that sensorineural hearing loss (77%) and heterochromia iridis (47%) were more common in type II than in type I. On the other hand, white forelock and skin patches were more frequent in type I.

Reynolds et al. reviewed their collection of 26 type I and 8 type II families. Deafness was more frequent and more severe in the type II individuals than had been found previously. No one in either group had neural tube defects or cleft lip and/or palate. However, 12 individuals in five families had some signs or symptoms of Hirschsprung megacolon. Their data led the authors to conclude that use of the W index to discriminate between affected type I and type II individuals may be problematic since (1) ranges of W-index scores of affected and unaffected individuals overlapped considerably within both type I and type II families, and (2) a considerable number of both affected and unaffected type II individuals exhibited W-index scores consistent with dystopia canthorum.

Hughes et al. found that whereas some families with type II are linked to DNA markers at 3p14.1–3p12.3 (type IIA, 193510), other families do not show this linkage, indicating the existence of at least one other form of type II, designated type IIB. In general, type II shows autosomal dominant inheritance, sensorineural hearing loss, heterochromia iridis, white forelock, and early graying. Unlike type I, type II shows no dystopia canthorum or facial dysmorphism and does not show linkage to 2q35 or mutation in the *PAX3* gene. To evaluate the presence or absence of dystopia canthorum, a critical differential feature of types I and II, Hughes et al. used the average W index in all affected members of the family. A W value less than 1.95 was taken as evidence of no dystopia. The W index was proposed by Arias and Mota.

Type IIB maps to 1p21–p13.3. Type IIA maps to chromosome 3 and is due to mutations in the microphthalmia-associated transcription factor (*MITF*; OMIM 156845).

Looking for locus heterogeneity, Farrer et al. typed microsatellite markers within and flanking *PAX3* in 41 type I kindreds and 26 type II kindreds (defined on the basis of the presence or absence of dystopia canthorum according to the W index of patients). Evaluation of heterogeneity in location scores obtained by zmultilocus analysis indicated that in 60% of all families and in 100% of type I families, the syndrome was linked to *PAX3*. None of the type II families was linked to *PAX3*.

The diagnosis is often made on first observation of the patient or during the slit-lamp examination, when telecanthus is noted to be associated with some of the other features of the disorder.

The white forelock has been noted at birth but may disappear in the first year of life.

Definite segmental or total heterochromia first becomes apparent in Caucasians at 3 to 6 months of age, but a definite statement about the presence or absence of heterochromia in infants should be delayed until after the end of the first year of life.

Normal values for intercanthal and interpupillary distances for infants have not been reported. In an infant with the syndrome, Feingold et al. reported the following measurements at age 3.5 months: medial intercanthal distance (MID): 26 mm, interpupillary distance (ID): 42 mm; at age 6 months: 27 mm MID, 44 mm ID; and at age 1 year: 27 mm MID, 48 mm ID.

The differential diagnosis includes congenital Horner syndrome due to damage of the cervical sympathetic nerves. Other causes of congenital deafness should be considered, especially in the absence of associated white forelock or telecanthus. The diagnosis is suspected if there is no lateral displacement of the inner canthi. Klein syndrome is another hypopigmentation disorder with congenital sensorineural deafness. Waardenburg syndrome is differentiated from Klein syndrome by the absence of arthromyodysplasia, from pseudo-Waardenburg syndrome by the absence of synkinetic ptosis, and from the dominantly inherited piebald trait by the absence of ataxia and mental retardation and the presence of heterochromia.

OCULAR FINDINGS

The diluted iris stromal pigmentation in the heterochromia may be bilateral and total, unilateral and total, or segmental either bilaterally or unilaterally.

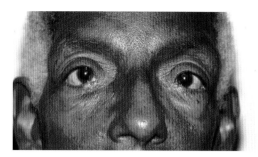

Waardenburg syndrome Telecanthus and premature graying of the hair in a black patient with Waardenburg syndrome type I.

Segmental or total depigmentation of the choroid frequently follows the distribution of the hypopigmentation in the iris, although this is by no means invariably true.

Vision is not reduced, as might be seen in ocular albinism.

Transillumination of the iris is also not a usual feature.

The lacrimal puncta characteristically rest against clear cornea in this disorder because of the lateral displacement of the medial canthi. As a result of the displacement, true telecanthus exists in most these patients. The estimated penetrance for the canthal dystopia is 0.75 for each affected individual.

THERAPEUTIC ASPECTS

The syndrome is consistent with good vision.

A hearing aid may be helpful for individuals with hearing impairment.

The ocular prognosis is excellent.

In some patients, the hair may become white or gray early in life.

REFERENCES

Arias S, Mota M: Apparent non-penetrance for dystopia in Waardenburg syndrome type I, with some hints on the diagnosis of dystopia canthorum. *J Genet Hum* 1978;26:103–131.

Bard LA: Heterogeneity in Waardenburg's syndrome. Report of a family with ocular albinism. *Arch Ophthalmol* 1978;96:1193–1198.

Delleman JW, Hageman MJ: Ophthalmological findings in 34 patients with Waardenburg syndrome. *J Pediatr Ophthalmol Strabismus* 1978;15:341–345.

DeStefano AL, Cupples LA, Amos KS, et al: Correlation between Waardenburg syndrome phenotype and genotype in a population of individuals with identified *PAX3* mutations. *Hum Genet* 1998; 102:499–506.

Farrer LA, Amos KS, Asher JH Jr, et al: Locus heterogeneity for Waardenburg syndrome is predictive of clinical subtypes. *Am J Hum Genet* 1994; 55:728–737.

Feingold M, Robinson MJ, Gellis SS: Waardenburg's syndrome during the first year of life. *J Pediatr* 1967;7l:874–876.

Goldberg MF: Waardenburg's syndrome with fundus and other anomalies. *Arch Ophthalmol* 1966; 76:797–810.

Hageman MJ, Delleman JW: Heterogeneity in Waardenburg syndrome. *Am J Hum Genet* 1977;29: 468–485.

Hughes AE, Newton VE, Liu XZ, et al: A gene for Waardenburg syndrome type 2 maps close to the human homologue of the microphthalmia gene at chromosome 3p12–p14.1. *Nat Genet* 1994;7:509–512.

Lalwani AK, Mhatre AN, San Augustin TB, et al: Genotype–phenotype correlations in type 1 Waardenburg syndrome. *Laryngoscope* 1996;106:895–902.

Liu XZ, Newton VE, Read AP: Waardenburg syndrome type II: phenotypic findings and diagnostic criteria. *Am J Med Genet* 1995;55:95–100.

Pantke OA, Cohen MM Jr: The Waardenburg syndrome. *Birth Defects* 1971;7:147–152.

Reynolds JE, Meyer JM, Landa B, et al: Analysis of variability of clinical manifestations in Waardenburg syndrome. *Am J Med Genet* 1995;57:540–547.

Shah KN, Dalal SJ, Desai MP, et al: White forelock, pigmentary disorder of the iris, and long segment Hirschsprung disease: possible variant of Waardenburg syndrome. *J Pediatr* 1981;99:432–435.

Waardenburg PJ: A new syndrome combining developmental anomalies of the eyelids, eyebrows and nose root with pigmentary defects of the iris and head hair and with congenital deafness. *Am J Hum Genet* 1951;3:195–253.

Watanabe A, Takeda A, Ploplis B, et al: Epistatic relationship between Waardenburg syndrome genes *MITF* and *PAX3*. *Nat Genet* 1998;18:283–286.

RESOURCE

Hereditary Hearing Loss Homepage
dnalab-www.uia.ac.be/dnalab/hhh

Wagner Disease

OMIM NUMBER
143200

INHERITANCE
Autosomal dominant

GENE/GENE MAP
WGN1
5q13–14

EPIDEMIOLOGY
Very rare

CLINICAL FINDINGS
See Ocular Findings.

OCULAR FINDINGS
In 1938, Wagner reported 13 members in two generations of a Swiss family. They were reexamined and revisited by Bohringer in 1959, Ricci in 1961, and Maumenee in the 1980s. The family was last revisited by Graemiger et al. in 1995. They examined 60 members of one family, 28 of whom were affected. The most consistent finding was an empty vitreous cavity, with avascular strands or veils.

Chorioretinal atrophy and cataracts increased with age and occurred in all patients over age 45.

Four patients had a history of a rhegmatogenous retinal detachment in one eye, which occurred at a median age of 20 years.

Peripheral traction retinal detachments were found in 55% of eyes among patients older than 45 years.

Glaucoma was present in 10 eyes (18%), in 4 of which the glaucoma was neovascular in nature.

Sixty-three percent of patients had elevated rod and cone thresholds on dark adaptation, and 87% showed subnormal b-wave amplitudes of the rod and cone systems on electroretinography. Thus, clinical expressivity of the disorder varied from unaffected carriers to bilateral blindness. Progression of the chorioretinal pathology was paralleled by electrophysiologic abnormalities.

Erosive vitreoretinopathy is allelic to Wagner disease and maps to the same gene locus. Both disorders are distinct from *COL2A1*-associated Stickler syndrome.

THERAPEUTIC ASPECTS

Patients should be monitored for retinal breaks and detachments, with frequent dilated fundus examinations.

Retinal breaks should be treated prophylactically.

Cataracts should be extracted if they impair vision significantly.

Genetic counseling should be recommended.

REFERENCES

Brown DM, Graemiger RA, Hergersberg M, et al: Genetic linkage of Wagner disease and erosive vitreoretinopathy to chromosome 5q13–14. *Arch Ophthalmol* 1995;113:671–675.
Graemiger RA, Niemeyer G, Schneeberger SA, et al: Wagner vitreoretinal degeneration: follow-up of the original pedigree. *Ophthalmology* 1995;102:1830–1839.
Maumenee IH, Stoll HU, Mets MB: The Wagner syndrome versus hereditary arthroophthalmopathy. *Trans Am Ophthalmol Soc* 1982;80:349–365.
Wagner H: Ein bisher unbekanntes Erbleiden des Auges (degeneratio hyaloideo-retinalis hereditaria), beobachtet im Kanton Zurich. *Klin Monatsbl Augenheilkd* 1938;100:840–858.

RESOURCES
None listed

WAGR Syndrome

WAGR = *W*ilms' tumor, *A*niridia, *G*enitourinary abnormalities, and mental *R*etardation

OMIM NUMBER
194702

INHERITANCE
Contiguous gene syndrome

GENE/GENE MAP
Deletion of 11p13

EPIDEMIOLOGY
No good data available

CLINICAL FINDINGS
Turleau et al. reported three patients with the 11p/aniridia complex and reviewed 37 cases from the literature. They found the following:

1. There were twice as many affected males as females.
2. The chromosome rearrangements were extremely variable and included familial insertions, translocations, and interstitial deletions.
3. Aniridia appeared to be the only constant clinical feature of the complex.
4. Tumors developed in about one-third of cases.
5. Genital abnormalities were present in the majority of male patients and included cryptorchidism, hypospadias, and abnormalities of internal organs.
6. Mental retardation was a constant feature of the complex but was variable in severity.
7. Growth retardation was present in 9 of 14 reliable observations.
8. Additional malformations were rare and included renal abnormalities, tetralogy of Fallot, microcephaly, and polydactyly.

In addition to aniridia, genitourinary malformations (resulting in ambiguous genitalia in male patients), mental retardation, and Wilms' tumor, patients with 11p13 deletion syndrome have rather characteristic dysmorphic facial features, with a long narrow face, high nasal root, ptosis, small palpebral fissures, and low-set, poorly lobulated ears.

OCULAR FINDINGS
See **Aniridia.**

THERAPEUTIC ASPECTS
Patients with sporadic aniridia require karyotyping to look for deletions of 11p13, especially if other malformations or mental retardation is present.

REFERENCES

Fryns J, Beirinckx J, DeSutter E, et al: Aniridia-Wilms' tumor association and 11p interstitial deletion. *Eur J Pediatr* 1981;136:91–92.

Turleau C, de Grouchy J, Tournade MF, et al: Del 11p/aniridia complex: report of three patients and review of 37 observations from the literature. *Clin Genet* 1984;26:356–362.

RESOURCE

International WAGR Syndrome Association
www.wagr.org

Weill-Marchesani Syndrome

OMIM NUMBER
277600

INHERITANCE
Autosomal recessive with partial expression in heterozygotes in most cases

An autosomal dominant form exists that is allelic to Marfan syndrome

GENE/GENE MAP
The recessive form maps to 19p13.3–p13.2 and is due to mutations in the ADAMTS10 gene that codes for a disintegrin and metalloprotease with thrombospondin motifs.

A 24 nt in-frame deletion within a latent transforming growth factor-β1 binding protein (LTBP) motif of the fibrillin-1 gene was found in an autosomal dominant (AD) Weill-Marchesani syndrome family (exon 41, 5074-5097del).

This deletion cosegregated with the disease and was not found in 186 controls.

EPIDEMIOLOGY
1 in 100,000 individuals

CLINICAL FINDINGS
The presence of dislocated lenses and congenital short stature, with stubby spade-like hands and feet, is needed to permit a diagnosis.

OCULAR FINDINGS
The lens is 6.5 to 7.5 mm in diameter and tends to move anteriorly, resulting in a shallow anterior chamber and pupillary-block glaucoma. Dislocation into the anterior chamber is possible.

Glaucoma is a frequent accompanying finding and is probably due to pupillary block and the formation of peripheral anterior synechiae.

High myopia most frequently results from an anteriorly displaced round lens.

THERAPEUTIC ASPECTS
Pupillary block requires a peripheral iridectomy or lens extraction. Mydriatics are preferred to miotics. In one series, glaucoma was controlled in six of seven eyes after lens extraction. Frequent monitoring for the presence of glaucoma is mandatory. The author has successfully

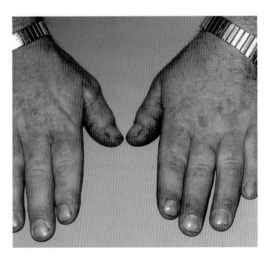

Weill-Marchesani syndrome Brachydactyly (short, stubby fingers) in this man with Weill-Marchesani syndrome.

performed trabeculectomies without removal of the lens in one patient with this condition.

Patients have a normal life span and intelligence, but the visual prognosis may be poor.

REFERENCES

Dagonneau N, Benoist-Lasselin C, Huber C, et al: ADAMTS10 mutations in autosomal recessive Weill-Marchesani syndrome. *Am J Hum Genet* 2004;75:801–806.

Faivre L, Gorlin RJ, Wirtz MK, et al: In frame fibrillin-1 gene deletion in autosomal dominant Weill-Marchesani syndrome. *J Med Genet* 2003;34–36.

Faivre L, Megarbane A, Alswaid A, et al: Homozygosity mapping of a Weill-Marchesani syndrome locus to chromosome 19p13.3–p13.2. *Hum Genet* 2002;110:366–370.

Jensen AD, Cross HE, Paton D: Ocular complications in the Weill-Marchesani syndrome. *Am J Ophthalmol* 1974;77:261-269.

Kloepfer HW, Rosenthal JW: Possible genetic carriers in the spherophakia-brachymorphia syndrome. *Am J Hum Genet* 1955;7:398–419.

Megarbane A, Mustapha M, Bleik J, et al: Exclusion of chromosome 15q21.1 in autosomal-recessive Weill-Marchesani syndrome in an inbred Lebanese family. *Clin Genet* 2000;58:473–478.

Rennert OM: The Marchesani syndrome: a brief review. *Am J Dis Child* 1969;117:703–705.

Wirtz MK, Samples JR, Kramer PL, et al: Weill-Marchesani syndrome: possible linkage of the autosomal dominant form to 15q21.1. *Am J Med Genet* 1996;65:68–75.

RESOURCE

Coalition for Heritable Disorders of Connective Tissue
382 Main St.
Port Washington, NY 11050
516-883-8712
800-862-7326
c/o Priscilla Ciccariello

Williams Syndrome

OMIM NUMBER
194050

INHERITANCE
Autosomal dominant

GENE/GENE MAP

Mutations in the elastin gene are responsible for the disorder in a majority of cases. LIM kinase-1 (*LIMK1*) has also been implicated in the pathogenesis of this disease, and hemizygosity for the *LIMK1* gene has been proposed as the basis for impaired visuospatial constructive cognition in this disorder.

7q11.2

EPIDEMIOLOGY
Frequency is 1 in 10,000 newborns

CLINICAL FINDINGS

The full-blown form of the syndrome includes supravalvular aortic stenosis, multiple peripheral pulmonary arterial stenoses, elfin face, mental and statural deficiency, characteristic dental malformation, and infantile hypercalcemia.

A wide variation in the presence and severity of clinical features is characteristic.

OCULAR FINDINGS

Holmstrom et al. examined external eye photographs of 43 children with the syndrome and 124 control subjects. A stellate pattern was noted in the irides of 51% of the Williams pa-

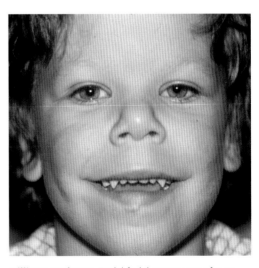

Williams syndrome Typial facial appearance of a patient with Williams syndrome.

tients and 12% of controls. The pattern was easier to detect in lightly pigmented irides.

In a study of 152 patients, Winter et al. found that 54% had strabismus and almost all had esotropia. In Europeans, blue irides were present in 77%, green in 7%, and brown in 16%. A typical stellate iris pattern of the anterior stroma was found in three-fourths of patients. Wolfflin-Krichmann whitish spots were also detected in brown irides. Retinal vascular tortuosity was found in 22% of patients, and three patients had cataracts. There were no ocular abnormalities that could be attributed to hypercalcemia.

THERAPEUTIC ASPECTS

Esotropia and amblyopia are treated as appropriate with surgery and patching.

REFERENCES

Holmstrom G, Almond G, Temple K, et al: The iris in Williams syndrome. *Arch Dis Child* 1990;65: 987–989.

Winter M, Pankau R, Amm M, et al: The spectrum of ocular features in the Williams-Beuren syndrome. *Clin Genet* 1996;49:28–31.

RESOURCE

Williams Syndrome Association
P.O. Box 297
Clawson, MI 48017-0297
248-541-3630
Fax: 248-541-3631
TMonkaba@aol.com
www.williams-syndrome.org

Wilson Disease

OMIM NUMBER
277900

INHERITANCE
Autosomal recessive

GENE/GENE MAP
ATPB7
3q14.3–q21.1

EPIDEMIOLOGY
1 in 30,000 individuals worldwide, with a gene frequency of 0.56% and a carrier frequency of 1 in 90

Prevalence is higher in Sardinia, where 10 to 12 new cases are identified each year.

CLINICAL FINDINGS
The main manifestations of the disease are related to liver and basal ganglia dysfunction. Patients have neurologic manifestations, such as chorea, spasticity, dysarthria, dystonia, flapping intention tremor, and complications of cirrhosis.

There is no mental retardation.

Deteriorating handwriting and speech are often first noted in school.

There is low serum ceruloplasmin, which functions in enzymatic transfer of copper to copper-containing enzymes such as cytochrome oxidase.

Hypercalciuria and nephrocalcinosis are common. Hypercalciuria may lead to renal stone formation and may be due to a tubular defect in calcium reabsorption. It can be treated with penicillamine.

There appear to be racial/geographic differences in age of onset and severity of the disease, with Eastern European Jewish patients having a later onset and milder disease.

Three forms appear to exist in Canada: Slavic, juvenile, and German-Mennonite.

Arab patients show an earlier age of onset and a more severe course than Jewish patients.

There seems to be intrafamilial consistency in age of onset and severity of the disease.

Chondrocalcinosis and osteoarthritis may be due to copper accumulation, but most patients are asymptomatic.

Magnetic resonance imaging scans show abnormalities of the basal ganglia in generalized cerebral atrophy. Also noted are subtle white matter abnormalities in some patients, particularly at the dentatorubrothalamic, pontocerebellar, and corticospinal tracts.

Free radical formation and oxidative damage, probably mediated via mitochondrial copper accumulation, are important in pathogenesis and provide a rationale for studying the use of antioxidants in the disease.

Excessive deposition of copper and oxidative stress increase the risk of liver cancer.

The diagnosis can be made on clinical grounds if patients have the characteristic clinical triad of Kayser-Fleischer ring, cirrhosis, and basal ganglia disease.

Patients have low serum copper, low serum ceruloplasmin, and excessive excretion of copper in the urine.

Molecular genetic testing can be done, and mutations in the *ATPD7* gene can be detected (Milunsky Laboratory at Boston University).

OCULAR FINDINGS

The Kayser-Fleischer ring is a deep copper-colored ring in the periphery of the cornea at the level of Descemet's membrane and is thought to be due to copper deposition. Azure lunulae of the fingernails probably have the same significance as the Kayser-Fleischer ring and possibly arise by the same mechanism.

The ring is absent in asymptomatic patients but is always present in patients with significant neurologic disease. Its absence in such patients rules out the disease.

The copper deposits are best visualized with a Goldmann three-mirror gonio lens. They first appear as an arc superiorly and gradually spread toward the horizontal meridian as the arc widens. An inferior arc forms later and the two meet, forming a ring that continues to increase in density and width with progression of the disease.

The corneal ring is not pathognomonic of the disease and has been described in patients with cryptogenic cirrhosis, active chronic hepatitis, and neonatal hepatitis.

Patients with advanced disease can develop nonvisually significant anterior lens capsular cataracts, which have been described as sunflowers, resembling those from chalcosis due to copper intraocular foreign bodies. They are, however, disc-shaped anterior capsular opacities with fine stellate extensions tapering toward the periphery. Oculomotor problems have been described and include loss of accommodation, loss of the near response, and transient external ophthalmoplegia.

THERAPEUTIC ASPECTS

Treatment with chelating agents may induce disappearance of the corneal deposits.

Treatment with penicillamine leads to faster disappearance of the cataracts than of the corneal deposits.

Oral *D*-penicillamine (1 g/day in two doses) has been reported to result in the removal of excess copper and the disappearance of copper deposits in the cornea and lens.

Another mode of therapy, if penicillamine either fails or is toxic as an initial modality, is zinc acetate, which works by inducing hepatic metallothionein and the sequestration of copper in a nontoxic pool.

Trientine is a third agent that has been successfully used.

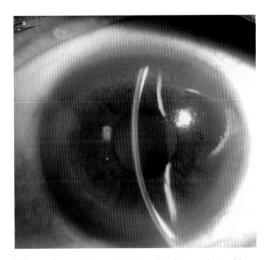

Wilson disease Kayser-Fleischer ring in a patient with Wilson disease.

Neurologic and hepatic complications of the disease can be reversed if the diagnosis is made promptly and therapy is instituted early in the course of the disease.

REFERENCES

Brewer GJ, Dick RD, Johnson VD, et al: Treatment of Wilson's disease with zinc, 15: long-term follow-up studies. *J Lab Clin Med* 1998;132:264–278.

Bull PC, Thomas GR, Rommens JM, et al: The Wilson disease gene is a putative copper transporting P-type ATPase similar to the Menkes gene. *Nat Genet* 1993;5:327–337.

Cairns JE, Walshe JM: The Kayser-Fleischer ring. *Trans Ophthalmol Soc UK* 1970;90:187–190.

Cartwright GE: Diagnosis of treatable Wilson's disease. *N Engl J Med* 1978;298:1347–1350.

Dobyns WB, Goldstein NP, Gordon H: Clinical spectrum of Wilson's disease (hepatolenticular degeneration). *Mayo Clin Proc* 1979;54:35–42.

Frommer D, Morris J, Sherlock S, et al: Kayser-Fleischer-like rings in patients without Wilson's disease. *Gastroenterology* 1977;72:1331–1335.

Sussman W, Scheinberg IH: Disappearance of Kayser-Fleischer rings. *Arch Ophthalmol* 1969;82:738–741.

Tso MO, Fine BS, Thorpe HE: Kaiser-Fleischer ring and associated cataract in Wilson's disease. *Am J Ophthalmol* 1975;79:479–489.

Walshe JM: Penicillamine: the treatment of first choice for patients with Wilson's disease. *Movement Disord* 1999;14:545–550.

Wiebers DO, Hollenhorst RW, Goldstein NP: The ophthalmologic manifestations of Wilson's disease. *Mayo Clin Proc* 1977;52:409–416.

RESOURCE

The Wilson's Disease Association (WDA) www.wilsonsdisease.org

Wolf-Hirschhorn Syndrome

OMIM NUMBER
194190

INHERITANCE
Chromosomal

GENE/GENE MAP
Partial deletion of 4p16.3. Deletions are extremely variable in magnitude. Some patients with a characteristic clinical diagnosis may not have a microscopic deletion in this region.

EPIDEMIOLOGY
Incidence at birth is 1 in 100,000.

CLINICAL FINDINGS
Patients have severe growth retardation, mental defects, microcephaly, *Greek helmet* facies, closure defects (including cleft lip or palate and coloboma), and cardiac septal defects.

An autopsy study of five patients with severe intrauterine growth retardation showed typical craniofacial dysmorphia without microcephaly. Renal hypoplasia was the only constant visceral anomaly. Midline fusion defects were found in

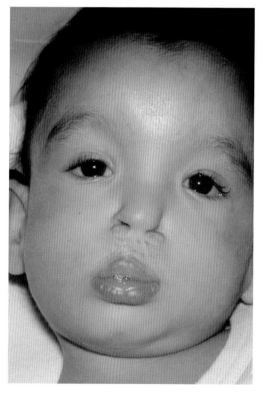

Wolf-Hirschhorn syndrome Characteristic facial appearance of a patient with Wolf-Hirschhorn syndrome. (Reprinted with permission from *Ophthalmic Genet*)

all fetuses. Zollino et al. suggested that a "minimal" phenotype consisted of the typical facial appearance, mild mental and growth retardation, and congenital hypotonia.

OCULAR FINDINGS
Variable with colobomatous microphthalmia and anterior segment dysgenesis, including Rieger anomaly and Peters anomaly.

THERAPEUTIC ASPECTS
Individual medical problems are treated as necessary.

If anterior segment dysgenesis is present, patients should be monitored for the development of glaucoma.

REFERENCES
Battaglia A, Carey JC, Cederholm P, et al: Natural history of Wolf-Hirschhorn syndrome: experience with 15 cases. *Pediatrics* 1999;103:830–836.
Kozma C, Hunt M, Meck J, et al: Familial Wolf-Hirschhorn syndrome associated with Rieger anomaly of the eye. *Ophthalmic Paediatr Genet* 1990;1:23–30.
Tachdjian G, Fondacci C, Tapia S, et al: The Wolf-Hirschhorn syndrome in fetuses. *Clin Genet* 1992;42:281–287.
Zollino M, Di Stefano C, Zampino G, et al: Genotype–phenotype correlations and clinical diagnostic criteria in Wolf-Hirschhorn syndrome. *Am J Med Genet* 2000;94:254–261.

RESOURCES
Wolf-Hirschhorn (4P-) Parent Contact Group
  913 Herons Run Lane
  Woodbridge, VA 22191
  703-497-2807
  TombecR@aol.com
Wolf-Hirschhorn Syndrome (4p-) Support Group and Newsletter
  c/o Brenda Grimmett
  5536 Virginia Court
  Amherst, OH 44001
  440-282-1460
  blgrimmett@centuryinter.net
  www.members.aol.com/lbent503/whs

Wolf-Hirschhorn Syndrome Support Group
  2B Harvesters Close
  Rainham
  Kent, ME8 8PA
  United Kingdom
  01634372218
  Fax: 01634372218

Wolfram Syndrome

OMIM NUMBERS
222300 for type 1
604928 for type 2
598500 for mitochondrial form

INHERITANCE
Autosomal recessive

GENE/GENE MAP
WFS1 gene at 4p16.1
WFS2 gene at 4q22–q24 in three of four families in one report

EPIDEMIOLOGY
The frequency of DIDMOAD (*d*iabetes *in*sipidus, *d*iabetes *m*ellitus, *o*ptical *a*trophy, and neural *d*eafness) among patients with juvenile diabetes varies between 1 in 148 and 1 in 175. The incidence may be significantly higher in populations with consanguineous marriages, such as those in the Middle East. The percentage of the heterozygous carrier state may be as high as 1% in Europe and the United States.

CLINICAL FINDINGS
This syndrome is an autosomal recessive genetic disorder. It is also known by the acronym DIDMOAD, which represents its major complications. However, not all components are found in all patients.

The disease results in noninflammatory degeneration of the visual pathways, brain, and posterior pituitary. The defective gene codes for a transmembrane protein found in the brain and the pancreas.

The association of juvenile diabetes mellitus and optic atrophy in four of eight members of a sibship was first described by Wolfram and Wagener. Autosomal recessive inheritance was documented in numerous subsequent articles.

Only insulin-dependent diabetes mellitus and bilateral progressive optic atrophy are necessary for the diagnosis of DIDMOAD. Diabetes mellitus is often detected first, and onset may be in childhood, adolescence, or adulthood.

Microvascular complications are less frequent and develop more slowly in patients with Wolfram syndrome than in those with classic type 1 diabetes. In one study, 5 of 35 Wolfram patients had merely background diabetic retinopathy, even though their initial diagnosis occurred on average 24 years earlier.

Like nonocular symptoms and signs, hypophyseal diabetes insipidus and sensorineural deafness usually develop during the second decade of life. Urinary abnormalities, most commonly dilated renal outflow tracts and neurogenic bladder, tend to occur in the third decade. In the fourth decade, patients develop neurologic signs such as truncal ataxia.

Patients usually die at approximately age 30 from respiratory arrest as a result of brain stem atrophy.

Lessell and Rosman described anosmia, tonic pupils, and disc cupping. Swift et al. also associated urinary tract atony, peripheral neuropathy, mental retardation, dementia, and psychiatric illness, while Rando et al. added ataxia, nystagmus, and seizures. Swift et al. reported that 25% of homozygous patients had severe psychiatric illness resulting in hospitalization or suicide, and that heterozygous carriers were also at greater risk of severe psychiatric disturbance.

Conditions that involve both diabetes mellitus and optic atrophy include Wolfram syndrome, juvenile diabetic papillopathy, Leber hereditary optic neuropathy, thiamine-responsive anemia with diabetes and deafness, Friedreich ataxia, Refsum disease, Alström syndrome, Kearns syndrome, and congenital rubella.

OCULAR FINDINGS

In a small number of patients, optic atrophy is the initial presenting sign. Examination of the visual fields usually reveals bilateral paracentral scotomas with early peripheral constriction. The atrophy of the optic nerves, chiasm, and tracts is progressive but variable. The median age of onset is 11 years, but the range is from 6 weeks to 19 years. The atrophy can progress over a period of 1 to 25 years.

The prognosis for vision is relatively poor. Seventy-seven percent of patients develop a visual acuity of 20/200 or worse in their better eye after about 8 years.

Visually evoked cortical potentials are abnormal, and abnormal electroretinograms have been described.

Optic atrophy in children with diabetes may also occur in the absence of Wolfram syndrome or may be secondary to papilledema or to severe proliferative diabetic retinopathy. However, in the absence of other factors in children and adolescents with type 1 diabetes mellitus, the presence of optic atrophy should be considered highly inferential.

THERAPEUTIC ASPECTS

Patients with diabetes mellitus and optic atrophy should be investigated regularly for dia-

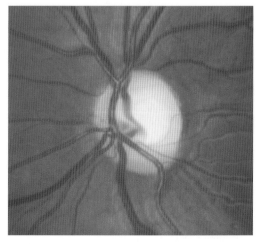

Wolfram syndrome Optic atrophy in a patient with Wolfram syndrome.

betes insipidus or other forms of hypothalamic dysregulation. Diabetes insipidus may be confirmed by using a water-deprivation test for 8 hours and measuring serum and urine osmolalities. Intravenous pyelography, voiding cystourethrography and ultrasound may reveal dilation of the urinary tract. It is important to diagnose diabetes insipidus, because patients can develop dilation of the urinary tract, varying from mild hydroureter to severe hydronephrosis; all such abnormalities improve with treatment of the diabetes insipidus.

Magnetic resonance imaging studies may show widespread atrophic changes throughout the brain, some of which correlate with the major neurologic features of the syndrome.

REFERENCES

Barrett TG, Bundey SE: Wolfram (DIDMOAD) syndrome. *J Med Genet* 1997;34:838–841.

Barrett TG, Bundey SE, Fielder AR, et al: Optic atrophy in Wolfram (DIDMOAD) syndrome. *Eye* 1997;11:862–868.

Barrett TG, Bundey SE, Macleod AF: Neurodegeneration and diabetes: UK nationwide study of Wolfram (DIDMOAD) syndrome. *Lancet* 1995; 346:1458–1463.

Gunn T, Bortolussi R, et al: Juvenile diabetes mellitus, optic atrophy, sensory nerve deafness, and diabetes insipidus: a syndrome. *J Pediatr* 1976;89: 565–570.

Inoue J, Tanizawa Y, et al: A gene encoding a transmembrane protein is mutated in patients with diabetes mellitus and optic atrophy (Wolfram syndrome). *Nat Genet* 1998;20:143–148.

Lessell S, Rosman NP: Juvenile diabetes mellitus and optic atrophy. *Arch Neurol* 1977;34:759–765.

Rando TA, Horton JC, Layzer RB: Wolfram syndrome: evidence of a diffuse neurodegenerative disease by magnetic resonance imaging. *Neurology* 1992;42:1220–1224.

Strom RM, Hortnagel K, et al: Diabetes insipidus, diabetes mellitus, optic atrophy and deafness (DIDMOAD) caused by mutations in a novel gene (*wolframin*) coding for a predicted transmembrane protein. *Hum Mol Genet* 1998;7:2021–2028.

Swift RG, Sadler DB, Swift M: Psychiatric findings in Wolfram syndrome homozygotes. *Lancet* 1990; 336:667–669.

Wolfram DJ, Wagener HP: Diabetes mellitus and simple optic atrophy: report of four cases. *Mayo Clin Proc* 1938;13:715–718.

RESOURCE

Worldwide Society of Wolfram Syndrome Families www.wolframsyndrome.org

Wyburn-Mason Syndrome

OMIM NUMBERS
Not included

INHERITANCE
All cases are isolated

GENE/GENE MAP
Not applicable

EPIDEMIOLOGY
Unknown

CLINICAL FINDINGS
Retinal and systemic arteriovenous malformations (AVMs), which involve predominantly the central nervous system, ocular adnexa including the conjunctiva, lids, face, and oronasopharynx. Eighty-six percent of AVMs are supratentorial and are supplied by the middle cerebral artery.

Central nervous system AVMs lead to a variety of clinical signs or symptoms, depending on their location and extent, including headaches, seizures, and cranial nerve palsies, as well as a variety of sensory and motor defects.

Intracerebral and subarachnoid hemorrhages may occur.

Nasopharyngeal AVMs can lead to epistaxis and oral hemorrhages.

OCULAR FINDINGS
Ocular complications of orbital AVMs include proptosis and dilated conjunctival vessels.

Bruits can be heard on auscultation.

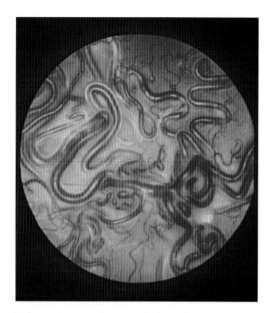

Wyburn-Mason syndrome Retinal arteriovenous communications in Wyburn-Mason syndrome.

Retinal AVMs are usually stable and have a predilection for the superotemporal quadrant. Visual loss can occur from retinal ischemia or vascular occlusive disease, especially in patients with generalized dilation of the retinal vasculature.

Intraretinal macular hemorrhage, neovascular glaucoma, and vitreous hemorrhage have also been reported.

THERAPEUTIC ASPECTS

Workup for central nervous system and oropharyngeal AVMs is necessary in patients with characteristic retinal vascular malformations.

REFERENCES

Font RL, Ferry AP: The phakomatoses. *Int Ophthalmol Clin* 1972;12:1–50.

Mansour AM, Walsh JB, Henkind P: Arteriovenous anastomoses of the retina. *Ophthalmology* 1987; 94:35–40.

Mansour AM, Wells CG, Jampol LM, et al: Ocular complications of arteriovenous communications of the retina. *Arch Ophthalmol* 1989;107:232–236.

Wyburn-Mason R: Arteriovenous aneurysm of midbrain and retina, facial naevi, and mental changes. *Brain* 1943;66:163–203.

RESOURCES

National Aphasia Association
156 Fifth Ave., Suite 707
New York, NY 10010
800-922-4622
Fax: 212-989-7777
Klein@aphasia.org
www.aphasia.org
NIH/National Eye Institute
31 Center Dr., MSC 2510
Building 31, Rm. 6A32
Bethesda, MD 20892-2510
301-496-5248
Fax: 301-402-1065
2020@B31.nei.nih.gov
www.nei.nih.gov
NIH/National Institute of Neurological Disorders and Stroke
31 Center Dr., MSC 2540
Building 31, Rm. 8A16
Bethesda, MD 20892
301-496-5751
800-352-9424
Fax: 301-402-2186
www.ninds.nih.gov

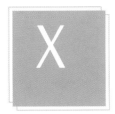

X-Linked Congenital Stationary Night Blindness, Incomplete or Type 2

See Retinal Dystrophies and Degenerations

X-Linked Congenital Stationary Night Blindness, Complete or Type 1

See Retinal Dystrophies and Degenerations

X-Linked Juvenile Retinoschisis

See Retinal Dystrophies and Degenerations

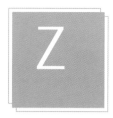

Zellweger Syndrome

OMIM NUMBERS
214100
170993

INHERITANCE
Autosomal recessive

GENE/GENE MAP
Several genes for the syndrome exist, and all are involved in peroxisome biogenesis. They are *PEX1* on 7q21, *PEX2* on 8q, *PEX3* on 6q, *PEX5* on chromosome 12, *PEX6* on 6p, and *PEX12*. A discussion of them is beyond the scope of this book; the reader is directed to OMIM to read entry number 214100.

ZWS3 is due to a defect of peroxisomal membrane protein 35K or *PXMP3* on 8q21.1.

EPIDEMIOLOGY
Very rare

CLINICAL FINDINGS
Zellweger syndrome is the model for, and most severe form of, a group of disorders that affect the peroxisomes, subcellular organelles

TABLE 25. Classification of Peroxisomal Disorders

Disorder	Enzyme Defect
Deficiencies of Peroxisomal Assembly	
Zellweger syndrome	Generalized
Neonatal adrenoleukodystrophy	Generalized
Infantile Refsum disease	Generalized
Zellweger-like syndrome	VLCFA oxidation, THCA oxidation
	DHAP-AT, phytanic acid oxidation
Rhizomelic chondrodysplasia punctata (classical and atypical phenotypes	DHAP-AT, alkyl-DHAP synthase, phytanic acid oxidase, unprocessed peroxisomal thiolase
Deficiencies of Single Peroxisomal Enzymes	
Rhizomelic chondrodysplasia punctata*	Isolated DHAP-AT or alkyl-DHAP synthase
X-linked adrenoleukodystrophy	VLCFA-coenzyme A (CoA) synthetase transport
Pseudoneonatal adrenoleukodystrophy*	Acyl-CoA oxidase
Bifunctional enzyme deficiency*	Bi(tri)functional enzyme
Pseudo-Zellweger syndrome*	Peroxisomal thiolase
Classical Refsum disease	Phytanic acid oxidase
Hyperoxaluria type I	Alanine:glyoxylate aminotransferase
Acatalasemia	Catalase

DHAP-AT = dihydroxyacetonephosphate acyltransferase; THCA = trihydroxycholestanoyl; VLCFA = very long chain fatty acids.

Source: Weleber RG: Peroxisomal disorders. In: Traboulsi EI, ed: *Genetic Diseases of the Eye*. New York: Oxford University Press; 1998:663–696.

*Disorders in which clinical manifestations resemble those of the group with deficiencies of peroxisome assembly.

involved in oxidative reactions that use molecular oxygen and produce hydrogen peroxide. The peroxisomopathies can be divided into two major groups: one of peroxisomal biogenesis and one of individual peroxisomal enzyme defects (see Table 25). Zellweger syndrome belongs in the former category.

The major features of the syndrome include a characteristic facial appearance, deformations of the extremities and joints, abnormal cartilage calcification, hypotonia, seizures, profound psychomotor retardation, hepatomegaly, hepatic fibrosis, and renal cortical cysts.

Histologic examination of the brain shows abnormal neuronal migration and cerebral dysgenesis. Peroxisomes are absent in liver cells and decreased in fibroblasts. Serum levels of very long chain fatty acids (VLCFAs), pipecolic acid, phytanic acid, pristanic acid, and bile acid precursors are elevated. Plasmalogen levels are severely reduced.

Most patients die within a few months of birth.

OCULAR FINDINGS

Ocular findings include upslanting palpebral fissures, epicanthal folds, cataracts, glaucoma, corneal clouding, retinal degeneration, and optic atrophy

The electroretinogram is nonrecordable.

THERAPEUTIC ASPECTS

Treatment is usually supportive.

Cataract surgery does not need to be performed because these patients have severe retinal degeneration and die very early in life.

REFERENCES

Cohen SM, Brown FR, Martyn L, et al: Ocular histopathologic and biochemical studies of the cerebrohepatorenal syndrome (Zellweger's syndrome) and its relationship to neonatal adrenoleukodystrophy. *Am J Ophthalmol* 1983;96:488–501.

Weleber RG: Peroxisomal disorders. In: Traboulsi EI, ed: *Genetic Diseases of the Eye*. New York: Oxford University Press; 1998:663–696.

RESOURCE

National Organization for Rare Disorders (NORD) www.rarediseases.org

AUTHOR INDEX

SUBJECT INDEX

ROYAL VICTORIA HOSPITAL
MEDICAL LIBRARY